Mapping the Sociology of Health and Medicine

Also by Fran Collyer

SO WE WRITE STAR AUTHORS: Anthology of the Society of Women Writers South Australia 2006 (*editor*)

PUBLIC ENTERPRISE DIVESTMENT: Australian Case Studies (*with J. McMaster and R. W. Wettenhall*)

Mapping the Sociology of Health and Medicine

America, Britain and Australia Compared

Fran Collyer
University of Sydney, Australia

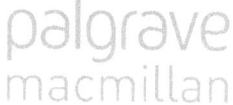
palgrave
macmillan

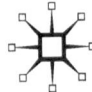

First published 2012 by
PALGRAVE MACMILLAN

Palgrave Macmillan in the UK is an imprint of Macmillan Publishers Limited, registered in England, company number 785998, of Houndmills, Basingstoke, Hampshire RG21 6XS.

Palgrave Macmillan in the US is a division of St Martin's Press LLC, 175 Fifth Avenue, New York, NY 10010.

Palgrave Macmillan is the global academic imprint of the above companies and has companies and representatives throughout the world.

Palgrave® and Macmillan® are registered trademarks in the United States, the United Kingdom, Europe and other countries.

ISBN 978–0–230–32044–4

This book is printed on paper suitable for recycling and made from fully managed and sustained forest sources. Logging, pulping and manufacturing processes are expected to conform to the environmental regulations of the country of origin.

A catalogue record for this book is available from the British Library.

A catalog record for this book is available from the Library of Congress.

10 9 8 7 6 5 4 3 2 1
21 20 19 18 17 16 15 14 13 12

Transferred to Digital Printing in 2014

This book is dedicated to Claire Williams, who taught me to be rigorous with methodology but passionate about facts; Bryan S. Turner, who provided my first opportunity to explore medicine and health and showed me the enduring value of a good yarn; Evan Willis, who has stood by as a constant mentor, colleague and friend; Anna Yeatman, who showed me how to get on with my work while keeping my head below the trench wall; my mate Kevin White, who always says we should never let facts get in the way of a good story, but agonises over every word and date nevertheless; Stephanie Short, who has always believed in me; Raewyn Connell, whose fearlessness continues to inspire; and of course, Peter, without whom . . .

Contents

Tables

Introduction

This volume is a contribution from within the sociology of knowledge to on-going debates about the history of sociology, about the way academic disciplines are formed, and how resilient they might be in the face of rapid (and radical) changes in the university environment. It poses questions about sociologists – the people who inhabit the discipline – and the work they do. It furnishes answers to such questions through a comparative study of the discipline in three countries, offering a history of the sociology of health and medicine and an investigation of the current terrain of this speciality field.

The sociology of health and medicine is a currently viable and flourishing arena of intellectual activity found in many countries, including Australia, the United Kingdom and the United States. As a specialist field within the universities, it has developed institutionally since about 1950 and currently represents about a quarter to one-third of the membership of these countries' professional associations. Despite being a major area of both research and teaching, few histories of the field have been offered. As one might expect, some countries have been more comprehensively studied than others, but to date the only monograph on the history of medical sociology is about its formation in the United States. Even more rare have been substantial cross-national comparative analyses. This monograph fills the gap, providing the growing population of health and medical sociologists with a book about themselves, their colleagues, their discipline, and their history.

What's in a name?

Sociological enquiry into the nature of health, illness and medicine is known by different names across the globe. In the United Kingdom the term 'medical sociology' is preferred. In Australia, the terms 'the sociology of health and illness' and 'health sociologists' are more common. These names may reflect variation in the kind of sociological work being produced in each country, the political preferences of the more vocal or elite members of the profession, or even, as Irving Zola (1991:12) has suggested, the labels we prefer when presenting ourselves publicly and professionally. Until the publication of this monograph, we have known very little about what our name might represent.

The most appropriate name for the speciality field has been debated, at times fiercely, among sociologists from several countries. For Virginia Olesen (1974:6) and others (Stacey and Homans 1978:295; Russell and Schofield 1986:xi; Levine 1991:827), the use of the term 'medical sociology' is thought to inhibit the capacity of sociologists to conceptualise problems of health and health care which do not fall under the aegis of the institutions of biomedicine. Less constrictive terms, such as the sociology of health, the sociology of health and illness or the sociology of health care systems, might encourage greater consideration of the full range of potential subjects. It would, they argue, broaden the analysis beyond those 'things medical' to encompass other health workers and other factors impacting on a society's health status, including traditional healing systems and the many forms of knowledge, beliefs, experiences and practices associated with well-being, sickness and treatment.

Names of speciality fields are important to the individuals working within them, and sometimes considerable energy is expended in seeking to change these within professional associations. In the United States, various attempts to alter the designation of the Medical Sociology Section of the *American Sociological Association (ASA)* have been unsuccessful, even though some, such as Sol Levine (1991:827), regard the title 'medical sociology' as a misnomer. In Australia, the medical sociology group, first formed in 1967, became the Health Section during the 1980s, perhaps reflecting the concerns of the leaders of the group to more accurately reflect the research and teaching interests of members.

The choice of 'the sociology of health and medicine' as the title for this speciality is made partly as a compromise between the 'sociology of health', commonly used in the Australian setting, and the 'medical sociology' of our British and American counterparts. The title is also, and much more importantly, offered as a plea to sociologists – in all countries – to return to an interest in the institutions of medicine. Several decades ago in the British context, Anne Murcott (1977:167–8) suggested the field should not be called a sociology of *health* because this might maintain, rather than challenge, the boundaries between the medical and the non-medical. With hindsight it seems neither name has encouraged sociologists to focus on these boundaries, whether this be in Britain, America or Australia. The greater proportion of contemporary sociological studies in each country now – in contrast to the 1960s and 1970s – address issues of illness and the experiences of patients in the health care system, rather than analyses of the institutions of medicine. While there are some attempts to broaden the sphere of research interest beyond the illness experience, the scope of most studies remains *defined by the institutions of biomedicine*. What do I mean by this? It means most sociologists assume the most important aspect of the health care system is the patient–doctor dyad. This is the arena medical doctors regard as central to the health care system. Yet the clinic, with its patient–doctor interactions, is only one, and increasingly small, component of the system. The majority of health care activity is informal, occurring in the private, domestic setting, and much of it concerns not doctors and the clinical context but pharmaceutical consumption, technological testing and self-medication. Moreover, when we turn our gaze to the public, and more formal aspects of the system, a much larger proportion of expenditure and social activity takes place in research laboratories, bio-pharmaceutical corporations, electronic-engineering firms, health insurance companies, universities and the administrative and political offices of government. Yet, as sociologists, we continue to accept the labels, categories, divisions and distinctions laid down in the interests of the medical institutions and direct our gaze towards the very small arena of action held to be important by biomedicine, the same one promulgated by the medical sociologist Talcott Parsons over sixty years ago.

The selection of the title 'the sociology of health and medicine' is therefore, in large part, a plea to my colleagues to broaden their orientation to the field, focus on the social action beyond (and beneath) the clinic, refrain from treating the medical context merely as background, pay greater attention to the construction of boundaries between the medical and non-medical, and take up some of the *other* pressing issues relevant to our research and teaching. Enough about the title!

The intellectual heritage of the sociology of health and medicine

This book is offered to readers at a time when sociologists have begun to take an interest in the origin of intellectual fields and disciplines. One branch of this new genre focuses on the history of the discipline by putting forward significant individuals and their writings, perhaps noting the similarities between past ideas and those of contemporary studies. Within the sociology of health and medicine, Uta Gerhardt's (1989) *Ideas About Illness*, is one example of a whole monograph within the genre, though it is more common to find overviews of the discipline presented as introductory chapters in edited collections (e.g. Scambler 1987; Turner 2000). Favoured *individuals* in such historical accounts more often than not include the nineteenth-century figure Rudolf Virchow (1978/1859), and his efforts to show 'social misery' as a cause of disease. Edwin Chadwick (1842) is another popular figure, given his building of a system of sanitation within industrialising Britain. Favoured historical *writings*, on the other hand, may embrace the seven volumes on the 'medical police' by Johann Peter Frank (from 1798, see Lesky 1976); Henry Mayhew's *London Labour and the London Poor* (1985/1861); Frederick Engels' (1969/1845) revelations about the condition of the working class in England; the social surveys of London life by Charles Booth (1902); the histories of medicine and studies of hygiene by John Shaw Billings (1888); and the turn-of-the-century texts on medical sociology by Elizabeth Blackwell (1902) and James Warbasse (1909). Also popular within this literary genre are the social science works of the early twentieth century, including investigations into mental disorder by Robert Faris and Warren Dunham (1939); the first American community study by Robert and Helen Lynd (1929); the histories of medicine of Henry Sigerist (1937); the problems of immigrant health unearthed by Michael Davis (1971/1921); and the studies of medical innovation by Bernard Stern (1968/1927).

Such studies serve to remind current generations that few ideas are truly new. Most have been considered before, often in some depth, and we must know our history if we wish not to repeat its many mistakes. In offering an overview of the field, these texts give members of a discipline an insight into the discipline's intellectual progress and provide the field with a form of 'cognitive identity'. These are both essential for attracting new members, orienting students within a large and growing discipline, and distinguishing between intellectual fields in an increasingly competitive academic marketplace.

There is nevertheless a danger in assuming the history of a discipline can be adequately documented by tracing its intellectual precursors and a set of key ideas or theories. *Intellectual* histories can be quite ahistorical in their approach to the past, for without adequate contextualisation of ideas and persons, the connections between past and present are often assumed rather than historically factual. The result may be a view of past developments which have not actually occurred, and of linkages between ideas or persons which are largely imposed on the past by our twenty-first-century perspective. Known in the trade as *presentist* approaches to history, these are an ever-present concern for scholars interested in the early formation of a discipline, and offer particular traps for sociologists of health and medicine.

For instance, if we presume to discuss the works of Virchow, Booth or Chadwick *as if* they were part of the heritage of the sociology of health and medicine, we would be offering a presentist view of history; for their works were not produced under the rubric of the discipline, nor would they comfortably fit within the body of knowledge now regarded as sociology. If, on the other hand, we were to make it clear that our intention was not to produce 'history' but rather to reveal the 'missing voices' of the past, then the works of Florence Nightingale (1871) or Ludwick Fleck (1979/1935) may indeed have relevance and scholarly interest, for much has been excluded from the historical record, whether through mishap or the structures of racism, sexism or imperialism.

There is another sense in which *intellectual* histories may represent a problem for scholars of the past. Too often, studies within that genre name individuals with an interest in the social aspects of medicine – perhaps Virchow, Nightingale or Chadwick – and contrast these with the heroic individuals of medicine and medical science, perhaps Louis Pasteur, Marie Curie or Robert Koch. The problem of course is in the creation of two distinct categories, with *sociological* history separable from *medical* history. These categories rest on a presumption that the modern categories of the 'social' and the 'medical' can be applied to the past, when in fact they are distinctions born of a modern disciplinary structure. From a nineteenth-century perspective, when medicine was yet to throw its future in with the emerging experimental laboratory sciences (and when sociological perspectives had not yet been purged of their psychological, organicist or physiological roots), health and disease were not clearly defined as biological and physiological processes but more commonly discussed in broader terms better encapsulated within the concept of well-being.

From a twenty-first-century perspective though, it is tempting to view the past as containing two independent 'histories', and envisage distinct lines of development stretching backwards in time, one tracing ideas about 'the social' and the other concerned with our 'biological' health. It *is* difficult to consider our heritage in other ways, for when we are informed, for instance, that the sociology of health and medicine is a derivation of three major concepts – medicine as a social science, social medicine, and the sociology of medicine (Bloom 2002) – it is almost impossible not to take on the message that the sociology of health and medicine was the product of 'sociology' on the one hand and 'health and medicine' on the other.

This problem of imposing a contemporary perspective on the past increases the difficulty of writing the history of the specialist field. The current separation of 'medicine' and 'sociology' into two distinct (and often antagonistic) disciplines continually finds its way into all aspects of sociological analysis. It often colours discussions about the sociology of the classical period, suggesting there were few early efforts to theorise health and disease. Graham Scambler's (2005:1) introduction to a history of medical sociology, for example, discounts Durkheim's work on suicide, asserting the theorist's interest was 'not in health or suicide *per se'*, and looks instead to Blackwell and Warbasse as providers of 'the earliest texts' of the sociology of health and medicine. This view is widespread within the discipline: our texts are littered with statements about the classical scholars' lack of interest in health or medicine and how its theorising did not have a place in sociology until the 1950s. William Cockerham (2005a:11) tells us: 'None of the classical theorists – Comte, Spencer, Simmel, Marx, Durkheim, and Weber – concerned themselves with medical sociology'. Likewise, Cockerham (2005a:5) speaks of Parsons' book as the 'pivotal event' which 'was the first time a major sociological theorist included an analysis of the function of medicine in his view of society'.

It would be quite wrong to suggest that all sociological writings have fallen into this trap. There have been some very important exceptions, including Michel Foucault, whose theories suggest a common past for both medicine and sociology. In the *Birth of the Clinic* (1973), Foucault theorised the formation of modern medicine and sociology as the consequence of epistemic change. Drawing on the broader theory of knowledge propounded in *The Order of Things* (1970) and *The Archaeology of Knowledge* (1972), Foucault proposed a profound change with the birth of a new 'archaeological system' underpinning, and making possible, a new form of language and a new way of seeing and knowing. This system, he argues, was qualitatively different from that of the previous epoch:

> At the beginning of the nineteenth century, doctors described what for centuries had remained below the threshold of the visible and the expressible ... [and a] new alliance was forged between words and things, enabling one *to see* and *to say* ...
>
> (Foucault 1973:ix–xii).

In other words, at a particular historical juncture, both knowledges – medicine and sociology – developed as surfaces or sites of emergence for the technologies of surveillance and discipline. Both also began to operate, hand in hand, to make the (individual and social) body and its diseases 'legible'. For Foucault, their commonalities as forms of knowledge and practice are more important than their differences.

It is the dominance of biomedicine – in its twentieth-century alliance with the natural sciences – which frames and determines our perspectives on the history of our discipline, and it is almost impossible to envisage a past in which scholars, policy makers, reformers, and even the healers themselves, did not make such distinctions. Indeed, without the modern partitioning of knowledge into the 'medical' and the 'social', individuals such as Florence Nightingale, Frederich Engels and Henri Saint-Simon saw, more clearly than we do today, the interconnections between poverty, environmental squalor, the lack of human rights and the sufferings of the physical body.

What does this mean for a history of the discipline? It means the very categories of 'biological health' and 'the social' are modern ones. Sociology and medicine, which are now presented as two very different ways of looking at well-being and suffering, both began to take their modern (antagonistic) form only in the opening decades of the twentieth century. And, as I have argued elsewhere (Collyer 2010), these modern disciplines developed in relation to one another, with proponents of each field beginning the process of differentiating and defining their knowledge bases and giving shape to their disciplines as professional projects. Acknowledging *this* aspect of the past has implications for our history, for it suggests we should look to the formation of disciplines as a process which includes interaction and competition across scarcely defined and mutually emerging fields; even those which might today appear unrelated (such as medicine, chemistry or the other sciences). It also suggests the importance of considering our approach to the past. Given the problems of presentism and of intellectual histories, are there other – and better – ways of examining the days of yesteryear?

Institutional histories

An alternative to putting forward an intellectual history, with all the attendant risks of offering a presentist view of the past, is to examine the institutional history of the sociology of health and medicine. *Institutional histories* document the formation of the bodies through which ideas and practices have been nurtured, developed and transmitted: social networks, societies, university research centres, schools, departments and so on. Although a discipline's cognitive and institutional trajectories are entwined and only fully separable at the analytic level, a focus on *institutional* development is an analysis of the processes through which important ideas become embedded in social practices and structured into more resilient and permanent arrangements. Unlike intellectual histories, *institutional* histories can demonstrate actual contact or influence between specific social actors (or generations of actors), and divulge the social and political struggles through which disciplinary goals are furthered and bodies of formal knowledge protected from oblivion.

Surprisingly, many sociologists, otherwise meticulous in their scholarship, do not distinguish institutional from intellectual developments when they are discussing the distant past. The literature is full of potential confusion, with many statements about the origin of the field which do not define precisely what *it* was that developed at that time. For example, we find the Australian Sol Encel (1970:147) stating: 'Historically, the growth of the sociology of medicine began in response to medical interest in the social background of certain diseases'. In the British case, Margaret Stacey and Hilary Homans (1978:282) assert:

> The major impetus for the development of the sociology of medicine was practical rather than theoretical. Furthermore it came from outside sociology rather than from any recognition on the part of mainstream sociologists that it is important to understand health care institutions if the society as a whole is to be understood.

Statements such as this do not provide sufficient detail for the reader to know whether the author is referring to the birth of an idea, a programme of research, a set of social practices, the first time a university course was taught bearing the title of 'the sociology of medicine', or even the formation of a department or professional association. Part of the problem of course is that the term 'sociology' can refer to a body of formal scholarly knowledge, a theory or perspective, but also to a discipline. As a discipline, sociology may be a body of knowledge, but it also might be a set of practices, or an organisational entity such as a university department. This simply compounds the larger problem of failing to specify differences between the intellectual and institutional development of the discipline, and the result is a significant level of confusion about our historical past.

The current study seeks to overcome the problem by taking an institutional approach to sociology's past. This involves an investigation of the processes through which certain social practices, bodies of knowledge and forms of organisation became woven into the social fabric. Taking a sociology of knowledge approach, questions are asked about the history of the specialist field, the actors and the groups they formed, and the relationships between this and other fields. Moreover, we examine the nature of disciplines in the rapidly changing university system of the twenty-first century and the impact of departments, universities and geography on the production of sociological knowledge. These questions, and these answers, result in new ways of understanding disciplines and the relations they have with their specialities.

One sociology or many?

Sociologists have long been pre-occupied with examining the nature of their discipline (Small 1903, 1924; McLaughlin 1926; Ogburn and Nimkoff 1964/1947; Parsons 1970/1951; Merton *et al.* 1959; Coser 1965; Naegele 1965a; Nisbet 1967; Tiryakian 1971; Fletcher 1971). Recent decades, however, have witnessed a surge of interest, particularly with the growing popularity of the sociology of knowledge. Two somewhat entangled themes can be noted in these debates and discussions: one concerned with the discipline's knowledge base and the other its political or institutional development. The first of these is the more common, with a focus on defining sociological knowledge. These accounts vary a little, depending on *when* they were written, and to some extent, their country of origin. Back in the late nineteenth century, for instance, sociology was considered by many intellectuals to be a 'countervailing point of view and a moral disposition rather than a specialised academic discipline' (Sigerist, in Bloom 2002:12). By the 1920s, sociology was more likely to be described as the 'science of society'. In 1926, American sociologist Isabella McLaughlin (1926:392–3), when comparing history with sociology, assumed sociology to be a natural science because it observes, tests, compares and classifies, aims to locate the typical and the universally true, and offers explanation rather than interpretation. By 1982, Frank Lopez, writing many kilometres away in Australia, considered it problematic to regard sociology a *science*. Instead he saw sociology as 'a body of information about society and the interactions of individuals and groups within it' (Lopez 1982:8).

The specialist field of the sociology of health and medicine has been subjected to similar conjecture. Unlike sociologists from the parent discipline, we find amongst sociologists of health and medicine an initial emphasis on the scientific nature of their field. For example, in 1894

Charlie McIntire, in the *Bulletin of the American Academy of Medicine*, defined medical sociology as:

> ... the science of the social phenomena of the physicians themselves as a class apart and separate; and the science which investigates the laws regulating the relations between the medical profession and human society as a whole; treating of the structure of both, how the present conditions came about, what progress civilisation has effected and indeed everything related to the subject

> (McIntire 1894).

By the 1980s, the notion of sociology as a science had been dismissed, and the *sociology of health and illness* was described by Australians Gillian Lupton and Jake Najman as the sociological approach to health care that tests 'taken-for-granted' assumptions and examines the symbolic and cultural components of society, the health needs of various categories of people, and the way social relationships shape health needs, processes and outcomes (Lupton and Najman 1989:366).

These few examples attest to the changing cognitive focus and methodology of the discipline and its speciality field. Such transitions have not always occurred without tension in the sociological community. For instance, dissatisfaction with Talcott Parsons' programmatic statements about the unity of the discipline and its 'core' sociological concerns (as propounded in *The Structure of Social Action* of 1937, and *The Social System* of 1951) were evident by the 1970s. Alvin Gouldner (1970:331–3) was one of many who condemned Parsons' theoretical synthesis as fundamentally conservative, indifferent to inequality and compatible with the maintenance of elite power. As such, Gouldner and others saw attempts to offer 'one sociology' as ideological and an attempt to repress radical voices.

For Gouldner (1970:21), there were *two sociologies*, American academic sociology and Marxism, developed for different purposes and different audiences. The former was a programme of reform directed at the established middle class, and the latter the official science of the Soviet Union, where the task was to consolidate the processes of industrialisation. Gouldner's criticisms were directed at American sociology in general and Parsons' functionalism in particular.

Alan Dawe's (1970) 'two sociologies' represents another enquiry into sociology's knowledge base and also addresses the question of whether there might be *one sociology or several*. Dawe argued against the prevailing view of sociology as centrally concerned with the problem of social

order. Debunking this as a 'doctrine' about the origins and development of sociology, he sought to reconfigure our views of the discipline,
proposing two forms of sociology: a sociology of social system and one
of social action (Dawe 1970:214). Dawe suggests it has been the tension between these very different views of human nature and society
which have underlain the development of the discipline, for one posits
an autonomous individual and the other a socially constrained and
determined being. This model of sociology was, in turn, countered by
Ted Benton (1978) with a proposal for three rather than the more common binary division. Benton suggested Dawe's positivist and humanist
(or hermeneutic) forms of sociology should be supplemented with a
modified, Althusserian reading of Marx as an additional form, resting
upon a realist and materialist foundation.

The issue raised by Dawe and Benton about whether sociology might
contain a central, defining perspective has occupied numerous sociologists over the decades, both prior to their discussion and since (Parsons
1968/1937; Stark 1961/1937; Shils 1965; Ritzer 1990; van Krieken 2002).
Some have sought to treat this as a 'technical' issue about the logical
possibilities of the sociological knowledge base, but others, such as
Gouldner, have taken the view that sociology *should* not attempt to
be a universal science, but instead reflect a broad range of perspectives and experiences. This acknowledgement of the ethical and political
complexity of the issue figures prominently in debates over the possibility of autonomous forms of sociology, with proponents suggesting
the selection of concepts and problems for analysis might be unique to
each culture and society (Pieris 1969; Den Hollander 1971:205; Sanda
1988; Loubser 1988; Langer 1992; Alatas 2001, 2006a). From a sociology of knowledge perspective, such debates have brought into focus the
European, British and North Atlantic domination of sociological knowledge and its consequences for other countries, particularly the post-
colonial nations of Africa, Singapore and Australia. These debates have
subsequently encouraged further study into the 'Southern' sociologies of
the periphery (Akiwowo 1999; Alatas 2006b; Connell 2007; Keim 2011).

Tumbling around within these debates about the discipline and its
composition – and rarely teased apart – have been views on the other
theme of this literature: the appropriate professional strategies or *roles*
of sociologists. Parsons (1959:547, 559) articulated his view on the latter
on various occasions, identifying the twin responsibilities of sociologists to develop the knowledge of the discipline and engage in practical
affairs. A more recent effort, this time from Michael Burawoy (2005a),
employed the concept of *four* sociologies to address the four roles of

the sociologist: (1) the professional, (2) policy, (3) public and (4) critical dimensions. The institutional and professional roles of sociologists have also been the subject of scholarly investigation. For example, Eric Thompson's (2006) survey of four countries (three of them in South-East Asia) examines diverse patterns of professional communication, and shows the lack of a 'level playing field' within global academia. Similarly, Raewyn Connell's studies of intellectual workers raise questions about whether the labour process differs for those in postcolonial situations (Connell 2006:7; also Connell and Wood 2002; Connell *et al.* 2005).

The notion of one or more sociologies has thus been employed in an assortment of ways to point to the coherence or otherwise of socio-logical knowledge, on the one hand, and the diverse disciplinary roles, ethics and professional strategies of sociologists on the other. There are two important elements missing from these studies which have relevance for our discussion here.

In the first place, there are too many sociological studies which offer 'a view from nowhere', failing to locate their debate in a spe-cific national or geographic context and instead presenting it *as if* such knowledge were universal. Yet proponents of the sociology of knowl-edge have demonstrated the links between the ideational and material worlds, and it has become increasingly important to be more, not less, reflexive about the cultural context of one's knowledge-making. This makes it imperative to engage in empirical, comparative studies to ensure we can be better informed about the extent of variation in sociological knowledge in different countries. In this volume we direct our queries towards only a handful of countries: Australia, the United Kingdom and the United States. These countries share a similar lan-guage, some significant aspects of culture and social structure, and, according to the conventional histories of sociology, their disciplines stem from a common origin in Europe and the Industrial and French revolutions (Nisbet 1943; Wardell and Turner 1986; Alexander 1997). This limited selection reduces the size of the research task and the potential for cross-cultural misunderstanding, but nevertheless offers an opportunity to explore the possibility of a common sociological project.

The second element missing from the sociological literature is an attempt to bridge the institutional and cognitive worlds of sociologists, *and* to do so from a comparative, cross-national perspective. There are some comparative studies of sociological knowledge (Crane and Small 1992; Abend 2006; Clair *et al.* 2007; Seale 2008), but these lack an insti-tutional dimension and so preclude an analysis of *why* there might be national differences in orientation or method. As Gabriel Abend (2006:29) points out at the conclusion of her study of the sociologies of Mexico and the United States, additional studies need to be designed to investigate *how* epistemologies and theories might be shaped by their national contexts.

Abend's proposal for such a task is tackled in this book. The chapters provide an analysis of the connections between the institutional context of sociological workers and the sociological knowledge base, and consider the extent to which the former has an impact on the kind of sociological knowledge sociologists help to create. And by investigating these connections *comparatively*, this study provides material for significantly advancing the debate of whether there are one or three – or more – sociologies to be found in these three countries.

Inside this book

This monograph offers a comparative history of the specialist field of the sociology of health and medicine in three countries. It begins with a theoretical chapter, introducing the reader to the sociology of knowledge, and shows how this programme of research can be employed in the examination of disciplines, regardless of whether these are conceived as bodies of knowledge, occupational groups, professions or systems of regulation or control.

Central to an analysis of disciplines and disciplinary formation is the literature on intellectual and scientific change. This is a large and exciting literature, and it raises questions about whether the development of new knowledge might result from cultural processes *internal* or *external* to the sciences (or indeed, the social sciences). On the one hand, we can see the logic of an internalist approach: the intense conflicts over sociological knowledge between social scientists, the cognitive problems arising from new discoveries, new trends associated with the borrowings between disciplines, the formation of new alliances between previously disparate disciplines, and the constant re-organisation of disciplinary boundaries. Any such events should have ramifications for the production of academic knowledge. On the other hand, it is not hard to see how *external* events might drive disciplinary change: alterations in the funding regimes of the social sciences, growth in the global publishing market, the contracting-out of knowledge work or perhaps the declining support for public sector institutions.

There are problems, however, with these two views. Neither internalist nor externalist theories of intellectual change are in themselves sufficiently robust to explain the formation of disciplines and their historical shifts. Thus we find, in Chapter one, an alternative theoretical framework for capturing the dynamics of intellectual change. Rejecting the conventional view of disciplines as merely discrete 'parcels' of formal knowledge or cognitive products that immanently 'emerge' or 'unfold' over time, disciplines are re-configured as sites of social action and as institutions which structure, regulate and control that action. As institutions, disciplines are themselves situated within a broader social field and thus subjected to the organising effects of other social structures, including those of capitalism. This theoretical framework takes into account intellectual products and intellectual change, but also the processes of institutionalisation through which human actors come together to build departments, schools, journals and professional associations. It therefore constructs pathways between the worlds of actors and institutions, and between knowledge products and social structures.

For readers who might be otherwise unfamiliar with the institutional history of sociology, Chapter one is where you will find a brief overview of the formation of departments and schools in the university systems of the three countries, as well as information about the timing of the creation of their journals and professional associations. These three different, though connected, narratives about the institutionalisation of sociology provide the groundwork for later discussions about the sociology of health and medicine, for the two developmental trajectories – of the specialist field and its parent – were not independent.

In Chapter two, the focus is on the processes of institutionalisation of the sociology of health and medicine rather than of its parent discipline. Similarities and differences between the histories of the three national sociologies of health and medicine are examined to reveal the way sociologists have dealt with both friendly and hostile relations with other disciplines, how specialities have been formed and constrained through professionalisation processes, and how external bodies (including governments, foundations and corporations) have shaped the fortunes of disciplines and regulated and controlled the behaviour of members.

The processes of social action and institution-building within the three national sociologies of health and medicine are dissected in greater depth in the third chapter. Drawing from what has been learned about the historical achievements and struggles of the sociologists of health and medicine in each of the three countries; this chapter extends the theoretical work of Chapter one to develop new ways of conceptualising the relationship between disciplines and their specialities. Expanding the notion of disciplines as multi-dimensional social forms, and arguing for sociology to be understood as both a discipline *and* a profession, the sociology of health and medicine is demonstrated as a field produced primarily through the historically located, internal and external boundary activities of sociologists.

The empirical study is the focus of the fourth chapter. Rather than describe the specialist field of the sociology of health and medicine *a priori*, readers are offered a comparative, empirical study of the production of sociological knowledge in three countries: Australia, the United Kingdom and the United States. The research is essentially an analysis of health and medical sociology articles from major international journals since 1990. The chapter begins with a justification for the study, a summary of its research questions, reasons for the method and descriptions of its variables.

Two kinds of information are taken from these journal publications. On the one hand, the sociological knowledge within the publications is investigated to indicate the major trends in methodology, topics, theoretical orientation and citations in each country. On the other hand, information from the publications about the authors themselves is taken into consideration: their gender, differing work environments, their access to research grants, efforts at research collaboration, and also variations in the labels they adopt to identify themselves as scholars and knowledge workers.

This approach to the field does not impose a researcher's view of sociology and sociologists, but takes at face value the definitions of sociology found within the journal materials. Sociology is what sociologists produce. Equally, sociologists are those scholars who identify themselves as such, and those so identified by others. This is not a standard approach to the discipline, for it allows the boundaries and terrain of the field to be discovered rather than pre-determined by the researcher. One of its consequences, immediately evident from a perusal of the study's findings in Chapter five, is that we become aware of how diverse sociology is. There are many approaches and forms of analysis, methods, topics and paradigms, even though this is work produced by individuals identifying as sociologists and describing their work as sociological. Even the label 'sociologist' is adopted by a very diverse group of people. Such findings raise questions about the transferability of sociological concepts and theories between countries such as the United States, Britain and Australia, where the sharing of the English language may otherwise obscure important differences in outlook and culture. Imagine the diversity if the study was able to be truly global in its approach to sociology!

Chapter five thus offers a discussion about the findings from the Content Analysis, showing the statistical results in illustrative tables. Combining the two forms of information – about the publications and about the authors – reveals some similarities, but also surprising differences between the three sociologies. Most apparent are contrasts in the way sociologists prefer to identify themselves (e.g. as a sociologist, a social scientist, a sociologist of medicine), the disciplines they are aligned with, the departments, schools and institutions they work within and the funding of their research. There are also differences in what they say about medicine and health, the methods they use and who they cite.

The analysis of this data, in combination with the historical materials from the earlier chapters, is employed in the final, sixth chapter to draw conclusions about disciplinary knowledge, disciplines and disciplinary specialities. The chapter highlights a number of significant national differences in the way sociology is practised. For instance, each country has its own set of 'rules' about who might identify as a sociologist and what they might legitimately study within the discipline. There are also profound variations in the placement of disciplinary boundaries in each country, meaning the relations between sociology and other intellectual fields (such as epidemiology and psychology) might be hostile in some instances but co-operative elsewhere. These varying patterns are associated not only with different political, socio-cultural and economic configurations of the national context but also with rather diverse ways of organising the work of sociologists. In some countries, it is more common to find sociologists in departments of medicine or to have their research funded by medicine; and in others, we find greater levels of collaboration with other disciplines, be they psychologists or epidemiologists. The focus of the final discussion is on the implications of these similarities and differences for the discipline, its practice and its future. Under processes of globalisation, and in a context of the global marketing of universities and escalating competition in the sale of 'knowledge products', what does it mean if there are three independent sociologies, or one, united (even if geographically dispersed) intellectual field?

Limitations of the study

The study's emphasis on providing a *sociological* understanding of the sociology of health and medicine as a discipline necessarily means that readers seeking comprehensive histories of sociology will need to look elsewhere. This book will offer a form of history – because the contemporary world of the sociology of health and medicine cannot be adequately understood without its past – but the focus is not a compilation of facts and figures, nor an in-depth analysis of specific historical moments. Instead it is a study adhering to the principles of the sociology of knowledge and aiming to ask sociological questions about the relationship between ideas and the social context; specifically, how the production of formal, scholarly knowledge is shaped by socio-cultural practices, forms of organisation and social structure.

The study's focus on the relationship between knowledge, disciplines and institutions, and its approach to understanding sociologists and sociology through archival and statistical research, inevitably prevents a full investigation of the world of sociologists. These methodologies provide a systematic 'snapshot' of the discipline from 'outside', but cannot reveal any of the subtleties of what the discipline might mean to individual sociologists or the processes through which sociologists adopt a sociological identity, construct a sociological career and make their way in the world. For these insights, we need to delve into our methodological armoury and talk to, and observe, sociologists in action. That, of course, will be another project.

Why this book?

When I was an undergraduate studying sociology for my Bachelor of Arts degree in Australia, I became increasingly captivated by the underlying logic of the discipline. It seemed that irrespective of the topic or problem at hand, an alternative, sociological perspective could be found. I kept waiting for this magic to peter out, for a new problem to emerge for which it would have no answer, but the solutions kept rolling in. These days, when my honours and post-graduate students enter a period of (temporary) despair with the lack of progress in their theses, I tell them, 'Believe in your discipline. There *is* another way of looking at this. There *is* another answer. Keep looking'. And there always is.

I have not lost my curiosity over this form of 'sociological magic'. The idea that there may be some underlying 'essence' to sociology – an 'it' which can always be found with sufficient effort – has remained with me. The question has since become how this 'essence' might be constructed and shaped through social practices and institutions, and then persist (in some form) over time: through war, migration, the efforts of governments to purge or marginalise oppositional views; the resistance of other powerful disciplines to an interloper into their 'patch'; and more recently, the vicissitudes of the modern university system with constant threats of budget cuts and amalgamations, all in the name of institutional efficiency and reform. Pondering over these matters – at some length – eventually led to this study of the discipline, to a consideration of its current form, how it has travelled from the past to the present, and whether or not it matters.

1
Theoretical Frameworks and Beginnings

There have been numerous contributions to the debates about sociology, its origins, and how the discipline has altered over the decades. Some of these offerings have been scholarly and highly analytical, proffered by sociologists of marked professional standing, though others are remembered more as notes of concern about the present and future course of the discipline. And, of course, there has been a parallel debate shared with other disciplines about precisely *how* we should view the past and write disciplinary histories.

This book promises to contribute a little to each of these discourses. It will investigate aspects of sociology's past. It will engage with sociological ideas about how we should account for the past. It will offer a view of the specialist field of the sociology of health and medicine in a manner which simply hasn't happened before. It will also address long-running concerns about the future of the discipline and its specialist field. It even promises to do these things within the established traditions of scholarship. Just as importantly though, one of the aims of this study is to journey into the world of academia and explore some facets often taken for granted in histories of sociology: just what *is* a discipline? What is a speciality? What is a sociologist? What is a sociologist of health or medicine? What kind of knowledge-making do they undertake? Where do they work? What factors shape their working lives? And is there one or several sociologies of health and medicine?

Theoretical and methodological approaches to the field

This book was always planned to have, at its core, an *empirical study* of the specialist field of the sociology of health and medicine. It seemed important to explore sociology in its current manifestation rather than define, *a priori*, its terrains and boundaries, tensions and debates, its people and forms of organisation. And it soon became evident that such a study must be comparative, for this is a tried and true method of investigating the nature of any beast.

Making *sociological sense* of this empirical and comparative study, on the other hand, requires a robust, theoretical framework. The choice of such a framework, I must admit, has been associated with more than one restless night. In the end, the issue was resolved with thoughts of Edward Shils and Elliot Freidson. Shils (1982:10) reminds us that from a sociology of knowledge perspective, disciplines are not mere creations of their intellectual processes, but bodies of knowledge produced and developed by human agents in specific social and institutional contexts. The message from Freidson (1986a) is similar, for he tells us that any investigation of a body of knowledge means taking into account its relationship with the social context or social structure. Yet Freidson's emphasis is not on the body of ideas or theories of the agents, but the social institutions within which these grow and develop. This means looking beyond much of what has been written about the sociology of health and medicine, its major theoretical developments and shifting sociological conceptions, and, from a sociology of knowledge perspective, considering sociology primarily as a discipline, a profession, and an institutional form.

A discipline is necessarily a multi-faceted phenomenon. It can be a formal body of knowledge; a community of scholars, intellectuals, teachers, policy makers and practitioners; a social practice; a labour process; a profession; a regime of socialisation and training; or even a system of regulation and control. As a discipline, sociology straddles the material world of institutions and the symbolic world of ideas. A focus on sociology as a discipline within an institutional context enables questions to be posed, and addressed, about the body of knowledge and how it formed, about changes over time, its relationship to other formal bodies of knowledge, and the extent to which it varies cross-culturally. The same focus however sets in motion a series of questions about the group of scholars and practitioners associated with this body of knowledge. Who are the sociologists of health and medicine? When did they become an identifiable intellectual community, and when a discipline? How are they employed, and what social forces shape their working conditions, their capacity to innovate and extend the discipline's boundaries? Moreover, to what extent might they share their discipline with scholars from other countries?

The sociology of knowledge

With this central focus on sociology as a discipline, the sociology of knowledge becomes an obvious choice for the research process. The sociology of knowledge is essentially the study of the social conditions that produce knowledge, and of the social and cultural processes and institutions within which knowledge is produced, exchanged, legitimated, and transmitted. It offers a focus on the causal relations between society and knowledge, that is, between the varied social arrangements and the ideational sphere of beliefs, values, concepts, and theories.

The sociology of knowledge is considered to have its origins in the works of Max Scheler (1874–1928) and Karl Mannheim (1893–1947), with Peter Berger and Thomas Luckmann (1984/1966) more recent proponents. In its early manifestation it was the field of *Wissenssoziologie*, composed of the German word *Wissen*, meaning knowledge (of an indeterminate kind), and *Soziologie* or social philosophy, which includes, but is somewhat broader than the field of sociology (Wolff 1970:32). Under Scheler, the field was very much a *philosophy of knowledge*, but with Mannheim it began to pose a somewhat different set of questions, becoming less concerned with the nature of truth and more focused on the social location of ideas within the social structure. The field was re-named the *sociology of knowledge* when it made its way to the United States – after Mannheim's early death in 1947 – and Robert Merton claimed it as a new field (Sica 2010:175). In this act of geographical transportation, the phenomenological (Scheler) and Marxist (Mannheim) origins of *Wissenssoziologie* were partially replaced with a Durkheimian emphasis on the categories of thought and their relation to social organisation. It was combined with the American traditions of pragmatism, instrumentalism and behaviourism, largely abandoned the historical frame or reference, and became more future-oriented (Wolff 1970:33, 47). In its American form, the sociology of knowledge also became more aligned with the natural science model (Wolff 1970:32), was denuded of its political edge, and offered a reformulated relationship between knowledge and social forces (Sica 2010: 175–6).

In the present study, the sociology of knowledge is employed to ask questions pertinent to twenty-first-century readers, rather than those initially formulated by its German founders. It also re-emphasises the European tradition of the programme where the works of Karl Marx and

Frederich Engels were central, for within their schema all knowledge is produced for the benefit of the ruling class:

> In so far, therefore, as they rule as a class and determine the extent and compass of an epoch, it is self-evident that they do this in its whole range, hence among other things rule also as thinkers, as producers of ideas and regulate the production and distraction of the ideas of their age: thus their ideas are the ruling ideas of the epoch
> (Marx and Engels 1976:64).

Mannheim did not fundamentally disagree with this proposition. He too theorised a connection between the social order and the ideas of the period, and assumed intellectual production could be stimulated by specific social developments. He phrased the connection somewhat differently:

> In fact, it is one of the most striking features of history that a given economic system is always embedded, at least as to its origin, in a given intellectual cosmos, so that those who seek a certain economic order also seek the intellectual outlook correlated with it
> (Mannheim 1971:108–9).

Yet Mannheim's (1960) theories challenged the Marxian view of all knowledge as derivative of class. He argued for the inclusion of other factors shaping the formation of knowledge, and gradually expanded *Wissenssoziologie* to include the study of other social structures, institutions, and settings. Subsequent scholars have offered many studies within this programme (Touraine 1971; Chomsky 1972; Bell 1974; Konrad and Szelényi 1979; Knorr Cetina 1981a, 1981b, 1999; Shils 1982; Bourdieu 1984; Freidson 1986b; Shumway and Messer-Davidow 1991; Martin and Richards 1995; Collyer 1996a, 2010; Lynch and Bogen 1997; Connell *et al.* 2005).

This body of scholarship, and the sociology of knowledge, brings to the study of sociology and sociologists a level of reflexivity and scepticism crucial in an arena where the very phenomenon one is seeking to analyse is not well understood. After all, sociologists have been much better at studying other forms of social life than turning their gaze to their own territory. This shouldn't be seen as resulting from a lack of effort, for there is a considerable literature on 'the sociology of sociology'. However little 'discipline' has been invested in studying the 'discipline'. Its explorations have been insufficiently empirical, and much of it fails to 'have something plainly sociological to say about sociologists' (Peek 1971:447).

The current study aims to fill some of this gap, and the sociology of knowledge is the vehicle through which 'discipline' will be introduced. Here, the sociology of knowledge is taken up as a contemporary research programme with a set of objectives to guide investigation into the myriad of connections between the ideational and material worlds. Its programme raises questions about the origin of ideas and how these are produced, transmitted and exchanged. Historically, proponents of *Wissenssoziologie*, and subsequently the sociology of knowledge, have not entirely succeeded in stipulating specific social theories nor epistemologies for the programme, and the field has remained relatively eclectic. This offers contemporary sociologists of knowledge the freedom to adopt theoretical tools according to the nature of their research questions or, as Gouldner (1970:28–9) might suggest, their background assumptions. In this case, our questions concern the nature of disciplines, the social action of disciplinary actors, and the importance of professions and institutions in the history of the sociology of health and medicine. Aiming for at least a modicum of rationality in the process of selecting a theoretical armoury (and ignoring Gouldner's concern with our ideological predilections for the present), the rest of this chapter takes a journey through the sociological landscape and the theories which have assisted others in their attempts to understand sociology and its past. It builds a new, more sociological approach to the field, and develops a new theory of disciplines and the processes of institutionalisation. This theoretical framework will be applied in later chapters to document and analyse the story of the sociology of health and medicine.

Intellectual or institutional histories?

The compiling and interpretation of history – *historiography* – is always a fraught process. Many of the early histories of chemistry, mathematics, medicine (and not a few histories of sociology) were 'Whig' histories, emphasising progress and implicitly glorifying the present (Jones 1997:143). The focus of their narratives were the 'great' individuals and 'great' deeds of the past, ignoring evidence of previous developments, collaborations, networks, and the support of institutions. Often written by 'insiders', retired medical doctors or chemists, the very nature of creativity and innovation went unquestioned, and these histories left a false impression that discoveries, inventions, and radically new theories were the sole production of particularly talented or creative individuals.

Yet the notion of 'creativity' has its own history, for it gained salience in eighteenth-century Europe, and became in the nineteenth a celebration of scientists and artists as romantic heroes who drew upon almost mystical forces for inspiration (Collyer 1996b). Contemporary studies of inventiveness and creativity have differed considerably, offering a diverse range of explanations. For instance, psychological studies have invested in the idea of *personality types*, where certain groups of individuals have a greater psychological propensity towards creativity (Rothenberg 1990:10). Business and economic disciplines have, in contrast, looked to the creative capacities of *market forces*, proposing these can produce and control innovative technological trajectories (Abernathy and Utterback 1978; Rothwell and Zegveld 1985). Sociological perspectives on the creation of new ideas and knowledge have also been wide-ranging. For instance, McKinlay (1981) has pointed to the importance of the sponsors of research, where their influence and power override any intrinsic worth of the idea or technology itself. Dahrendorf (1980:15) has come to a very different set of explanations, proposing the existence of a large, socially organised, chaotic 'reservoir' of ideas: a phenomenon which hegemonically defines the ideational world according to relevance, validity, and reward. And others, including Knorr Cetina (1981a), Whitley (1977) and Callon (1995:44), emphasise the *cultural context* as a support for learning and the formation of knowledge, particularly in the laboratory. New forms of knowledge – and even creativity itself – are shown in these sociological studies to be produced through social processes. As Bernard Stern, a sociologist *and* medical practitioner, noted with regard to medicine:

> Spontaneous creation can no more explain medical discovery than it can the origin of life. An invention or a discovery is invariably a product of the intellectual, technical, scientific and specifically medical traditions from which it emerges, and of the multitude of accretions, important and seemingly insignificant alike, which have preceded it. Certain specific medical discoveries are epoch-making in that they are milestones which mark new directions and paths for inquiry, diagnosis and treatment, but the road along these milestones cannot be ignored in realistic, as distinct from romantic, medical history
>
> (1941:41).

Stern's point is well made. Too often the history of medical discovery is told in a 'Whig' form, and it continues as a popular genre with many films and books devoted to the heroic inventors of anaesthetics or insulin or the genetic code. Yet 'Whig' accounts of the past endanger their very *historicity* or historical authenticity, for they over-estimate the role of individuals and consider the present to be a consequence of the thoughts and intentional actions of a few key individuals. To tell history in this way is to give the impression, for instance, that Marx alone conceived of the evils of capitalism or only Durkheim showed an interest in primitive cultures. But few individuals at any period of history are lone voices with singularly unique ideas: even if many are notable for the clarity or brilliance with which they put words to the concerns of the period. The fact that their ideas are noted – rather than those of another – should be the beginning of the historian's investigations rather than their end.

'Whig' histories also fail the test of good scholarship for the way they tell history as if the road from past to present has been a tidy succession of achievements. Such approaches are characteristically evaluative, dismissing many past forms of knowledge as untrue in the light of current theories and developments: rather than showing that the knowledge 'made sense' within the given state of technological development and its social context. These accounts are also problematic in the impressions they give of social change, offering individuals as the 'engines of history' (Nisbet 1967:5). While it may be true that some individuals play a relatively larger, or even pivotal role in social change, historical change is not reducible to the psychology, skills or intentions of individuals.

The majority of 'histories' of sociology – in contrast to those of medicine's past – are essentially *intellectual histories*, concerned with locating the origin of the sociological *tradition*. These are histories of ideas, with individuals being given an explicit role, but emphasising the interconnections between individuals and the ideas being put forward. Its method is the construction of intellectual threads through paradigms and often schools, which, over time, grew, prospered and perhaps faded from view. According to Cherkaoui, this form of historiography has the benefit of recognising the way a:

> ...system of thought or a school is a relatively consistent set of elementary and fundamental ideas. It can by no means be reduced to ideas put forward and defended by a given sociologist: a system of thought is the overall product of one or more generations
>
> (1997:iii).

In this approach to sociology's past, many turn to the era of the Enlightenment, to Scotland (Halsey 2004:55), or the turmoil of the Industrial, American and French revolutions (Nisbet 1943, 1967; Naegele

1965a; Wardell and Turner 1986; Alexander 1997). They focus on the philosophical ideas of many intellectuals, sometimes bringing into prominence men such as Ibn Kaldun (Alatas 2006a), or women such as Florence Nightingale or Beatrice Webb (McDonald 1994); but more often keeping to the male gender and the products of Christian Europe (perhaps Locke, Hume, Vico, Montesquieu, Hobbes, Ferguson, Smith or Rousseau). These writings, reflections and debates of the Enlightenment period are put forward as having offered a new perspective on the social order, human rights and widespread injustice, and to have constituted a new set of standards for public discourse and scholarship. In brief, they are said to have established the essential principles upon which the social sciences were later constructed (Hamilton 1997; MacPherson 1997).

Histories of ideas and intellectual histories are essentially *presentist* in their approach, seeking out possible connections between past and present ideas (Seidman 1983, 1985). They perform an important function for the discipline, giving it a 'cognitive identity'. Nevertheless, it is important to keep in mind these are *constructed* histories, and that:

> ... historians, like all scientists, always write from the standpoint of the present, must base their judgements entirely upon presently existing documents, and necessarily impose their own, present criteria of what is rational, significant, and interesting
>
> (Jones 1978:178).

As constructed histories, they are very selective interpretations of the past, offering a form of communication about the past but framed according to present concerns. As Ann Rigney (1992:86) argues, there can be no singular 'History', but only multiple 'histories', each a revision or re-interpretation of the past. Among historiographers there are few words which invoke such intense polarity as 'revisionism', for it conjures a frightening image of history as endlessly open, a minefield of ideological positions and perspectives. Yet revisionism is an essential cornerstone of historiography, for it is how we correct the distortions of previous scholars, and reconsider scholarship that has been neglected or dismissed from the historical record. This is the method taken by Charles Camic for example, in his re-examination of the works of the Utilitarians (1979). Although much of Camic's scholarship is *historicist* in orientation (e.g. Camic 1987, 1997), and thus explains past ideas or actions in terms of the social contexts of their own periods, we find also an acknowledgement of the importance of presentism and approaching 'the past with a very contemporary concern, understanding the process whereby theories of the social emerge, grow, and change' (Camic 1981:1142). The matter is also taken up by Robert Jones (1997:168), who suggests both historicism and presentism have a place in sociological work. Historicism, with its detailed analyses of past scholarship, might lead us to revise our knowledge and increase self-awareness of what those classical theorists may have meant. Presentism, with its repetition of claims about the classics which serious scholarship has often shown to be erroneous, nevertheless mimics the efforts of those past scholars, for they too were involved in seeking out a language and developing a set of tools to find solutions to pressing, everyday concerns.

These insights tell us that the choice of historiographic method should be made according to the goals of our research and the tasks it must fulfil. Of particular relevance to the current study is the notion of *contextualised* histories. This form of historiography takes on board the inescapable fact of history as always written from a particular spatio-temporal location. It's the approach to the past advocated by David Livingstone in his investigation of the discipline of geography. Here, Livingstone seeks to lay aside the mere cataloguing of people, publications and institutions, and offer a social history of the context of these ideas and persons (Livingstone 1992:11). In rejecting the notion of some 'eternal metaphysical core to geography independent of historical circumstance', Livingstone proposes a *situated* geography, suggesting it has meant 'different things to different people in different places and thus the "nature" of geography is always negotiated' (Livingstone 1992:28).

Livingstone's point is, of course, central to one of the research questions of the current study: the possibility that sociology takes not one but several forms in the world today. Hence our historiographical approach must be capable of uncovering the extent to which sociology is geographically as well as temporally 'situated'. And given our concern with social structure, and the extent to which individuals, ideas, and schools of thought have been supported and nurtured within specific time periods and societies, the most appropriate methodology for this historical analysis is to undertake an *institutional* history.

An institutional history documents the formation of the bodies through which scholarly ideas are nurtured, developed and transmitted. It offers a focus on the social networks, societies, university research centres, schools, and departments within which individuals work, develop their arguments, debate, collaborate and compete for resources. Unlike intellectual histories, institutional histories can demonstrate actual contact or influence between specific social actors (or generations of actors). In this sense they fulfil one of the principles of historicism. They can also contextualise the divergent voices and perspectives of the past, and so provide the reader with a greater sense of historical change, as well as of intellectual accumulation and its opposite: the systematic silencing of persons or perspectives. As an approach to the past, institutional histories offer an antidote to the misconception that disciplines might automatically result from a record of successful discoveries or intellectual accomplishments. The case of biochemistry in nineteenth-century Germany versus America, where the former country failed and the latter succeeded in establishing a discipline, indicates intellectual achievement to be hardly sufficient in itself to result in institution-building (Kohler 1982:3–4).

There are additional benefits to institutional historiography. The method doesn't prevent the exploration of the cognitive content of disciplines. This is important, because cognitive development and the formation of institutions are entwined in complex ways. Nevertheless little effort is expended in this study on tracing the earliest known examples of sociological perspectives on health or medicine: for that is the task of a history of ideas. Instead, an institutional historiography treats the cognitive realm primarily as a set of claims, and focuses on the processes whereby certain ideas and perspectives have become embedded in social practices and structured into more resilient and permanent arrangements. This means it concentrates attention on a much shorter period of history – the formation of departments of sociology, academic journals, and associations – and focuses on social and political struggles, on material resources and the events enabling the sociology of health and medicine to develop as a sub-discipline and become a fixture within the university systems of the three countries under our purview.

For a closing note on the importance of institutional histories we might turn to Pierre Bourdieu (1984), who uses the concept of 'habitus' to discuss features of social behaviour which have become part of an individual while living in a particular culture. For Bourdieu, the *habitus* is the set of dispositions attuned to a particular field or culture, which ensures the individuals concerned have the capacity, inclination, and interest to be part of its institutions and practices (Bourdieu 1993:18). Thus we might talk of a discipline's *habitus*; for a discipline can also be associated with relatively unique forms of social and cultural behaviour and a set of characteristics which have, over an historical period, become part of its very structure. And if we are to comprehend a discipline's *habitus*, we must understand its history, particularly the processes through which it comes to have a home in the academy. This is because, for sociology as a body of knowledge and set of social practices, its association with the university system has been a critical aspect of its development. As Talcott Parsons noted (in 1959:552), a 'secure position in university faculties... is the structural base from which a scientifically oriented profession can most effectively operate'. In keeping with this viewpoint, the emphasis is not on sociology as an intellectual tradition but *an institutional form* within the university system.

On the processes of intellectual change and disciplinary formation

It would be neglectful of anyone examining intellectual fields or disciplines to ignore theories of how these form and change over time. An area of social theory which deals specifically with the historical processes of intellectual change is inter-linked with the sociology of knowledge via the sociology of science (e.g. Barnes 1977; Fuchs and Ward 1994; Camic 1995; Fuller 1995; Fourcade-Gourinchas 2001; Groenewegen 2002). For our purposes, where the empirical focus is primarily on disciplines in the recent period, and our historical investigations aimed largely at revealing national differences in sociological practices and the content of sociological knowledge, we need to engage with this body of work only where it can assist with explaining the connections between knowledge and varying institutional forms.

Prior to the work of Thomas Kuhn (1970), which theorised radical, revolutionary changes in science as the consequence of an accumulation of anomalies within the scientific community, a standard approach to scientific change assumed the ideational sphere to be an immanent driver of change. In other words, some ideas and theories were thought to be sufficiently fertile to beget new knowledge, and eventually these matured into a coherent system of thought through a process of 'unfolding' and 'emergence'. Aspects of Talcott Parsons' (1968, 1970) approach to the discipline follow this model. Parsons favoured the methodology of neo-classical economics and of Pareto, and promoted the idea of sociological knowledge as a bounded and logical system produced in a process of 'discovery' and progressive movements towards 'truth'. This pre-Kuhnian conception offers an essentially passive view of science (Camic 1987:434–5). It is knowledge-making almost without social actors, for although Parsons acknowledged the influence of norms and values on sociological knowledge, these were generally thought to be over-ruled by the logical requirements of the system. It was also very much a positive conception of sociology, because it proposes that 'action itself... is not conceivable without some degree of correctness in observation of facts' (Parsons 1968:58).

More recent sociological efforts generally regard such models of cumulative progress and rational selection as unrealistic (Fuchs 1993:933). Attention has been re-focused on the interaction of actors, institutions or other elements of the social context in a search for the 'drivers' of intellectual change. This is a significant shift from the 'Great Men and Great Deeds' approach to examining history, where individuals were assumed to be behind intellectual change. It is also a move away from the heroic histories of discovery which were reliant on an orthodox epistemology of private processes of cognition. Instead, a renewed focus on the sphere of social action insists that we 'see through the personalities... [and] dissolve them into the network of processes which have brought them to our attention as historical figures' (Collins 1998:4).

This growing body of literature has largely polarised into two camps: internalist versus externalist approaches to intellectual change. The internalist perspective may, like some of the less recent theories, focus on the ideational sphere as an immanent driver of change; but more often theorises *cultural mechanisms of change*, with an emphasis on social practices, social networks and social interaction. Externalist explanations, in contrast, theorise the drivers of intellectual change to be primarily economic and political. This means 'knowledge is somehow wed to power and power propels change' (Abbott 2001:4).

In practice, few contemporary studies conform to either a purely internalist or externalist model of intellectual change. Most offer a composite, and few veer towards the latter. The decreasing interest in externalist theories of social change within the sociological community is associated with the broader demise of structuralism, particularly frameworks of Marxism and Structural Functionalism. The 'cultural turn' of recent decades and the growth of post-structuralism have had their impact on how we have come to understand intellectual change, ensuring the favouring of the internalist framework. Nevertheless, most sociological explanations of intellectual change acknowledge the interconnections between culture and social structure, and can best be differentiated by their emphasis or bias towards, on the one hand, the cultural sphere, with its focus on social action and meaning; and on the other hand, the social system and its structures of power. These differences become particularly apparent when we examine the way they theorise the influence of 'external' factors (such as the market) on the cultural production of knowledge.

Andrew Abbott's (2001) thesis of intellectual change in the social sciences is an example of an internalist approach. Proposing processes of 'fractal cycles' and 'fractal differentiation' and using the language of chaos theory, Abbott focuses on the cognitive products of the knowledge base, as well as the debates and disputes of the academic community. He argues these disputes, which might be over forms of measurement, social constructionism, labelling theory, or even Marxism, recur over generational time and eventually dissipate, producing a re-mapping of the issues and concerns and shifting the leadership of the field from one group to another (Abbott 2001:20–5). It is a theory which puts fractal conflict at the centre of intellectual change:

> The fractal cycle is at heart a profoundly traditional mechanism. Like any good ritual, it unites opposites. On the one hand, it generates perpetual change. Old ideas are always being thrown out. Intellectual autocracy is perpetually overthrown. On the other, it produces perpetual stability. The new ideas are always the old ideas under new labels. The new people are the old people in new roles…on the whole, the ritual is profoundly useful. We get to keep our best concepts forever and yet can retain our belief in perpetual intellectual progress
>
> (Abbott 2001:26–7).

This approach to change explains, to some extent, the noticeable patterns of borrowings between disciplines, their mutual take-up of ideas, perspectives, and methods (e.g. the spread of post-modernism and post-structuralism in the most recent period). It also highlights an important characteristic of the discipline of sociology: its many schisms re-appearing in scarcely altered form, sometimes after several generations of neglect. Abbott offers us a cyclical rather than cumulative theory of intellectual change, for we see the constant re-invention of old ideas rather than the extension of knowledge. The potential for the thesis to contribute to the current study of the sociology of health and medicine is somewhat curtailed by its lack of attention to the structures and relations of power. While it is true that Abbott discusses the 'external' pressures on academic life (perhaps from the global publishing market, budget cuts on educational resources, or repeated assaults on the system of university tenure); these are not well-developed or integrated into the theory of fractals. This means it can tell us only part of the story of intellectual change. It says little about how, or why, some ideas are systematically ignored or marginalised. Its says little about how, or why, some groups – such as Anglo-Saxon men from prestigious universities – might more often lead these disputes. And it says little about how, or why, specific intellectual or methodological disputes are taken up at particular times and places.

Randall Collins presents another example of an internalist approach. Primarily offered as a sociology of philosophies rather than of the social sciences, Collins (1998:5–7) nevertheless examines the structure of intellectual networks, proposing these as composed of inter-generational groups, made up of 'chains of eminent teachers and pupils'. These networks concentrate intellectual creativity, and at their centre, face-to-face encounters pass 'emotional energy and cultural capital from generation to generation' (Collins 1998:379).

For Collins (1998:534), intellectual change occurs differently across the spectrum of discipline areas, and there are even two kinds of intel-lectual networks operating within the natural sciences. In the latter, there is science 'in the making': a form of scientific network which produces emerging forms of knowledge. There are also traditional sci-entific networks dealing with established areas of science, that is, science 'behind the line'. Networks where science is 'in the making', are characterised by their emphasis on re-visiting and revising old posi-tions, while those where science practices are 'behind the line' have a broader level of consensus. In this schema, networks of science 'in the making' have similar organisational properties to philosophical net-works, and thus to social science networks, for they are more prone to dispute and even past disputes and theories are re-visited (Collins 1998:876).

Collins' (1998:380–1) thesis is that in networks where science is 'in the making' (and thus also in social science), intellectual change oper-ates according to 'the law of small numbers', where there is a continual struggle for intellectual attention space, and only a limited number of competitors in any given speciality – usually between three and six – can successfully propagate their ideas across the generations. Any attempts beyond this to capture attention will not be successful, and actors must instead form alliances and re-combine to fit in with other factions. These processes driving intellectual change mean that debate is always structured and contained by the availability of 'attention spaces'. Net-works are fragmented into a small number of opposing and contested positions, providing members with intellectual content. New ideas, cre-ativity, occurs only through refutation and the processes of clarification, and these 'structured rivalries constitute the successive moments of intellectual history' (Collins 1998:379).

Over the long term, the major intellectual driving force is the dynamics of organisationally sustained debate. Factions which keep their identities during many generations of argument become locked into a long dance step with one another; increasingly impervious to outside influences and turned inward upon their mutually constituted argumentative identities, they drive the collective conscience of the intellectual attention space repeatedly to new heights of abstract self-reflection

(Collins 1998:818).

Collins' thesis offers at least a partial explanation of why intellectual workers might expend so much energy on drawing attention to themselves and their work, and why they might continually situate their ideas in relation to existing traditions, schools and networks. This makes his thesis useful for examining some of the dynamics of intellectual interaction among sociologists of health and medicine, and thus will be revisited in later pages of this volume. As we found with Abbott's thesis, however, the connections between knowledge, the networks of intellectuals, and the social structure tend to be asserted rather than explained. Collins suggests there is a linking of 'outer conditions of social conflict with the inner shifts in the networks which produce ideas', for external changes (e.g. the rise or fall of a publishing market, or a material shift in institutional support for universities or monasteries), can bring about new spaces for individuals and new alliances can emerge (Collins 1998:380–1, 792). This, for Collins, is the association between 'the law of small numbers' and the social structure.

At the heart of this thesis is a conception of social structure as a form of constraint on social action. As Collins explains, these structures are the product of repetitive patterns of ritual behaviours which have the *feel of externality*, they seem 'thing-like, compulsory, resistant to change' (Collins 1998:28–9). We find, however, a curious disconnection between the intellectual world and the rest of the social system in this thesis. Intellectual knowledge and careers are determined by contests, but these contests operate according to patterns peculiar to the intellectuals themselves (Kurzman and Owens 2002:74). Are scientists, sociologists and other intellectuals not part of the class or gender system? Are they autonomous and unaffected by the structures of power, race, gender or class privilege? If it cannot incorporate the impact of global developments and shifts in the locus of power between nations (or between the state and the market as we have seen with the rise of neo-liberalism); how can the law of small numbers explain the rise of feminist theory in the 1960s, the post-modern turn of the 1980s, or the new interest in Terrorism or Security Studies?

A significant variation on these approaches comes from Thomas Gieryn's studies of science. Re-directing attention from the *contents* of the intellectual knowledge base to the cartographic *landscape* of intellectual work and the *activities* of intellectual workers; he focuses on the boundaries which gird and protect the divisions between disciplines. Gieryn (1983) initially produced his thesis of boundaries and boundary-work in an analysis of science and its demarcation from other intellectual activities (i.e. non-science). His subsequent work (Gieryn 1999) looks 'downstream' to the consumption of science and its 'credibility contests', to find answers to why science has been so successful as the legitimate arbitrator of reality (Gieryn 1999:xi). Both works investigate science using the same theoretical framework of boundaries.

Gieryn's thesis of boundaries challenges the philosophers and sociologists of science (particularly Karl Popper and Robert Merton), who spent considerable time seeking a set of principles for differentiating science from other forms of knowledge (e.g. Merton 1977). Gieryn (1983) radically proposes science as 'no single thing', for its boundaries are continuously drawn and re-drawn in a rhetorical attempt to manipulate its public image. In other words, the nature of science is flexible, and what science *is* depends on its representation at any historical point. Although Gieryn is fundamentally concerned with the boundaries between science and non-science, his concept of boundary-work has implications also for sociology, for it suggests that the demarcation of the discipline from other fields (such as anthropology and social psychology) may be equally as fluid and strategic as it is with science.

Gieryn regards scientific change as a process in which both culture and social structure are indistinguishable partners. Although his focus is on boundary-action and the realm of scientific practice, he argues that historical change cannot be reduced to either the internalist processes of cultural action, nor the externalist 'durable, distended, constraining stuff of social structure'. Neither ontological domain can permanently or unequivocally account for history, for they are 'mutually constitutive' (Gieryn 1999:12):

> Can boundary-work...be *reduced* to interests? Too crude by half: interests are not preformed and fixed forces (fully knowable and articulatable by cartographers or their audiences) that lie behind cultural maps, any more than the several embodiments of 'real

science' determine (in an unmediated way) the contents of its occasional representations. Boundary-work brings social interests and real science together in the mapping, and on these cultural maps both get articulated, altered, appreciated, denied, deployed, reconstructed, and translated in and through the cartographic process

(Gieryn 1999:23–4).

Given his emphasis on the terrain of the cultural field of science and the disputes of science rather than their stabilisation (Gieryn 1999:34), it is apparent that while this is an internalist perspective on scientific change, its conceptions of intellectual change and social structure are markedly different from those explored above. For Gieryn, intellectual change is produced through a process of constant interpretation and claims-making by social actors. This means the direction of intellectual change is relatively open, for although it is shaped by past and current practices, science is an arena in which there is little permanency or predictability:

There are just several of many coordinates used in the cultural cartography of science, but never consistently so. Nor is there a discernable direction in the long-run history of boundary-work toward one pole or other. Real science and its boundaries on cultural maps are supple and pliable things, like warm putty, but not so elastic that they may stretch endlessly in every direction

(Gieryn 1999:21).

The future trajectory of science is less determined and predictable for Gieryn than it is for either Abbott or Collins. In part this is because Gieryn (1999:12) conceptualises social structure as another field of cultural production, rather than a set of conventional constraints on social action. For Gieryn, structures are dependent on cultural meanings for their interpretation and operation. There is no 'real science' behind the claims-making processes, but several 'real sciences', none of which can be guaranteed to come into play and determine the next set of moves (Gieryn 1999:19).

Gieryn's (1999:27) approach to science draws from the interpretive sociological tradition which stretches 'from Weber to Mead to Schutz to Geertz – all of it focused on actors' understandings of things in their worlds'. It implicitly takes a Weberian (1949) approach to the production of knowledge and the processes of historical change. In Max Weber's view, knowledge production is a social process in which the social actor faces an *infinite* empirical context, and selects certain aspects of reality to create a view, theory and perspective (Weber 1949:78). The central organising principle of this process of knowledge selection is the system of values. These direct an actor towards what is culturally significant, *narrowing* the field and enabling the individual to 'make sense' of the empirical context (Zaret 1980:1183; Collyer 2008). This is not a passive model of the knowledge-making process – as we saw with Parsons – for in making his or her *selections*, the actor actively constitutes the object of study (Camic 1987:435).

This Weberian model is methodologically multi-causal (Turner and Turner 1990), meaning that it takes various historical and social factors into consideration when examining any given event, and weighs up the probability that the event could have resulted without the presence of any one of these factors. Weber's most notable use of this method was in *The Protestant Ethic and the Spirit of Capitalism* (1930), where he theorised Calvinism as one of several causes in the emergence of modern capitalism and thus offered a cultural interpretation of its origins to stand alongside Marx's historical materialist thesis. When applied to the realm of intellectual change, the methodology enables the inclusion of structural, cultural and ideational factors as causes. And when applied to an examination of the discipline of sociology (or its specialist fields), it suggests an alternative set of conclusions to that presented by Talcott Parsons: sociology as a product of the historically conditioned interests of its members, as open to the forces of the market place, but also shaped by culture and cultural practices. As such, its trajectory is neither linear nor necessarily cumulative.

Situating Gieryn's analysis more firmly within a Weberian, multi-causal methodology provides us with the strengths of boundary-analysis (given its focus on social action) without the attendant weaknesses of an interactionist approach. The latter tradition has long been criticised for its tendency to focus on micro-interaction and avoid the relations and structures of power (Martin and Richards 1995). It is not adequate, in itself, to explain historical development, for it assumes knowledge can arise from, and be sustained within, temporally and spatially located social interactions. As a consequence, the interactionist tradition on its own is unable to address the global context of sociology and the mechanisms through which such 'external' factors might re-arrange and help construct the sociological landscape. As a tradition, it ignores 'the social world beyond the text, a social world which is the condition of the existence of the text' (Murphy 1986:170).

A strengthening of the Weberian element into our approach to the discipline, on the other hand, provides for the analysis of the immediate cultural site of social action, but simultaneously takes into account the processes through which this arena is structured by 'external' factors. In her studies of scientific practice in the laboratory, Karin Knorr Cetina (1982:102) points out that scientific practice occurs within a 'field of social relations' such that 'the situational contingencies observed in the laboratory are traversed and sustained by relationships which constantly transcend the site of research'. Likewise, our examination of the sociology of health and medicine will have an immediate focus on cultural interaction as sociologists construct and protect the boundaries of their speciality field; but will be mindful of the contextual organisation of this field by social structures, including the structuring of the discipline itself.

The nature of disciplines

The history of the sociology of health and medicine could be studied from a variety of angles, and the focus of analysis might be the body of sociological knowledge, the sociologists within the speciality field, or even the organisations within which they work. In this volume, the choice has been made to study sociology as a discipline, or more accurately, the sociology of health and medicine: a specialist field within a discipline. There are many reasons for *not* employing the 'discipline' as the conceptual focal point of the study. For one thing, disciplines can be highly permeable organisational units, with much intellectual activity taking place with complete disregard for their boundaries or territories. For another, disciplines are only one aspect of sociological work, and not all sociologists regard their disciplinary identity as a central or organising principle of their research or practice. Nevertheless the locus of this enquiry is the discipline, because this highlights those aspects of sociology which have been somewhat neglected: sociology as an arena of social action and as an institutional form rather than simply a body of formal, scholarly knowledge.

The study of disciplines is not an entirely new field of sociological study. The methodological differences between the disciplines were a matter of significant concern for Max Weber in the early years of the twentieth century. Weber wrote that medicine, biology, and physiology – the new laboratory sciences – were flawed bodies of knowledge, because their analytical logic required them to 'take out history', and focus their gaze on 'universal laws' which are not reality, but merely tools for understanding (1949:85–6). Weber also noted the hegemonic encroachment of these emerging disciplines, given their proponents' insistence on the virtues of a single method for all the disciplines, and saw the beginning of the new century as a critical moment for the cultural sciences and sociology in particular, calling it the 'final twilight of all evaluative standpoints in all the sciences' (Weber 1949:86).

Despite the well-argued concerns of Weber and many others of his generation (including Durkheim, see Chimisso 2000:56), disciplines failed to continue as a topic of major interest during the rest of twentieth century. When disciplines were discussed in sociology, it was assumed these were merely cognitive divisions of formal knowledge and their differences self-evident (e.g. Parsons 1968:765). In general, historians, scientists and others:

> ... did not inquire why the world of knowledge was divided up as it is, or how it got that way, any more than naturalists before Darwin's generation worried about the origin and extinction of the species. There was no particular reason for scientist historians to see how their disciplines were shaped by processes of social and economic adaptation and competition. Disciplines were the framework for descriptive natural histories of knowledge, not for analyses of the evolution and perpetuation of social forms
>
> (Kohler 1982:1).

The recent renewal of interest in disciplines has steadily undermined the view of these as essentially cognitive domains, differing only in subject matter, perspective or methodology. Certainly they can still be understood as historic deposits, where disputes over meaning, truth, epistemology, and method have congealed over time into disparate parcels of scholarly knowledge. However there are problems associated with viewing disciplines in this way, not least the issue of whether they *have* legitimate 'objects' of study and unique methodologies. This matter has been noted by Therborn (1976:424, 426) for instance, who observed the historical shifts in the disciplines and how some, such as political science, don't even appear to have an object of study. Though the notion of disciplines as discrete, cognitive divisions of knowledge continues to be a common one; from the perspective of the sociology of knowledge, there is much more to the story of disciplines.

As we shall see later in this volume, disciplinary divisions differ markedly from country to country, and were arranged, defined, and organised very differently in the past. Moreover, it is only in the recent historical period that universities have established a monopoly on the production of formal knowledge. The current pattern of disciplinary categories in Britain, for instance, began to shift towards its recognisably modern form only during the previous two hundred years, with the formation of the scientific societies, the separation of natural philosophy into several natural sciences at the end of the eighteenth century (Shumway and Messer-Davidow 1991:204), and the irreversible impact of the late nineteenth-century conflict between the natural and moral-cultural sciences (Veit-Brause 2001).

In this study, disciplines are conceived as multi-modal entities. Rather than discrete cognitive domains, emphasis is placed on disciplines as arenas of social action; as symbolic structures employed by social actors in their struggle for resources; and as social structures, which result in the arrangement of actors and relatively stable patterns of social relations. Moreover, as arenas of social action and structural forms, disciplines are subject to the organising processes of other social structures, including those of patriarchy, class and capitalism.

Disciplines as sites of social action and social practice

Many, though certainly not all intellectuals, operate within the social and intellectual space of disciplines. Disciplines, say Shumway and Messer-Davidow (1991), are 'forms of life'. They provide a world of meaning towards which, in the Weberian sense, social action is oriented. Belonging to a discipline can confer numerous benefits of membership, including the provision of a sense of identity and inclusion within a particular group (though they also operate to exclude individuals from the membership of other groups); opportunities for building and maintaining a commitment to certain values and perspectives; possibilities for the bestowal of social acceptance and legitimacy upon one's work; and a vehicle to secure resources and status for individuals and the discipline.

Disciplines are often spoken of, in the English language at least, with geographic metaphors of fields, territories, and frontiers. Their occupants are said to annex, map, and explore these arenas, grounds, or spaces (Becher 1989:36). These metaphors lend border activities an heroic and almost military quality. They stand in contrast to the stereotypical representation of academic life in terms of the *gentleman scholar*, but otherwise tend to maintain its masculine mantle. The metaphors remain apt however, because discipline boundaries need to be understood as sites of fierce struggle over both symbolic and social resources (in other words, life within them can be 'nasty, brutish and short'); and, despite some important recent developments, in most parts of the world they continue to be masculine dominions (cf. Cass 1983; Holmwood and Scott 2010:24).

Disciplinary terrains or territories can be established (and maintained) through a variety of border activities often perceived as largely discursive. Lectures, presidential addresses, public announcements, editorials and scholarly publications are all utilised to set out the parameters of the field; construct the discipline's core ideas, paradigms, and methods; determine the central problems of the 'field'; and outline its connections with, and distance from, other fields. Such discourse is likely to include statements and arguments about the kind of experts who should be trusted with significant social or technical problems, what kind of evidence should be sought, the methods of research for obtaining reliable and credible results, and why other disciplines are less likely to produce equally satisfactory solutions.

Yet disciplines are not only discursive spaces but sites of social action. Boundary analysis provides insights into disciplines using social actors – and the spaces within which social action occurs – as a central focus of enquiry. In this approach, disciplines are neither natural nor cognitively distinguished, but primarily the creation of social actors over historical periods of time. As Andrew Abbott (1995) points out, social entities (such as disciplines) 'come into existence when social actors tie social boundaries together in certain ways'. As members of a discipline, participants undertake a variety of boundary-activities. Boundary-action incorporates various forms of *social action* to maintain, build or breach disciplinary boundaries. Boundaries after all are about differences, and the 'creation of zones of difference within the social process or social space' (Abbott 1995:877). Hence boundary-action is about clarifying, establishing, defending, extending, entrenching or removing differences. It may take a competitive or more co-operative form, and may be intentional or unintentional.

In the still-growing literature on the history of sociology, the concept of boundaries has been effectively employed to examine many aspects of disciplinarity, including the historical processes of disciplinary formation. An illustrative example comes from the formative period of the discipline in the American, late nineteenth- and early twentieth-century context. In this period, the size of the sociological community was quite small and somewhat ill-defined (Camic and Xie 1994:791). Much of its financial support derived from its audience: a group of reform-minded individuals who attended lectures and purchased sociological books

(Buxton and Turner 1992:375). Moreover, university-based sociologists who undertook research and surveys were dependent on the community for the donation of time and money. This community was the one to which the sociologists addressed their survey reports, as well as the one from which the participants and questioners were drawn. Even where money came from foundations – such as the Russell Sage Foundation – the leadership was often composed of local elites who were part of the audience and at the same time the supporters and drivers of the social reforms (Buxton and Turner 1992:377–8).

By 1895, American sociology had divided into the 'irreligious academics' and the 'religious reformers'. Key texts were produced, some criticising the constraints imposed on sociology by religion (e.g. Lester Ward's *Dynamic Sociology*, 1883), and others proposing a sociology underpinned by religious principles and commitments (e.g. John Henry Wilbrandt Stuckenburg's *Christian Sociology*, 1880) (Evans 2009:10). Sociological leaders in the first group, including Frank Lester Ward, Albion Small, and Franklin Giddings, decided that an affiliation with religion was not in the best interests of the discipline, for allowing the 'religious public' to contribute to the production of sociological knowledge was undermining its credibility (Evans 2009:11).

In Evans' (2009) study, the concept of boundary-work is employed to demonstrate how these sociologists – and others – were able to break established alliances, prove their independence from religion, and reconfigure the 'sociological public'. Although not all boundary-work is deliberately strategic (Knorr Cetina 1981a:73), there is evidence in this case (in the form of letters and published papers), of a planned and conscious effort on the part of some of the leading sociologists from several universities to restrict the participation of religious reformers in the discipline and improve its reputation (Evans 2009:12–3). This 'deliberative boundary-work' involved a diverse range of strategies, including the presentation of the discipline to the public as unified rather than riven with cleavages and tensions; the provision of support to other sociologists by writing reviews of their work; the building of alliances with established university scientists who had previously been hostile to the 'new science of society'; and the inclusion of religious groups only as consumers of academically-produced sociology (Evans 2009:14). The success of this boundary-work became evident by the 1920s when sociology was no longer primarily conducted outside the university system by religious reformers but constituted by academic professionals employed in major universities (Evans 2009:5–6).

This case from early American sociology offers a good example of where boundary-work is directed at the deliberate *exclusion* of particular groups to re-shape its audience (Evans 2009:16). This was achieved in large part through the *removal* of one of the discipline's fundamental 'boundary objects': the *American Journal of Sociology* (*AJS*). The concept of a 'boundary object' is used here to denote a tool that brings individuals and groups together from diverse social sectors or *across* disciplines, principally by facilitating the production of knowledge and communication. Examples of boundary objects include societies and associations, conferences, journals (Evans 2009:19), and textbooks (Schrecker 2008; Lynch and Bogen 1997). However the concept of a boundary object is also useful for describing aspects of social behaviour *within* disciplines, for, as will soon become evident, disciplines are themselves internally structured and fractured. In this sense journals, departments and professional associations can be employed to bind members of disciplines together, and assist with solving common problems and achieving mutual goals. In the illustrative case examined by Evans (2009), the placing of restrictions on the journal – an important boundary object – provided a mechanism to exclude certain groups from the newly emerging discipline. When first produced in 1895, the *AJS* had effectively bridged the social worlds within and beyond the academy, including the religious sociologists and the scientific sociologists. However once it became the official journal of the *ASA* and available only through subscription, the religious content declined and it no longer served as a boundary object (Evans 2009:17–8). Employing the journal as a boundary object is one of the more critical means through which American sociologists have, over time, determined the boundaries of sociology and defined their discipline through strategically re-shaping their audience or 'public' (Evans 2009:19).

The concept of boundaries has become popular in sociological analysis in recent years, and been usefully applied to understand many aspects of disciplinarity, including the creation of internal boundaries within disciplines, where sub-specialities are created (e.g. with regard to Anthropology, see Stocking 1995); the building of credibility and the generation of authority for the discipline (Gaziano 1996; Mizrachi and Shuval 2005); the establishment and demarcation of territory through discursive struggle (Gieryn 1983; Cooke 1993; Amsterdamska 2005); the production of boundary 'objects' for the discipline (Star and Griesemer 1989; Huyard 2009); and the deployment of claims for legitimacy which alter or maintain the division of labour (Ritchey and Raney 1981; Norris 2001; Martin *et al.* 2009). The concept of boundaries is used in the current volume to examine the discipline as a site of social action. In the second chapter it is employed to assist with understanding the institutional formation of the sociology of health and medicine, and in the third chapter, to scrutinise the relationship between the discipline and its speciality field.

Disciplines as social structures

Disciplines have a structural presence. Sociologists and other intellectuals don't have to entirely re-fashion the boundaries or contours of their intellectual field each time they write or speak, but are able to rely on a relatively stable set of meanings, opportunities, restrictions and organisational arrangements to predict the probability of a given outcome from their actions. There are several traditional approaches to social structure in sociology, some of which are incommensurable. Social structures can be conceptualised as determining, stabilising forces, providing little room for human agency, yet able to produce or bring social action 'into being'. This is the sense of a disciplinary structure we receive from readings of Foucault, for he spoke of disciplines as 'repressive mechanisms'. For Foucault, a discipline is a system of control in which a set of methods and 'truths' are accepted and adhered to within the institution of the research university (Shumway and Messer-Davidow 1991:202). Disciplines produce expert discourses, and experts adopt the label of a discipline to provide their body of knowledge with a mantle of legitimacy (Foucault 1972:224). These discourses operate as mechanisms of power, for they are all-pervasive, preventing alternative ways of seeing, speaking, and understanding. Foucault writes:

> He who is subjected to a field of visibility, and who knows it, assumes a responsibility for the constraints of power; he makes them play spontaneously upon himself, he inscribes in himself the power relation in which he simultaneously plays both roles; he becomes the principle of his own subjection
>
> (1977:202–3).

Foucault's conception of a discipline is not suitable for our present task of compiling an organisational and political history of the sociology of health and medicine. Its rather broad and sweeping analysis of the epochs of history make it a poor tool for explaining how individuals and groups might respond to the discourses which surround them and act to establish or refashion a new branch of knowledge and social practice. This is because Foucault's history is a 'history without subjects' (Frank

1998:331), for he tells us little about the processes through which any given individual is produced within, and shaped by, the discourses of power. But it is also because Foucault's concept of structure speaks of disciplines as if 'they' were capable of bringing about innovatory ideas or re-ordering academic practices. It is a perspective that purposefully looks beyond the very social action we are seeking to examine and record.

A more constructive approach to envisaging the structural qualities of a discipline – and the way intellectual ideas, social problems, methodologies, and social practices are taken up and captured within a resilient social form – is to focus on structures as human constructions. In this notion of structure, Berger and Pullberg reject the idea of structures existing apart from the human activity that produces them:

> Any specific social structure exists only insofar and as long as human beings realise it as part of their world ... social structure can be understood as an expansion of the field within which life makes sense to the individual ... an open horizon of possibility for all its members, a medium for the production of a world, while at the same time it is itself a produced moment of that world ... social structure is produced by man and in turn produces him. In sum, man produces himself as a social being through social structure
>
> (Berger and Pullberg 1966:63).

Berger and Pullberg acknowledge that this is not how most humans experience structure. Due to the fundamental linking of alienation and sociation, social structure appears to the individual as a given 'external' reality which constrains and narrows the possibility for movement. As such it prevents reflective action and the appreciation of one's role in its creation (Berger and Pullberg 1966:63–4).

Applying this conception of social structure, disciplines can be explored as social forms which, on the one hand, regulate, constrain, and *make possible* the action of individuals; and on the other, are the products of the repetitive, interpretive, political action of individuals. Disciplines are said to be:

> ... political institutions that demarcate areas of academic territory, allocate the privileges and responsibilities of expertise, and structure claims on resources. They are the infrastructure of science, embodied in university departments, professional societies, and informal market relationships between the producers and consumers

of knowledge. They are creatures of history and reflect human habits and preferences, not a fixed order of nature

(Kohler 1982:1).

In the current study, questions about the structural qualities of the discipline of sociology (and its sub-disciplinary field of the sociology of health and medicine) are best approached through a focus on the intermediary vehicles through which these twin processes take place: institutions. Institutions are:

> ... *building blocks of social order*: they represent socially sanctioned, i.e., collectively enforced expectations with respect to the behaviour of specific categories of actors or to the performance of certain activities. Typically they involve *mutually related rights and obligations* for actors, distinguishing between appropriate and inappropriate, 'right' and 'wrong', 'possible' and 'impossible' actions and thereby organising behaviour into predictable and reliable patterns
>
> (Streek and Thelen 2005:13).

As a general rule, most studies of institutions emphasise their constraining features rather than the social action envisaged in producing these *as* structures. This occurs regardless of the type of social institution under scrutiny. In Streek and Thelen's analysis for instance, informal, 'anthropological' institutions – such as rising from one's seat to greet another person, or the practices of shaking hands and introducing oneself – are distinguished from formal, legal–political institutions, such as the Federal Reserve Bank or marriage. In the former type, conformity to rules is encouraged in interaction through the moral disapproval of offenders, whereas in the latter, third parties (such as the courts, the unions, or other agents representing the community as a whole) can impose sanctions and ensure compliance (Streek and Thelen 2005:14–5, 18).

'Disciplines', as institutions, sit somewhat uneasily between these two forms. While conformity to disciplinary rules, norms and practices are not legally enforceable, and infringements are unlikely to attract sanctions from *third* parties (except perhaps with regard to plagiarism), disciplines are nevertheless not merely social conventions or habitual sets of expectations, but have an enduring, structural quality which is beyond the immediate capacity of specific groups of actors to modify.

The constraining effects of institutions are emphasised, in part, because much of the literature on institutions has come from the inter-disciplinary arena of organisational studies, where policy solutions are more of an imperative than the building of social theory. Even where theory-building is on the agenda, organisational studies have not managed to find a way around the 'theoretical fault line' of agency and structure (Reed 1996:46). As a consequence, institutions are offered as deterministic structures which in theoretical terms either ignore agency or under-theorise it. In the first instance we are presented with a conception of institutions as self-enforcing, rule-imposing mechanisms (DiMaggio and Powell 1983:148; Liang *et al.* 2007). In the second, institutions are composed of individuals engaged in the rational calculation of costs and benefits, or 'oversocialised' and unquestionably following the prescribed set of social norms (Tolbert and Zucker 1996:176).

Less prevalent within the institutional literature is an analysis of how these institutions are themselves produced. The closest we get to this is the recognition that institutions provide an 'arena' within which constructive activity might occur:

> An institution is a social structure … made up of a collection of individuals or organisations within which collectives exercise action or orientations
>
> (Weerakkody *et al.* 2009:355).

Some aspects of this constructive side of institutions are captured in the idea of institutionalisation. To institutionalise a practice or a set of rules is *'to infuse with value* beyond the technical requirements of the task at hand' (Selznick 1957:16–7). The concept also refers to the 'processes by which social processes, obligations or actualities come to take on a rule-like status in social thought and action' (Meyer and Rowan 1977:341). When applied to disciplines, processes of institutionalisation can be understood as a qualitative as well as quantitative change in the manner of conducting intellectual activity. Prior to institutionalisation, participants in an intellectual community or network are forced to rely on persuasion and personal worth to obtain cultural authority, and there is a high probability of bureaucratic, corporate or religious intervention in the activities themselves. Through the processes of institutionalisation, material supports and cultural resources become concentrated; formal mechanisms for communication and interaction are established; the legitimacy of a set of rules and sanctions is accepted; and there is increasing public or community recognition and support.

Despite the potential for the concept of institutionalisation to be used to explore the creation of structure, the emphasis is more often on the *final stage* of the process. Institutionalisation is assumed to be the point at which an end is brought to the otherwise discontinuous and non-cumulative processes of intellectual activity (Oberschall 1972:4). Attention is therefore centred on the 'end-point', that is, where a set of social practices or rules have 'become institutionalised', and not on the question of how institutions *form and change*.

An example of this prevailing approach is Shepherd's (2003) analysis of the development of archaeology in South Africa. Here the formation of archaeological societies and systems of patronage are put forward as historically important aspects of institutionalisation, but there is no discussion of the concept of institutionalisation itself. This lack of attention to where institutions come from, their internal structures, and the processes through which they are produced, has been widespread within the social sciences (Zucker 1987:460; Weerakkody *et al.* 2009). Although conceptual scrutiny has been building, questions about the emergence and survival of institutions remain 'frontier issues' (Weingast 2002:692).

Paying greater attention to the *formation* of institutions means examining the *cultural production of structures*. It means considering social structures – such as disciplines and institutions – as coming into existence through a process of constant interpretation and sustained social action (Gieryn 1999:12). As *cultural* products, institutional structures can take diverse forms, and are potentially amenable to reform and renewal, even if, as Collins (1998:28–9) points out, they seem 'thing-like, compulsory, resistant to change'.

There are a handful of theories which can be used as a basis for examining how institutional structures – such as disciplines – are socially and culturally produced. Unlike most of the studies above, which focus on the institutionalisation of organisations, the external or internal pressures on these units (Zucker 1987) or the institutional linkages between them (DiMaggio and Powell 1983); there are a few which pay greater attention to the actions of individuals and social groups.

We can begin with Berger and Luckmann (1984) and Schultz (1967), for whom the process of institutionalisation in its earliest phases occurs as regular interaction between actors, bringing about shared meanings and practices. This shared reality can be taken up in other areas of society in a process of habitualisation, where social life becomes habitual, needing little immediate thought, and hence predictable (Berger and Luckmann 1984:53–7). Whenever there is a 'reciprocal typification of habitualised actions' by social actors over the course of a shared history, institutionalisation may result. This simply refers to the process whereby the meanings of habitual actions become independent of the original context and available to others. These shared social forms are passed on to new generations, and because the underlying reasons for the creation of the institution are no longer transparent, they appear to actors as self-evident and 'objectively real'.

The institutions, as historical and objective facticities, confront the individual as undeniable facts. The institutions are there, external to him, persistent in their reality, whether he likes it or not. He cannot wish them away. They resist his attempts to change or evade them. They have coercive power over him, both in themselves, by the sheer force of their facticity, and through the control mechanisms that are usually attached to the most important of them

(Berger and Luckmann 1984:59–61).

For disciplinary institutions to be created (those which are halfway between the anthropological and the formal–legal type), the analysis of Berger and Luckmann is less useful. Indeed there has been very little attention paid to the processes through which organisations and the formal bodies associated with disciplines are produced. These bodies, which are indicators of the final stages of institutionalisation, include departments, professional associations, and academic journals. Each plays an important part in the process of disciplinary development.

The first of these, *academic departments*, are administrative units to which staff are generally attached by some form of employment contract. Through these, staff are recognised as legitimate actors in university affairs: a connection providing certain resources, defining and directing some of their activities (primarily those associated with teaching rather than research), and setting out administrative and legal responsibilities. This departmental system developed, according to Abbott (2001:123–4) in America, and spread to Europe and other countries from about the mid-twentieth century. It brought with it a shift from the arbitrary (though intense) research activity dictated by the interests of individual and important chairs in the university (evident in the old German system), to a new disciplinary landscape divided into distinct fields. Since that period, almost all social practices associated with the formation or maintenance of sociology (as a formal body of knowledge) have taken place within, or in association with academic departments. This includes both *formal* and *informal* social practices.

With regard to the *formal* social practices, discipline-based departments act as the engine of the academic labour market across the university system. They supply as well as employ new individuals, advertise positions through discipline-based networks, and organise academic careers (which are formed within disciplines rather than individual universities) (Abbott 2001:126). Discipline-based departments have most often been the place of employment for the editors and reviewers of the scholarly journals, presidents and members of the executive of the professional associations, authors of sociological materials and textbooks, as well as the teachers of the disciplinary canon. Few government departments, corporations or community organisations set aside the resources for such tasks, though there is, as we shall see in subsequent chapters, some country variation in this. Moreover it is within academic departments – and sociology departments in particular – that most debates and decisions are made concerning the limits and appropriate intellectual contents of the discipline. New appointments, new course proposals and even maintaining or updating the degree structures, all require representatives of departments in university committees to spend time considering whether new courses 'appropriately belong' to the discipline rather than another. In this way, departments are centres of sustained reflection upon the discipline, preserve its traditions and drive disciplinary change.

Informal social practices which assist with the development of sociological knowledge also generally occur in association with academic departments. Departments provide many members not only with an income, but an arena within which social ties can be established between staff. Given that an academic vocation necessitates geographic mobility and tends to disrupt both family life and friendship networks throughout one's career, the department often serves as a major locus of social ties for the sociologist. These friendships and associations sometimes lead to joint intellectual or professional projects but also enable individuals to expand their social networks and find mentors who might assist with the challenges of academic life. These social ties are particularly important for academics in the social sciences, as most have a unique academic career in which its pathways have been actively constructed by the individual rather than directed by institutional requirements.

The formation of *professional associations* is another indicator of institutionalisation, and their role has been critical in this process:

> ...the importance of strong, well-managed professional associations should not be underestimated. Through their meetings, publications, and various other channels they form the most important single type of medium through which sociologists over the country communicate with one another. Furthermore they provide a means

for concerted action in promoting interests and discharging the responsibilities of the profession... The professional association can be especially helpful in mediating our 'citizenship' relations to neighbouring disciplines as well as to the public at large

(Parsons 1959:558).

An additional sign of institutionalisation is the formation of the *academic, scholarly journals*. These bring together individuals and groups from diverse social sectors, based on their common interest in sociology. Journals facilitate the production of knowledge and communication and propose a commonality of perspectives and values that differentiate the discipline. They also help forge a disciplinary identity for the participants (authors, readers, reviewers, and editors) and promote the discipline as a profession.

Despite the centrality of these organised social forms, the processes involved in their production have been largely neglected. Preference has been given to the examination of the broader social processes which shape and encourage their growth, for instance, the processes of rationalisation, bureaucratisation, surveillance, and governance (Weber 1948; Foucault 1977; Ritzer 1990). A few attempts have been made to theorise some of the precipitating factors critical to the eventual institutionalisation of disciplines. Although it would be difficult to describe these as systematic, theoretical frameworks, they can assist with the task of building one.

Ben-David (1965:49) offered one of the earlier efforts. In an analysis of the establishment of the scientific community in Europe, he points to the requirement for sufficient financial support to enable continuity in research and publication. Once achieved, this brought an autonomy from the non-scientific culture and the development of a scientific identity. In their study of the origins of psychology, Ben-David and Collins (1966) explained the emergence of new disciplines as a consequence of three factors: (1) the existence of an academic rather than amateur role for intellectuals, (2) a competitive situation allowing individuals to move into the emerging area, and (3) an hierarchical difference between discipline areas. Other precipitating factors are also mentioned within the same text, including the lack of opportunities outside the university to ensure innovation occurs *within* the system, institutions of sufficient size to allow for specialisation, and facilities for research and reasonable salaries (Ben-David and Collins 1966:465). Oberschall (1972), in investigating the institutionalisation of empirical sociology, considered the importance of certain 'historically present' conditions, including intellectual and scientific interest, social demand, sponsorship, and resources. Finally, Bloom (2002:41), drawing on Oberschall (1972) as well as Ben-David (1965), outlines a model of four stages of sociology's institutionalisation. First, the marking out of a distinct intellectual area which is different in method, subject matter or technique. Second, establishing this subject matter as culturally meaningful. Third, formalising the processes of training and recruitment into the discipline, as well as its means to attract resources, and thus ensuring its growth, continuity and stature. And finally a process of consolidation of the discipline, with its own subculture, publication outlets, means of communication and networking, and professional associations.

None of these studies can be characterised as fully theorised or systematic explorations of the processes of institutionalisation. Some, such as Oberschall's (1972), are based on market models of supply and demand which explicitly exclude individuals or groups from participating in the creation of institutional structures. Bloom's (2002) history of American medical sociology offers a rare example of discussion of the concept of institutionalisation, though this discussion is brief and largely ignored in the remaining pages of his book.

Theories of the formation and growth of sociology require a theory of institution-building which takes social action as a central feature of disciplines and yet does not ignore their structural features. Such a theory would have to take into account the temporal and cultural context of this process, for discipline-building in late nineteenth-century Japan is likely to vary from 1950s Australia. It would also have to take into account whether the discipline was forming for the first time in the world, or whether it was appearing in a new geographic and temporal location. In the case of sociology in the United States, Australia, and the United Kingdom, the discipline had already made an appearance in Europe (even if some of its features were quite different). This makes our study of discipline-building a case of *transcontinental borrowing* rather than a project beginning from first principles. A theory of institutionalisation would also outline the series of stages through which new disciplines develop, with sufficient flexibility for the fact that disciplines institutionalise at different rates, in slightly different ways, and perhaps in a different order in each geographic and organisational context. One of the reasons for these varying trajectories can be found in the broad array of possible inter-disciplinary relationships, because disciplines do not emerge independently, but in relation to others. This has been noted in Dorothy Ross' (1979:124) history of the social sciences, and also by Charles Camic (1995, 1997). The latter's suggestion is to introduce the notion of *localism* into institutional histories to explain such variations. He points to the fact that at each university, and in each discipline, there were different patterns and sets of relationships. Each academic field was positioned differently with respect to the others; there were variations in the administrative policies in each location; different histories with regard to intellectual and institutional contacts; and different levels of access to material and symbolic resources (Camic 1995:1011–2). Taking these points into consideration, the following model of discipline-building is offered:

1) Initial phases are characterised by a focus on *connectivity and communication*. Groups or gatherings are essentially informal meetings among friends and colleagues who are well-known to one another. There is usually one or a small handful of individuals at the 'core' of the group, without whom the process would probably falter. These individuals are likely to have experience of the discipline in another country (either as a migrant or whilst a student). General members/supporters come from a variety of disciplines and outside the university as well as within, and group discussions may be focused on a set of problems or mutual experiences of hardship or marginalisation rather than theoretical issues *per se*. Any form of organisation at this initial stage is likely to be non-hierarchical and tasks or roles are voluntary and transient;

2) The second phase is characterised by the *regularisation* of discourses, practices and forms of organisation. Meetings and other events have become more frequent; volunteers assigned roles as convenors, secretaries, or treasurers; and notes might be taken during meetings. Some research or teaching groups may have formed, and resources found for small projects or events. The endeavour continues to be dependent on the commitment of specific individuals and their capacity to secure resources (such as an office or regular meeting room). The assistance from members of other disciplines is critical, for these disciplines often provide members with a position within their faculties, opportunities for service teaching or a role in collaborative research programmes. Future members begin to be attracted to the field, though the graduate work of existing members is still generally completed overseas or in other disciplines because local post-graduate qualifications (in sociology) are not well established;

3) The third phase is characterised by a process of *embedding*, where efforts have been successful at obtaining a home of some form within the university, and a distinct identity is well under

construction. Professionalism has become a central feature, as has internal and external political action, particularly with regard to efforts to secure material resources and representation within the university. Such political activity is conducted by individual actors often now working within, or representing, organisational bodies, thus lending authority and credibility to forms of boundary-action. There is a strong emphasis on networking within and beyond the academy in order to acquire financial and other material resources. Friendship or networks of known individuals no longer constitute the main means to build membership. Distinct boundaries have appeared between this and other fields/disciplines, and the necessity of their support has begun to wane. Hierarchical and bureaucratic forms of organisation and practice have become the norm (e.g. office holders, editors), and places within the field have become exclusive, with members from other disciplines or outside the university sector no longer made welcome. A final feature of this phase is the level of introspection about the nature of the discipline, its current status and likely future. The subject is addressed in the discipline's newsletters, journal articles, and conferences; and

4) The fourth phase of *legitimation* completes the process of institutionalisation. In this final phase, any remaining informal practices or units have been converted into a legal form, such that the new discipline has all the relevant trappings, including journals, professional associations and departments. Boundary-action is now routine, predictable, and formalised. Distinct degree programmes have been established, and the discipline is represented on all appropriate boards and committees of the university. Credentialism is controlled by disciplinary leaders (often in consultation with the professional body), and senior members of the discipline have considerable autonomy to oversee and direct the appointment of new staff, the curriculum, and the academic offerings within their departments.

The completion of the institutionalisation process provides the discipline with a level of protection against its ready dissolution. Contrary to the internalist conception of disciplines, where it is presumed the foundational ideas laid down by Marx, Freud, Weber, Durkheim and the classical economists form the basis of the discipline and also the current disciplinary landscape (Abbott 2001:152); this alternative theory indicates the discipline's strength lies instead in its social relationships and thus its institutionalisation. Through the processes of institutionalisation, mechanisms have been developed to defend disciplines against encroachment and other forms of inter-disciplinary assault, but their institutional structure within the universities also gives them a significant level of autonomy and resilience in the face of system-wide changes (an issue which will be re-visited in the final Section of this chapter 'Situated disciplines: Other forms of social structure').

In the Section immediately below, 'The institutionalisation of three sociologies', the institutionalisation of the parent discipline of sociology in each of the three countries is shown to have broadly conformed to these four stages. We see the creation of disciplinary departments, professional associations, and the discipline's academic journals. Given the similar institutional trajectories of the parent discipline and its specialist field of the sociology of health and medicine, the brief overview provided below will remind readers of the major features of the process of the former before embarking on the analysis of the specialist field in Chapter two. These institutional histories, it should be noted, are stories of disciplinary 'success'. Each stage contributes further to the process of disciplinary development, facilitating a sociological identity and building the sociological community's capacity to attract, socialise and educate new generations of scholars. Yet there is nothing in this theory which says institutionalisation cannot be reversed. If institutions are, as suggested, dependent on social actors and their support, strong opposition might bring about a decline or de-institutionalisation of intellectual fields. History is potentially full of stories of institutional 'failures' (and needs to be explored by future researchers). It should also be noted that, in the cases below, there is variation in the institutionalisation of the discipline in each country, and some discussion of this can be found at the conclusion of the three histories.

The institutionalisation of three sociologies

Developments in Europe

The discipline of sociology is usually assumed to have taken root within the university system during the 'classical' era; a period beginning in the closing decades of the nineteenth century and ending in the early decades of the twentieth century. Yet closer analysis suggests there are few places in the world where this occurred. Peter Wagner (2001), who is primarily concerned with the essential rupture between the sociology of the classical period and its modern form; tells of the scholarly journals and academic societies which were established in the early twentieth century, but also about the general lack of representation of sociology in the universities of Europe until well after the Second World War. He points particularly to the paucity of university chairs of sociology: one of the few named chairs was held by Emile Durkheim at the *Sorbonne* in France from 1913 (Wagner 2001:55; also Aron 1971:159; Claus 1983; Jefferys 2001). The situation was even worse elsewhere in Europe, for there were no named chairs of sociology in Germany or Austria until 1919 (when one was accepted by Max Weber), and although several dozen were established in Germany by 1933 (Wagner 2001:8–11), these disappeared during the Nazi era as sociologists were killed or fled abroad (Collins 1985:46). Efforts to establish sociology in Europe at the end of the nineteenth or beginning of the twentieth century were therefore both sparse and short-lived.

After the Second World War, the reconstruction of Western Europe began, and this was also a period of re-establishment for sociology and the social sciences as 'an explosion of vitality and sentiments broke the existing structures' and overturned the conservatism of the people (Aron 1971:160). The 1950s were marked by an effort to investigate social issues and provide an underpinning for the new era of social planning for the welfare state. Sociology and the social sciences were part of this mid-twentieth-century movement to modernise and transform the war-torn societies (Cherkaoui 1997:xii). Thus it was only in the 1950s that chairs in sociology appeared in Italy and re-appeared in Germany (Wagner 2001:11, 56). Even Durkheim's chair at the *Sorbonne* did not represent the beginning of a growth in sociology in France, for it was a long time before others appeared, and there were still only four by the mid-1950s (Wagner 2001:55).

Developments in the United Kingdom

Institutionalisation for sociology in the United Kingdom was also very much a mid-twentieth-century affair. The discipline was first given a home in 1903 at the *London School of Economics* (or *LSE*) (Bulmer 1985:5; Abrams 1968). The *LSE*, a Fabian institution 'invented and fostered' by social reformers Sidney and Beatrice Webb, opened in 1895 as a night school for part-time students. It initially specialised in the social sciences and eventually became a college of the *University of London* (Halsey 2004:13–4). Sociology's place in the academy was given some reinforcement in 1907 with L.T. Hobhouse's appointment to the Martin White Chair (Bulmer 1985:5). This was the gift of Martin White, a Scottish philanthropist who provided ten thousand pounds for the founding of the first chair of sociology (Halsey 2004:3). Hobhouse was a philosopher and a journalist, and the focus of his work was the development of non-industrial societies. In this he offered a challenge to the Social Darwinism of Herbert Spencer (Cockerham 1983:1519–20). Other early figures associated with the *LSE* include Edward Westermarck, William Beveridge, Morris Ginsberg, T.H. Marshall, David Glass, and Alexander Carr-Saunders. Apart from the creation of a social science department at *Liverpool University* in 1909, the *LSE* was essentially the centre of British sociology until the 1940s; particularly of empirical sociology, which was conducted largely outside sociology departments and even outside the university system (Platt 2002:180; Halsey 2004:51).

In the 1940s there was some growth in British sociology, with five other universities creating new degree-level courses in sociology (Roberts and Woodward 1981:533).[1] Overall there continued to be little institutional change, with most British universities continuing to ignore sociology (Halsey 2004:51). By the end of the 1950s there were only about 40 sociologists teaching in British universities (Jackson 1975:19), but these eventually began to take part in a developing international, academic network of sociologists, with links established between Britain and the United States (Halsey 2004:92).

The post-war years witnessed a flurry of government activity, with the state providing free secondary-school education, free social and medical care, and policies of full employment. It was a radical expansion of state power, and greatly encouraged academic reflection on social policy and administration (Halsey 2004:96). A conservative government was in place from 1951 to 1964, and this provided for the setting up of *The Institute of Community Studies* in 1953 (assisted by the efforts of Richard Titmuss), with Michael Young as its first director (Oakley 1991:186; Willmott 1985).

With a Labour government from 1965, there was considerable new growth. Notable was the construction of the new 'plate-glass' universities, approved by the *University Grants Committee* in the later 1950s and early 1960s. This is a term referring to the construction of university buildings in glass, steel and concrete as opposed to the older 'red brick' universities of the Victorian-Edwardian era and the 'ancient' universities of *Oxford* and *Cambridge*. The new 1960s universities, which included *Sussex* (1961), *Warwick* (1965), *York* (1963), and *Kent* (1965), enabled 28 departments of sociology to be created (Halsey 1985:152). These included a chair at *Cambridge*, taken up by John Barnes in 1969 (Encel 2005:47), although it was 1983 before the chair was occupied by a sociologist (the first being Anthony Giddens, see Halsey 2004:96,101).

Important also was the *Social Science Research Council (SSRC)*, established in 1965 (Oakley 1991:186). The creation of so many new appointments and institutions was soon followed by a heightened level of activity among sociologists, with numerous investigations of the social impact of the newly expanded public services; for instance, Townsend's (1962) report on aged care, and Packman's (1968) analysis of child care services. Poverty and inequality also became favourite areas for sociological and social policy research during this period, commonly employing the concepts of a 'cycle of disadvantage' or 'inter-generational poverty' (Halsey 2004:97–8). In addition, the number of sociology courses being taught across the United Kingdom grew during these years (Cockerham 1983:1519).

The 1960s were also a period in which members of the small but growing discipline began to take action to professionalise. Various dissatisfactions fuelled this effort: with the 'old-fashioned, senior members' of the *BSA*, the lack of an effective public voice for sociology, the common practice of hiring university staff without sociological training, and the generally poor standard of the discipline (Horobin 1985:96; Platt 2002:183–5). This oppositional group of university teachers began to meet informally with the aim of assisting sociology to become a discipline with its own system of training. It eventually developed into a 'Teachers' Section' of the *BSA*, and largely responsible for forming the journal *Sociology* in 1967 in competition with the *LSE* journal (Platt 2002:183–5). The section flourished until 1975 when it was disbanded. By this date there were sufficient numbers of well-trained sociologists being produced in Britain, and the 'young Turks' had taken over the control of the *BSA* itself (Platt 2002:188).

The most significant period of growth in university student enrolments occurred in the later 1960s, and the social sciences and sociology received an important share of these new students (Roberts and Woodward 1981:533; Platt 2002:180). This led to a further eight chairs of sociology being added by 1974 (Platt 2002:181), bringing the number of departments to 39 by 1973 (Roberts and Woodward 1981:533). In fact, during the 1970s the number of sociologists in the system expanded considerably with departments appearing in all major universities including *Oxford*, as well as in the colleges and secondary schools (Jackson 1975:19). This expansion in teaching jobs for sociologists was accompanied by an expansion in sociological research, with 900 sociology graduates employed in full-time research occupations by 1973 (Platt 2002:181). The general expansion brought opportunities for women to enter the universities, and by 1974/5 women held

22 per cent of the positions in British sociology departments, though only ten per cent of the professoriate (Roberts and Woodward 1981:538). The later 1970s and throughout the 1980s were years of contraction, with fewer academic posts, particularly in sociology, the humanities and social sciences (Roberts and Woodward 1981:533). The 1990s were years of sustained growth in student numbers across the university sector but were not matched by increasing funds for teaching. Universities also experienced a marked increase in regulation and monitoring, and previous entitlements to research resources for all universities were removed. This occurred amidst a major transformation of the sector with the merger of the former polytechnic and college system into a single system. Such changes are claimed by some to have represented a process of proletarianisation. They certainly 'disrupted institutional cultures and practices on a dramatic scale' (Fulton and Holland 2001:301). By the late 1990s the membership of the *BSA* reached 2,500, about half of whom had teaching posts in sociology (Platt 2002:192). The shape of the workforce did not change as rapidly as some of the other elements of the university sector. By 1997, women constituted about 33 per cent of British academics, and continued to be found in the lower ranks, for only eight per cent of the professoriate of British universities were women (Fulton and Holland 2001:312). This percentage doubled over the next ten years, to 17.5 per cent (Lipsett 2008).

Developments in Australia

The institutionalisation of sociology in Australia closely parallels the British case.[2] Chairs and departments of sociology did not begin to appear in Australia until the 1950s, and hence sociologists took refuge in other disciplines, with sociology courses taught within departments of anthropology or philosophy, and often under the auspices of the *Workers' Educational Association (WEA)*. This latter was a model of education originating in Britain and brought to Australia in 1914. It operated in many of the states of Australia under the direction of a committee composed of representatives from the universities, the trade unions and various community groups. Classes were taught at the universities, with its tutors, lecturers, and a director appointed by the local university (see Bourke 2005:150). *Academic* sociologists of some note during this very early period include Francis Anderson, *Professor of Logic and Mental Philosophy* in 1890 at the *University of Sydney,* who, in 1909, was the first to offer sociology as a unit of study in an undergraduate degree in Australia (Zubrzycki 2005:219); Anderson's student, Clarence Hunter Northcott, who also taught sociology at the *University of Sydney* but left Australia after completion of his doctoral thesis to study under Franklin Giddings at *Columbia University* (Bourke 2005:148–9); George Elton Mayo, who was appointed to the chair of philosophy at the *University of Queensland* from 1919 to 1923 and later moved to the United States (Mitropoulos 2005:108); John Alexander Gunn, a scholar in French philosophy from *Liverpool* with prior appointments at *London* and the *Sorbonne*, who took up the directorship of the *WEA* at *Melbourne University* in 1924 to teach sociology (Crozier 2005:126; Zubrzycki 2005:220); and Meredith Atkinson, who offered sociology classes at the *University of Melbourne* from 1918 to 1922 as director of the *WEA*. Given that Atkinson accepted the role of director on condition he was given the title of professor and a seat on the Professorial Board, he became the 'first self-styled professor of sociology in Australia' (Bourke 1981:31; Crozier 2005:126; Western 2005:50).

Sociology took on a more secure institutional form from 1950 with the formation of a Department of Anthropology and Sociology at the *Australian National University* (*ANU*), in the *Research School of Pacific Studies* in Canberra. W.E.H. Stanner was appointed as Reader in September 1949, and S.F.S. Nadel to the position of Professor and Chair in August 1950. This department is often overlooked in the official histories of sociology because it did not provide for undergraduate students. (Undergraduate teaching was not allowed under the charter of the *ANU*.) Nevertheless, it *was* a department of sociology, and as such offered a home for sociologists and their research. The *second* department began life in 1959 at the *NSW University of Technology* (which became the *University of New South Wales* (*UNSW*) in the same year), and was chaired by Morven Sydney Brown (*ANZJS* 1965a:62). Sol Encel (1984:5) argues that the formation of this department of sociology was the outcome of the 1957 *Murray Report* on Australian universities. This enquiry, chaired by Keith Murray, was set up by Prime Minister Robert Menzies, and led to the formation of the *Australian Universities Commission* to co-ordinate university development in Australia (Gallagher 1982:53–4). The same report recommended the *University of Technology* expand its range of academic courses, and sociology benefited from this. These two early departments were followed by a separate Department of Sociology in the *Research School of Social Sciences* (*RSSS*) at the *ANU* in 1961, and not long afterwards, departments (with undergraduate teaching and often combined with anthropology, social work or social policy) were formed at the *University of New England* (1962), *Monash* (1964), *Queensland* (1965), *La Trobe* (1966) and *Macquarie* (1969), with many others emerging over subsequent decades (*ANZJS* 1965a; Zubrzycki 2005).

Early sociologists of the 1950s and 1960s included Jerzy Zubrzycki (a graduate of the *LSE*, a Research Fellow at *ANU* from 1953, and Professor of Sociology at *ANU*, *The Faculties* from 1971); Morven Brown (a graduate of the *Universities of Sydney and London*); Wilfred (Mick) Borrie (a New Zealander educated at the *Universities of Otago and Cambridge*, Research Fellow at *ANU* from 1947, and Professor of Demography from 1957); and Hans Mol (a graduate of *Columbia*).

These were followed in the later 1960s and 1970s by another group which included Sol Encel (a graduate of *Melbourne* and Professor of Sociology from 1967 at *UNSW*); Athol Congalton (a New Zealander, Associate Professor from 1963, and then Professor of Sociology *UNSW*); Owen Dent (a graduate of the *ANU* and *Brown*); Frank Jones (a graduate of the *ANU* and Professor of Sociology *ANU* from 1972); John Barnes (a graduate of *Oxford*), Leonard Broom (from *Texas* at Austin, and Professor of Sociology *ANU*, *RSSS* from 1971), Jean Martin (neé Craig); Colin Bell (Professor of Sociology *UNSW* in 1975, Professor of Sociology in 1980 *Aston*, Birmingham, Vice-Chancellor *Bradford*, 1998–2001, and *Stirling*, 2001–2003); John Western (a graduate of *Melbourne* and *Columbia*, Professor of Sociology *Queensland* from 1970); Jake Najman (graduate of *UNSW*, Professor of Sociology *Queensland*); Cora Baldock; Ken Dempsey; Ann Daniel; Lyn Richards; Lois Bryson (graduate of *Monash*, Senior Lecturer 1970s *Monash*, Professor from 1990, *Newcastle*); and Raewyn Connell (graduate of *Sydney*, Professor of Sociology *Macquarie* from 1976, later *Harvard, Toronto, California*, and currently *Sydney*).

In part, the slower institutionalisation of sociology in Australia (relative to Britain) might be attributed to the smaller population, for the country had only six universities in 1939 with 14,000 students in a total population of seven million. By 1964 there were ten universities, with several new ones under construction, and 72,000 students enrolled from a population base of 11 million (Mayer 1964:27). However, just as it had in Britain, sociology took an independent form with its own departments in Australia in association with the significant expansion of the tertiary education sector, large increases in student numbers and the creation of several new universities (Baldock 1994:589; Baldock and Lally 1974). These new universities brought many more career opportunities for academics, as did the second major wave of expansion during the 1980s. By 1980, enrolments had increased to 330,000; there were 20 universities; and the Australian population stood at more than 14.5 million (ABS 2002). This second change in circumstances was not only due to growth in the population and the establishment of new universities, but a major shift in government policy resulting in a restructuring of the system to eradicate the difference between institutes, colleges and universities. For instance, in 1987 the *Western Australian Institute of Technology* became the *Curtin University of Technology* (Baldock 1994:613). This 'stroke of the pen' added significant numbers of new institutions, staff, and students to the university sector, and brought more opportunities for the study of sociology.

Apart from the *University of Tasmania*, independent sociology departments were mainly created in the newer, more progressive universities, and not the long-established 'sandstones' of *Sydney, Melbourne, Adelaide* or *Western Australia*. This historical pattern is similar to the United Kingdom and the United States, where the discipline was not favoured in the elite universities of *Cambridge* or *Oxford*, nor the Ivy League universities of the United States (see Bulmer 1985 for the account of *Cambridge's* reluctance to accept sociology in the United Kingdom). In Australia, a department of sociology (combined with social work) was formed at *Sydney University* in 1991, but even today, independent, named departments remain missing from the *Universities of Western Australia, Adelaide* and *Melbourne*.

Developments in the United States

The exception to this pattern of twentieth-century institutionalisation is found in the United States. In that country, the first sociology course is said to have been delivered by William Graham Sumner in 1875 at *Yale University* (Williams 2006:2). Sociology began to make more regular appearances towards the end of the 1880s, when some universities and colleges offered courses on 'sociology' and the 'social sciences' (Turner and Turner suggest these terms were used interchangeably at the time, see 1990:22). This coincided with the founding of several new universities and a period of improvement for existing ones, including a flurry of curriculum reform, the introduction of modern subjects and the addition of graduate schools. In this period a number of new disciplines were given their own departments, including history and economics in the 1880s, followed by sociology, anthropology and political science in the 1890s. The first department of sociology was established in 1893 at the new *University of Chicago* (Cockerham 1983:1515). Others were established soon after this at the universities of *Columbia, Brown, Yale, Wisconsin, Nebraska* and *Michigan* (Collins 1985:41–2; Bloom 2002:27), as well as *Pennsylvania* and *Leland Stanford* (Wallace, in Camic and Xie 1994:791).

Unlike Britain and Australia, sociology departments were also established in industry, not just in the universities. One of the earliest was started in 1901 at the Colorado Fuel and Iron Company. Others were created in 1905 at the Cleveland-Cliffs Iron Company in Michigan, and in 1914 at the Ford Motor Company (Weed 2005:269). These industry-based departments suggest a level of frustration with colleges and universities as sites for sociology, given that universities in the United States were oriented, until the second decade of the new century, towards inducing 'mental discipline' and 'religious piety' in their students rather than pursuing scientific enquiry. It also reflects an attempt in the United States to proffer sociology as a practical field, associated with the study of urban and industrial social problems, in contrast to Europe, where sociology was considered more as a philosophy. Efforts to position sociology as a solution to the prevailing problems posed by industrial labour had also been made in Australia during the same period: by academics such as Francis Anderson, but particularly by Elton Mayo. Whilst still in Australia, the latter delivered a series of lectures under the auspices of the *WEA*, in which he posited the thesis of militant radicalism among the working class as a form of madness, similar to a war neurosis, where the individual is unable to see reason. For Mayo, the solution for this would be found in sociological research and industrial management, allowing universities to act as a 'rational influence in the social organism' (Mayo 1920:131; Mitropoulos 2005:108). During the same period, the *WEA* also provided most of the speakers in a lecture series for the *Ministry of Public Works* on national efficiency, all of whom credited sociology with the means to produce industrial efficiency (Mitropoulos 2005:106). In Australia, despite the heavily unionised workforce and the capacity of labour to effectively resist calls to increase productivity, such efforts did not assist with the establishment of sociology departments in either universities or the corporate sector.

To return to our narrative about the United States, early academic sociologists around the turn of the century included Frank Lester Ward, Albion Small, Franklin Giddings, Charles Ellwood, William Graham Sumner, Charles Horton Cooley, Edward A. Ross, W.E.B. Du Bois, and Harry Elmer Barnes. Less well-known today, but nevertheless productive at the time were Julia Lathrop, Sophonisba Breckinridge, and Edith Abbott who taught sociology at *Chicago* and undertook studies of the living conditions of workers and immigrants in the first decade of the new century (Ross 1991:227). In 1900, sociology was being offered to students in about one hundred universities and colleges across the United

States (Cravens 1978:125). Yet in 1908 there were only 50 full-time professors of sociology across the country (Bloom 2002:42), suggesting the size of the sociological community was still small and somewhat ill-defined (Camic and Xie 1994:791). These years were financially difficult for many sociologists. Although some such as Harry Barnes were successful 'public sociologists', others, including Frank Ward, found it difficult to sustain a living as a sociologist. All were dependent on a small community of reformers and students for their funding and even books had to be financially guaranteed by the authors (Buxton and Turner 1992:378–9).

Between the late nineteenth century and the early decades of the twentieth century, American universities underwent a significant shift as they shook free of their European roots, turned away from their dependency on Christian theological scholasticism, and were reconstituted as secular, science-based institutions (Bloom 2002:23). The transformation in the discipline became evident by the 1920s when sociology was no longer primarily conducted outside the university system by religious reformers but academic professionals employed in major universities (Evans 2009:5–6, 14). By the late 1920s and into the 1930s, this brought about a 'brutal' social division in sociology. The 'public' sociologists who could speak to a broad audience were usurped by the 'professional' sociologists who were subsidised – and thus dependent on the foundations and 'favour-granting' networks – and wrote only for a narrow audience of sociologists (Buxton and Turner 1992:379).

Despite the growing interest in sociology in the United States in the early decades of the twentieth century, academic sociology continued to have only a tenuous hold on the system. The supply of graduates was precarious: only about 20 graduates of sociology with doctoral degrees were produced each year (see Turner and Turner 1990:28). Despite the support of the Rockefeller foundations (particularly its *Institute of Social and Religious Research*), as well as the Russell Sage and Carnegie Foundations, and the spreading of sociology teaching to many colleges and universities (Lengermann 1979:191; Turner and Turner 1990:74–5; Bulmer 1992:327); when Talcott Parsons sought employment in the economics department at *Harvard* in the 1930s, sociology was offered in most colleges and universities only as an occasional course within other disciplines such as economics (Camic 1987:428). Though there had been growth in opportunities within sociology, this was not broadly based, for the years of the depression had a negative effect on those in the lower ranks of the discipline, for the recent PhDs, and for sociologists in the less well-endowed universities (Lengermann 1979:194).

The process of institutionalisation, which had been very promising for sociology, was interrupted again in the early 1940s due to the war, with a decline in student enrolments and a reduction in teaching staff (Rhoades 1981:34). Expansion resumed in the immediate post-war period, with a rapid rise in student enrolments and new opportunities for research funding. In part this was due to an increase in public funding. Bulmer (1992:336–7) offers another explanation for this expansion: the emergence of an educated public. This, he argues, became particularly evident in the post-1945 period, so that along with the spread of popular journalism and radio came an interest in the works of psychiatry, anthropology (e.g. Margaret Mead), and sociology (e.g. *Middletown*).

The post-war years through the fifties and sixties constituted the 'golden period' for sociology in the United States. By 1959 there were at least 35 departments producing PhDs, and a steady growth in the number and quality of graduate training programmes. (In Britain and Australia these are called *post-graduate* programmes, indicating the difference between under-graduate or bachelor degree courses and those provided for students undertaking masters or PhD-level studies.) New journals and periodicals were established, programmes developed for secondary schools, membership of the *ASA* increased and conferences were well attended (Rhoades 1981:42–4, 53–4). For Talcott Parsons (1959:552), the discipline had reached an admirable level of institutional development by this time, for it had produced a:

> ... growing body of solidly trained and competent people who provide in the aggregate a *cumulative* development of knowledge on which their successors can build and which is the most important hallmark of a relatively mature science.

Reflections on the institutionalisation process

The appearance of discipline-based departments, associations, and academic journals gives an indication of differences in the timing of institutionalisation across the three countries. Taking first of all the formation of departments, we find the first British department of sociology established in 1903, and one started in Australia in 1950, but no significant flourishing of departments in either country until the 1960s. In America, in contrast, departmental expansion began to become a feature from the late 1940s.

With regard to the second facet of institutional formation, the sociological associations, the *American Sociological Society* was founded in 1905, and had its first meeting in 1906 (Bramson 1971:73; Williams 2006:2). Its name was changed in 1959 to the *American Sociological Association*. The *British Sociological Association* (*BSA*) began its life much later: in 1951. There had been predecessors to this, such as the *Sociological Society* established in 1904 in London. These previous associations had generally operated without the participation of the university sociologists, perhaps because there were so few individuals of this kind, and none of the societies were still operating by 1950. The first chair of the *BSA* was Morris Ginsberg, and the association was supplied with offices and resources at the *LSE* (Platt 2002:180–2). In Australia, the earliest society was the *Australian Institute of Sociology*, formed in 1942 by Peter Elkin, Professor of Anthropology at the *University of Sydney* (Germov and McGee 2005:81). This association was short-lived, producing the journal *Social Horizons* for a few years. The second was the *Canberra Sociological Society* (*CSS*), set up in 1958, with the first formal meeting held at *Canberra University College*. This body was effectively disbanded when a meeting in 1963 resolved to form the *Sociological Association of Australia and New Zealand* (*SAANZ*). Leonard Broom, an American visitor to the *ANU* who attended the meeting to create the first society in 1958; later made the point that the creation of a professional association was not merely a change in nomenclature, but would take the discipline beyond meetings for scholarly exchange, assisting it to build a public image, propagate its teaching and research, and advance its standing (Broom 1964:2). The joint association grew substantially, but in 1988, after a period of dissent (see Crothers 2005:74), the Australians and New Zealanders sought a separation, and the Australians formed the current organisation, *The Australian Sociological Association* (*TASA*).

Finally, focusing on the academic journals, the *AJS* began in 1895 at the *University of Chicago*. For many years it functioned as the official journal of the *American Sociological Society*. In 1935 the Society established the *American Sociological Review* (*ASR*) in order to resolve an ongoing dispute over the domination of sociology by the Chicago School and created an alternative outlet for other forms of sociology (see Lengermann 1979:185; Calhoun and Van Antwerpen 2007). At the same time, greater autonomy from Chicago was provided by setting up an independent administrative office, and the election of a non-Chicago-based president and executive for the *American Sociological Society* (Lengermann 1979:188). By way of comparison, the *British Journal of Sociology* was established at a much later date – in 1950 – at the

LSE, but a rival journal was set up in 1967. In this case, the new journal, *Sociology*, was expected to overcome the overly conservative approach of the *LSE* journal, and stimulate greater discussion and communication among sociologists (Platt 2002:185). In Australia, one of the first efforts at producing a sociology journal occurred in 1942 when Peter Elkin founded the journal *Social Horizons*. However, a more permanent sociology journal was conceived at the same 1963 meeting that oversaw the establishment of the professional association. Participants agreed to develop a sociological journal to be called the *Australian and New Zealand Journal of Sociology*. George Zubrzycki was to be the first editor, and the first edition published in 1965. The editorship remained at the *ANU* until a 'coup' in 1972, when, at the annual meeting of the association, members voted for editors to be elected democratically and answerable to the membership (Bryson 2005:38). With Lois Bryson as the first *elected* editor, subsequent issues were not radically different, but the journal's scope was broadened, publishing the work of sociologists from outside the *ANU* network, and more contemporary issues were featured in the articles and commentaries. In 1998 the journal was given the new name of the *Journal of Sociology* (*JoS*).

From this brief summation, it can be seen that institutionalisation was completed first in the American context, but over an extended period, beginning in the nineteenth century and reaching an end stage at the close of the 1940s when departments became prevalent and the discipline sustainable. In Britain the process of institutionalisation took place over a shorter period, becoming evident in the first decade of the new century at the *LSE*, but showing little sustained growth until the 1960s. In Australia the process of institutionalisation occurred during a very brief and intense phase. Departments appeared primarily in the 1950s and early 1960s and the process was completed by 1970. This means institutionalisation featured at least two decades earlier in the United States than in Britain or Australia, enabling it to be influential in the development of sociology in these other countries. This occurred through world-wide dissemination of American publications, its capacity to play host to foreign scholars and provide research training for foreign post-graduates. The United States also offered funding for foreign sociological associations, journals and departments through several well-endowed American-based foundations. The maturation processes of the sociologies of both Britain and Australia were shaped in this context, and hence strong parallels can be seen in the developmental patterns of the two countries; with regard not just to the timing of their institutionalisation processes but in the similarity of their efforts to establish independent disciplines with their own national identities and locally produced materials.

Despite the disparities between the three countries, there are also many similarities, particularly in the matters of 'rebellions' and 'coups' over journals and efforts to maintain executive control over the professional associations. Where these touch upon matters of relevance to the sociology of health and medicine, they are taken up for discussion in later parts of this volume.

Situated disciplines: Other forms of social structure

This chapter has examined disciplines as sites of social action and as institutional structures. In this final section we need to briefly consider the way disciplines are themselves subject to the organising effects of social structures. These structures traverse the disciplines and give shape to the 'situatedness' or social context of disciplines. They are aspects of social life often not consciously noted by social actors, even though their actions have implications for the construction and continuation of these structures.

There are a variety of social structures cutting across, and framing the disciplines, including those of class, ethnicity, race, gender and sexuality. In an attempt to restrict the size of this study and keep its focus, only the structuring effects of class will be considered in any depth. This limits our analysis of the discipline's social context to those features shaped by capitalism, but also the processes of professionalisation. This section explains why these forms of social structure need to be included in an examination of disciplines and their specialities.

Disciplines and professions

Early efforts to understand sociology, and disciplines, were made by Talcott Parsons. Drawing on work conducted at *Harvard* by Henderson and Mayo in their 'industrial hazards project' in the 1930s, Parsons saw sociology as capable of contributing positively to society and producing well-being in the social system through its use of specialised knowledge. He proposed twin social roles for sociology. Primarily a *discipline*, its role was the advancement and transmission of empirical knowledge. Secondarily, as a *profession*, sociology's responsibility was to communicate knowledge to non-members and engage in practical affairs (Parsons 1959:547). Parsons' theory of the professions – as performing a valuable contribution to the social system as a whole – was drawn from the much earlier work of Émile Durkheim (1933:26), and others including

Carr-Saunders and Wilson (1964/1933), and Edward Ross (1969/1901). These scholars theorised the medical and legal professions as 'moral authorities', able to act as intermediaries between the client or patient and the less ethical demands of the capitalist market.

Parsons' (1970) conception of the professions is clearly a normative and conservative one. Each profession was said to belong to one sub-system of society, with its own set of norms – institutionalised rules – and patterns of relationships determined by culture (Devereux 1961:42–3). They applied their specialist skills and expertise by managing and controlling illness and other forms of social 'deviance'. Essential to this role is a capacity for building trust: important if they are to carry out their work, whether this be attending to the souls of the congregation or healing the bodies of patients. In this way, the professions protect their patients or clients from market forces when they are at their most vulnerable. These unique professional–client relationships are the exact *opposite* of the contractual business relationship: a relationship not motivated by personal or economic self-interest, but ethically oriented towards a set of institutionalised expectations and standards. And in undertaking this special function, the professions contribute to the social good of the whole by maintaining the equilibrium of the social system and reproducing the normative order of capitalist society. In this sense, the professions are a unique form of occupation, for they stand apart from other products of the class structure, and are an *anachronism* in capitalist society.

Parsons (1959) employed his conception of sociology as both a discipline and a profession to encourage sociologists to engage with the 'world of practical affairs'. This was not a 'call to arms'. Professionalism for Parsons was about taking up one's responsibilities as a public figure and assisting the authorities with maintaining social order. Parsons made this clear when he wrote that a:

> ... professional association differs in ideal type from a trade union in that it is not so much an 'interest group' as an agency for facilitating the development of a professional field and a guardian of the technical and ethical standards of its personnel
>
> (1959:558).

The notion of sociology's dual role – as a discipline and profession – has since been widely taken up within the discipline. Debates over the professional elements of sociology, often fierce and emotional, have been regular occurrences within departments, professional association meetings, and newsletters and journals. Some sociologists have been optimistic about sociology's potential contribution in the public sphere (Gouldner and Miller 1965; Lazarsfeld *et al.* 1967); while others see this as the source of fundamental tension (Buxton and Turner 1992; Calhoun 1992; Waitzkin 1998; Pels 1999, 2000; Holmwood 2007). The contentious issue of professionalisation remains with us today (Platt 2002:194; Burawoy 2005b; Roach Anleu 2005:316).

These tensions have arisen in one of those rare instances where sociological theories, developed by sociologists to make sense of the broader social environment, have also been perceived as applicable to their own lives and work context. By the 1970s, the earlier functionalist perspective with its list of 'traits' was condemned in the midst of widespread social dissatisfaction with the professions and the established institutions; and a new literature emerged challenging the right of the professions to set the standards, act with complete autonomy in the work place, and determine the hierarchical division of labour. This new literature proposed professions to be distinct from other occupations only in as far as they had successfully claimed a mandate to control their own work and the work of others. Many of the studies were concerned with the professions' access to power and hence their class location (Johnson 1972; Larson 1977). For many sociologists, the knowledge basis of the professions became an irrelevancy, for its expertise and apparent restraint on self-interest were said to be the very source of its economic, cultural and institutional power (Hafferty and Light 1995:134).

Elliot Freidson's (1970a, 1970b) early books echoed this view. In later years, grappling with the idea of the professions as powerful occupations and yet *also* organised around specific bodies of knowledge; it became imperative for Freidson (1986a) to study the institutionalised *occupational roles* of the knowledge-makers. Knowledge, he argued, is the:

> ... very point of any occupation, the very basis for its existence as an occupation. The concrete resources upon which we all depend for our survival are not produced by some abstract and global class called labour but rather by a variety of specialised workers who exercise different bodies of knowledge and skill in the course of performing their tasks
>
> (Freidson 1986a:688).

Freidson noted that some of the professional occupations, including sociologists, had been granted a primary role in university teaching in countries such as the United States (and, we might add, the United Kingdom and Australia). This teaching role offers the sociologist an economically viable employment position, for it produces income for the institution and can be combined with research and scholarship. This analysis led Freidson (1986a:688) to propose sociologists (and other professions) as 'the institutional vehicles' for the production and transmission of formal knowledge.

Freidson's work importantly re-instates knowledge and expertise as significant points of focus in the sociological analysis of the professions. It came about at the very time when the main alternative to theorising the salience of intellectuals was in decline. This alternative was 'new class theory', and it had proposed the rise of a new elite or new class of intellectuals in a struggle for power with the traditional 'old class' of the business elites. The 'new class', vocally announcing its political preferences for state regulation of the economy, equality of opportunity, and the pursuit of social justice, had become a radical critic of the social order and seemed to owe allegiance only to its own class (Lasch 1965; Gouldner 1979). As the Cold War ended and a new, post-communist era in Europe began, questions were asked about whether this intellectual class had been 'captured' by the establishment (Konrad and Szelényi 1979; Brint 1985). Others questioned the classification of educated, white-collar workers as a new class, suggesting the group simply reflected cultural shifts in attitude which were, in essence, society-wide (Bell 1979). With the Marxist branch weighed down by a concern with locating the precise historical moment of the emergence of the new class (Gouldner 1979), and the functionalists and symbolic interactionists wedded to the intellectually unsupportable proposition of the new class as the holder of universal, abstract values and lacking in self-interest (Coser 1965) (a notion not entirely dissimilar to the 'trait' and functionalist theories of the professions of the same period); the field was ripe for renewal.

Disciplines and capitalism

In the 1970s and 1980s the professoriate still had significant power to make and enforce decisions on subordinate academic staff members (though they were compelled, in some instances, to put proposals to the vote within their departments, and also to the student body, see Butler *et al.* 2009:124). By the 1990s, student representation had disappeared in many universities, and the staff election of the deans and other senior staff had given way to a system of appointments by vice-chancellors. Decision-making arrangements within the universities became centralised, and professors increasingly marginalised[3] (Butler *et al.* 2009:127–8). This constituted a significant transformation in the relations of power, and begs further explanation.

So too does the growing managerialism of the university system, which has changed the nature of the boundary-work performed by disciplines, opening them more directly to influences well beyond the universities. Where once disciplines were maintained largely through a system of peer control – and highly regarded professors in key locations of the university community able to enhance and expand their discipline, give shelter to an emerging discipline, or even prevent a rival discipline from being established – new elements within the university environment began to reduce the autonomy of the professoriate and shift the balance of power in favour of university management and its business administrators. Along with the declining power of the professoriate and the growing managerialism of the universities, the recent decades have witnessed a radical overhaul of the university sectors of many countries, with a new focus on minimising costs (efficiency) and maximising outcomes (effectiveness) (Currie and Vidovich 1998:114). In some locations, particularly those without strong academic unions, this has led to an increase in retrenchments for academic knowledge workers, a growth in casual (and part-time and untenured) staff (with fewer employment rights and benefits), the cutting of courses and disciplines according to their financial return, reduced autonomy, lower staff morale and greater alienation, less-participatory forms of decision-making, and a decline in collegiality (Currie and Vidovich 1998:115–6, 122; Rhoades and Slaughter 1998:43–8).

These radical changes to the university system have occurred over the past few decades. They begin to make sense when we consider universities as sites of fierce contestation over power and the creation of capital. Universities have for some time been characterised by worker resistance to the subjection of scholarship and learning to the requirements of profit. In previous decades, particularly those of the immediate postwar period, the nation state held a dominant position with regard to the market, particularly in the United Kingdom and Australia, though also in the United States. Numerous new research institutes and government departments and agencies were established during this period, and universities (and individual academics) given large amounts of funding to undertake projects of relevance to governments. Efforts were aimed at 'reconstruction', at nation-building, and the development of the social and physical infrastructure necessary for growing the workforce and shifting the economies from a military to a civilian focus. In this environment the professoriate was able to maintain its hold on the management of the university, and almost independently undertake the required boundary-work for their discipline by making decisions about the creation of a new department or journal, or the appointment or dismissal of academic staff (particularly where they had good relationships with government ministers, as many did). Senior academics, such as Sol Encel at the *UNSW*, Talcott Parsons at *Harvard*, or Ralf Dahrendorf at the *LSE*, were all very powerful individuals. They held chairs of flourishing departments, were often leaders of their professional associations and editors of the associated journals. From these positions of power, such individuals were equally capable of promoting as ruining the career of a more junior sociologist, and many such stories can be told.

With the 1960s and 1970s came rapid expansion of the university sector, and for Kurasawa (2002:327–8) the period is described as one of *democratic contestation*, where the 'academy was opened up to subaltern social groups from civil society'. Social movements, including the civil rights and women's movement, led demands for democratic and social change, challenging the established social order. In Australia, university fees were removed by the Whitlam Labor government, and student living allowances instigated. Although this did not bring many from the traditional working class into the higher education system (as some had hoped), the barriers were removed for those from the less wealthy sections of the middle-class, and it brought many women – both married and single – into the universities. Within the universities, the generally conservative academics were pressed by the growing student body for radical changes to reform the curriculum so it might begin to address contemporary questions and concerns. These demands brought a marked diversification to the traditional offerings of the university, opening up a space for new disciplines such as sociology and women's studies, and producing new employment opportunities for academics (Sheridan and Dally 2006). It was a period of radical change in social attitudes and social practices. Australian sociologists, reflecting (somewhat fondly) on the annual conferences of those years, remember the colourful 'bean bags' replacing the conventional rows of chairs before the speakers, papers given without a formal podium, and the 'sweet smell of marijuana' wafting from one room to the next. In the classrooms of the same period, decision-making processes became more democratic, with regular assessment methods often replacing examinations, and in university councils and committees the student representative bodies became *par for the course*. The professoriate, still powerful, had to share the podium with a cadre of others.

By the 1980s there were signs of a university system in transition towards another, and very different era. The current period, for Kurasawa (2002:327), is one of *colonisation by the market*, where the university sector is opened to the logic of capitalism. This process has not been apolitical, but characterised by the imposition of a specific neo-liberal world view and 'forcing compliance to the norms of profitability and instrumental efficiency' (Kurasawa 2002:335). My own experience as an undergraduate in the 1980s illustrates this very different environment. It was one, not of student solidarity and the fundamental right to a voice in the institution, but of individualism and marred by a nagging anxiety about the future. Academic staff could be heard talking of the financial pressures on students and how this restricted their capacity to read for intellectual enjoyment and prepare for classes. My fellow students had no time for protest marches or student newspapers: many rushed home to feed children or to a part-time job. On campus, religious groups began to flourish, and the army and security agencies – previously very unwelcome in the student food halls, union spaces, and activity rooms – began regular recruitment drives.

For the academics, other changes to the university system were noticeable by the 1980s. At sociology conferences, the rows of chairs and the podiums were returned, and even cigarette smoking started to be frowned upon. For Kurasawa (2002), this was the beginning of the transnational corporations as 'major players on the world stage'. Academic competition was no longer primarily contained *within* the nation but had shifted decidedly into the international arena, functioning between *trans-national corporations* (Kurasawa 2002:336). For universities, this heralded a new role. No longer envisioned as centres of scholarship, they became a source of human resources for national enterprises and trans-national corporations and a means to gain a competitive edge in the global arena (Kurasawa 2002:336). Moreover, decision-making within the universities was removed from the hands of academics to administrators, 'bean-counters', and a new breed of university managers. Restructuring and administrative 'reform' became commonplace. Academics began to talk of 'managerialism' and the threat to scholarship in a new environment which favours easily monitored and documented activities (Currie and Vidovich 1998:115–6).

One of the more notable effects of the university's new role as a 'platform for the generation of territorial wealth and corporate profitability' (Kurasawa 2002:336) has been the construction of ranking systems and performance reviews. These are essentially new systems of 'examination', allowing management, funding and regulatory bodies to quantify output and performance (Najman and Hewitt 2003; Cheek *et al.* 2006). Within such schemes, individual universities are given a place in both the national and international arenas, disciplines and departments are measured relative to other disciplines (in the national context as well as internationally), and the 'output' of individual scholars is monitored and ranked and taken into account for employment opportunities and promotion.

Citation systems, created and controlled by a few large international corporations (such as *Thompsons Institute for Scientific Information*), provide managers and regulators with the tools for intervening in the previously, peer- and discipline-controlled systems of knowledge production. Whereas boundaries were once largely maintained through the social action of the members of disciplines, knowledge workers are increasingly subject to external control. And although national, discipline-based professional associations may be consulted by the corporations or university management about the inclusion of appropriate journals or the classification of specialities within their disciplines, overall control of the system has been removed from the disciplines and power has been re-distributed.

This new era of the corporate university has had, and continues to have, significant ramifications for the production of scholarly knowledge. Although the *strength* of its impact varies from one country to another, as a phenomenon it has made its appearance across the globe. Sociologists and other academics are keenly aware of the pressure from university management to produce 'relevant' knowledge, which usually means, for university administrators, knowledge which can be used by private capital (Kurasawa 2002:337). The influence of the market can also be seen in the changing priorities of research programmes. Research directed at short-term commercial gain is favoured, projects requiring long-term investments (such as longitudinal studies of the chronically ill) are not, and the search for 'truth' and knowledge for its own sake, virtually abandoned (Graham 2000). With respect to the kind of knowledge produced, this too indicates the influence of the market and the new corporate environment. Independent publishers have given way to corporate chains in a flurry of mergers and take-overs, while national publishers have been swallowed up within trans-national conglomerates. In countries with small markets – such as Australia – most university presses have disappeared, and it has become a struggle to find outlets for works of local interest. The strength of commercial pressure and competition in this market environment has led publishers to adopt profit-driven strategies such as focusing on text books and well-known authors and foregoing the unusual in favour of established or 'fashionable' paradigms or topics (Agger 2000:261–2; Kurasawa 2002:340).

Across the university sector, claims are made that the new corporate environment places pressure on academics to avoid damaging the commercial interests of sponsors, and indeed refrain from criticising capitalism in general (Kurasawa 2002:338). Even more damaging are claims that academics conducting research under contract to commercial sponsors are more likely to offer results favourable to the sponsor (Smith 1977; Baker and Manwell 1981; Broad and Wade 1982; Glazer and Glazer 1989; Martin 1992). Such behaviour is contrary to the ideals of academic scholarship and an anathema to the pursuit of academic freedom (Kurasawa 2002:339). Most of these claims have been made in relation to the natural sciences. The extent to which sociological research has succumbed to the same market pressures is a question which has been raised, but few answers have yet been proffered. It is a matter taken up – though not fully resolved – later in this volume.

The chapters ahead

This chapter has offered a framework for theorising disciplines and the processes through which they become features of the institutional terrain. Travelling through the sociological literature on disciplines, these peculiar historical constructions have been theorised not only as arenas of formal knowledge but also sites of social action, institutional structures, professions, and as themselves structured by class and capitalism. Readers have also been treated to a brief overview of the institutionalisation of sociology in three countries: Australia, the United Kingdom and the United States. In each case, the four phase process of institutionalisation involved the social action of key individuals and groups, and resulted in the production of departments, journals, professional associations and other paraphernalia of modern, Western disciplines. This theoretical framework is employed in the next chapter in an examination of the history of one of sociology's specialist fields: the sociology of health and medicine.

2
Past and Present: Three National Sociologies of Health and Medicine

Each of the three countries studied in this volume were recipients of a set of ideas, social practices and institutional forms initially developed in Europe. This process of trans-national 'seeding' raises a number of intriguing questions about the discipline of sociology, and about disciplines in general. In what sense was 'sociology' – as an emerging intellectual field – *transplanted* from one country to another rather than *created anew* in each setting? Equally, were notions about health and medicine as fundamentally *social* concerns, *introduced* or *produced* in each new location? What factors shaped these processes of disciplinary 'seeding', and were the same social forces responsible for the specialisation of sociology into the new field of the sociology of health and medicine? Moreover, to what extent does the sociology of health and medicine in each of the three countries differ in its practices, its forms of organisation or its knowledge base, and what factors have created these differences?

In seeking to address these questions, this chapter begins our examination of the processes of disciplinary formation and change. Our focus is on the *institutional* development of the specialist field of the sociology of health and medicine in Australia, the United States, and the United Kingdom. The chapter follows the formalisation of the intellectual field as it developed into a set of structured practices with its own journals, professional and disciplinary associations, collegial networks and literatures. As we explore this historical process, and the connections between, and disconnections from, the parent discipline; a pattern of development for the specialist field is revealed which shows that in each country, the sociology of health and medicine followed a similar trajectory to that of the parent discipline. The goal here is not to present the entire history of the sociology of health and medicine but provide sufficient detail for readers to gain an understanding of the institutional differences between the three national sociologies, and an insight into the factors which have shaped, and continue to shape, their varying disciplinary practices and knowledges. We begin with the formation of the sociology of health and medicine in the United States, because it was the earliest of the three countries to undergo institutionalisation. The history of the field in the United Kingdom and Australia are examined in turn, and the chapter concludes with a brief comparative reflection on these developments.

The sociology of health and medicine in the United States

Well prior to the formation and institutionalisation of a specialist programme of the sociology of health and medicine in America, there was a body of research often considered an immediate, intellectual 'precursor' to the field. Among the individuals who took an interest in the social and sociological aspects of health or medicine were some university-based sociologists, though it was not a common practice for these individuals to *specialise* in the field. There were some exceptions, for a few university sociologists were very interested in health and medicine and rarely worked on other topics. One of these was Bernard Stern, a member of the sociology department at *Columbia* (Stern 1927, 1941), and another, Lawrence Henderson, a biochemist who lectured at the *Harvard Medical School* but made a late career change and took a position in sociology at *Harvard* in 1931 (Henderson 1917, 1935). There were also several individuals teaching courses in the sociology of health and medicine in the early decades of the twentieth century, including Stern at *Columbia* in the 1930s, Everett Hughes at *Chicago* in the 1940s, and Les Simmons at *Yale* (Bloom 2002:111).

The sociology departments were not the only spheres of activity during this early phase of the sociology of health and medicine. Another could be identified at some distance from the sociology departments, and was mostly an applied field of research, produced by psychiatrists and other doctors who sometimes also identified as sociologists. The projects they worked on were usually government-sponsored, and they examined problems set out by the doctors themselves, with the aim of improving medical practice and/or the health status of the population. In other words, it operated as a 'sociology *in* medicine', not a 'sociology *of* medicine'. For example, Elizabeth Blackwell, the first woman graduate of a medical school, wrote about medical sociology in 1902 (Bloom 2002:21), but worked as a medical doctor in New York State. Likewise,

James Warbasse, who wrote a book on medical sociology in 1909, was a surgeon and editor of the *New York State Journal of Medicine* from 1905 to 1909 (Warbasse 1909).

Another arena of action revolved around health reformers, statisticians and public health advocates, often under the banner of 'social medicine'. During the first third of the twentieth century, individuals such as William Ogburn, Michael Davis and Edgar Sydenstricker investigated the social and economic factors connected with illness, following a tradition established in Europe by the social hygienists and medical police of the previous century. Disciplinary boundaries at this time were less rigid than they are today, and sociology was not yet clearly differentiated from economics, social work, political science or anthropology (Bloom 2000:12). It appears Sydenstricker's expertise was in statistics, though Ogburn and Davis were graduates of sociology; and Bloom (2002:47) regards Davis' (1971/1921) work on immigrant health to be one of the first medical sociology monographs. At the same time however, Davis was an activist and instigator of the neighbourhood health centre movement. Moreover, both Ogburn and Davis were members of the *Committee on the Costs of Medical Care* (*CCMC*), an inter-disciplinary study funded by a consortium of eight private foundations and operating from 1927 to 1932 (Bloom 1986:270). Although this powerful and well-funded committee drew expertise from medicine, public health and the social sciences, the very public contribution of sociologists to its work eventually assisted the discipline to become a legitimate policy science and helped differentiate the sociology of health and medicine from these other fields (Bloom 2002:48).

Despite these various activities, the sociology of health and medicine did not become an institutionalised field until after 1950. This means it was not, prior to that time, an arena of research with its own academic journals or professional associations, nor were individuals likely to adopt the name 'medical sociologist' or 'sociologist of health' as a descriptor for a unique occupational grouping within or outside the university system. It also means there were no widely accepted programmatic statements delineating a set of principles, perspectives or methodologies to guide and shape future research efforts for the field. The first of these processes had already taken place in the broader discipline of sociology, for, as described in the previous chapter, the *AJS* had been established in 1895, the *American Sociological Society* founded in 1905, and departments of sociology had become widespread by the 1950s. The parent discipline also had a set of canonical statements prescribing a programme of research, notably those of Sumner (Sumner and

Keller 1927), Ward (1968/1883), and Small (1903, 1924); but there was nothing of a similar nature for the sociology of health and medicine at this time.

There had been a number of attempts at formulating a set of principles for the small field, but these had been neither widely accepted nor adopted. Many reasons could be offered for this failure, and while this is not the place for a full consideration of the issue, even a partial one throws some light on the social context of the first half of the century and some of the social forces which stalled the institutionalisation process. For example, in the case of Bernard Stern, attempts to produce a framework for a sociology of health and medicine (principles which were later echoed by Merton in *his* programmatic statements for the field) were marred by a prevailing ideological opposition to Marxism and the establishment of a fairer, publically-funded, national health system. Stern himself was a constant target of the congressional investigating committees from 1938 to 1953 (Bloom 2002:95–7).

Lawrence Henderson was another who should be considered in this light. Unlike Stern, Henderson was politically conservative, and, with Parsons, part of the functionalist antidote to the Marxism of the university campuses of the 1930s (Gouldner, in Bloom 2002:90). The efforts of Henderson to lay out a research programme were therefore not thwarted by politics as they had been for Stern. Nevertheless, Henderson, who delineated a programme of research that was soon to dominate the field, has not been recorded as a founder of the modern sub-discipline of the sociology of health and medicine. His proposed theoretical framework was based on his early work in physiology, and Henderson took from this the functional approach to the equilibrium of the body and the regulation of systems, and adapted these to the field of social behaviour and social relations. With this, his close focus on the doctor–patient relationship, and particularly his Pareto-derived concept of the social system, Henderson pre-empted and influenced the work of Parsons, his student Merton and many others of that generation. In the event, Henderson died in 1942, before the institutionalisation of the field could be completed, and he is not widely nor well remembered for establishing a set of parameters for the programme of medical sociology.

Part of the reason for this might be found in the turmoil of the society at that time, with many sociologists either serving in the military or co-opted into government for the duration of the war. While some activities and programmes continued to be funded by the private foundations, particularly some of the early studies of the professions and of medical education (Olesen 1974:7), the war produced a general halt to the growth of the university sector during the early 1940s (Rhoades 1981:34). This had a significant impact on sociology, as the discipline was still quite small (Bloom 1990:3). At the same time however, it brought about a period of intense collaboration between the universities, the military, and the government. Thus, as Bloom (2002:114–5) argues, the war was both a stimulant and an interruption to sociology and to medicine. When war broke out in 1939, although social research had become a normal response for government in the face of social problems, and social researchers had initially been drawn from the universities, the government's response to the war was to establish its own research agencies. In this process, social research lost its impetus as an independent academic pursuit with its own research questions and methods. An important consequence of this process was that when expansion resumed in the immediate post-war period, with a rapid rise in student enrolments and new opportunities for research funding, the role of general sociology had been stimulated but irrevocably altered, sowing the seeds for eventual conflict between 'basic' and 'applied' sociology.

The same factors – of slower university growth and heightened activity in the government sector – constrained the institutionalisation of the sociology of health and medicine at this time. In addition however, the advocates of social medicine, and sociologists on committees (such as the *CCMC*), seeking to curb the rising costs of medical services and establish a more equitable health system, were increasingly frustrated by the growing dominance of the private providers and the *American Medical Association*. These various medical interest groups and organisations were able to shape the legislative environment to attract legal protections and entitlements, build a cultural legitimacy and ensure their professional needs were favoured (Hafferty and Light 1995:132). Sociologists, social scientists working within social medicine, and a variety of social reformers seeking to strengthen the role of preventative and public health and establish a national health service, were all caught up in the 'irrationality' of McCarthyism: they were labelled 'political radicals' and the field denigrated as 'socialism' (Bloom 2002:118). Milton Roemer, for example, a sociologist, doctor of medicine, advocate of a national health insurance scheme and public health campaigner, found his appointment to the *World Health Organisation* withdrawn by the American government. He was forced to return from Geneva in 1953.

The 1950s and 1960s

The development of medical sociology as a distinct arena of intellectual and social practice would not have occurred during the 1950s if it had not been for a prior re-organisation of the institutions of medicine. This re-organisation involved a sustained process of social action directed at the re-drawing of the boundaries between the various spheres of knowledge and practice. In the previous chapter we discussed the turmoil of the late nineteenth to early twentieth century, where science was finally transformed from an activity undertaken by 'gentlemen' to a professional, occupational practice, and its knowledge base remodelled from its precursors of 'natural philosophy' and 'natural history' into an experimental, laboratory method (Warner 1995; Ilerbaig 1999; Veit-Brause 2001). These new laboratory sciences spread from Germany to the United States during the first decades of the twentieth century, boosted by the transmigration of scientists during and after the wars, and instilled a new respect and authority for science in the new location. This same process meant a down-grading and marginalisation of the cultural and social sciences, but also had implications for medicine, and ultimately for medical sociology, because proponents of medical reform made strategic use of the general disorder to build a new public image for the discipline of medicine and forge new territorial claims. As would occur in Britain a decade or two later (Lawrence 1994; Sturdy and Cooter 1998), American reformers in the first decades of the twentieth century switched their allegiance to the experimental sciences and began to professionalise, re-fashioning medicine from an 'art' into a 'science', transforming the field and constructing a completely new discipline.

A noteworthy event during this reform process was the publication of the report by Abraham Flexner, an educationalist who was asked by the *Carnegie Foundation* to undertake a survey of the 155 medical schools of the United States and Canada (see Flexner 1910). Flexner considered the general standard of medical education to be very poor, and argued that there was an over-supply of both medical schools and doctors. In conformity with the reformist spirit of the period, he recommended all schools adopt the new scientific format of the German institutions. The Flexner Report, as it is commonly called, did not have immediate impact, but over the next few decades nearly half the schools merged with other institutions or were closed, medical education was increasingly standardised, and admission procedures modified. The impact of the report, and the broader reform process, virtually eliminated alternative forms of therapy (without the need to legislate against them), had serious repercussions for the access of women and minority groups to medical training, and significantly increased the incomes of doctors.

The new emphasis on a *scientific* form of medical training and the re-organisation of the medical schools ensured the focus remained on the education and training of medical practitioners until the 1950s. After this period however, medical research became the dominant activity (Bloom 2000:16). The balance had begun to shift after the congressional act of 1937 enabled the *National Institutes of Health* to create specialist programmes of research on specific conditions and diseases, and provide funds for medical-scientific research to individuals and institutions (Bloom 2000:16). These government funds, which in this period outweighed the contribution from private sources, enabled research to become a much larger sphere of activity. *Scientific* medicine brought both symbolic authority to medicine as well as the capacity to acquire financial and other material resources. Legislative change, the influx of funding and the new cultural authority of science were all pivotal to shifting the balance between the teaching, research, and service functions of the medical institutions. The role of the scientist grew in prominence and prestige over teaching to the extent that by 1948 medical schools had developed the practice of independently budgeting for, and structurally separating, the functions of research and teaching. Moreover, the new emphasis on science and research, and particularly the relative proportion of income coming from research, had the unexpected effect of tying the medical schools to the state and ensuring their continual dependence on federal government grants (Stevens 1971:358; Bloom 2000:16).

What did this re-ordering of the medical landscape mean for sociology? The strengthening emphasis on the new experimental sciences as an underpinning for medical training, coupled with the depression years of severe cuts to medical education and training, meant that the 1930s were not amenable to the inclusion of sociology or the social sciences in the medical curriculum. Although there was more money for medical education during the war years, it was not until 1951 that this paid off for sociology, and the social or behavioural sciences were given a prominent place in medical education (Bloom 2002:112–4). This post-war period of growth for sociology occurred in conjunction with the expansion of the American university system. Returned soldiers, refugees from Europe, and young people without employment flocked to the universities and turned to the social sciences in an effort to understand the new social environment in a nation which had suddenly shed its cultural dependence on Europe and developed a new confidence in itself (Martindale 1976; Bloom 2002:125).

Growth for sociology followed the pattern of medicine. Prior to the 1950s, there was a similar lack of separation between the research and teaching functions within sociology, and any additional funding for research had come from private sources (Bloom 2000:16). This changed significantly for sociology with the creation of the *National Institute of Mental Health* (*NIMH*) in 1946, a central federal agency set up to fund research and the training of researchers (Hollingshead 1973; Cockerham 1983:1514). The founding director of the institute, Robert Felix, always had representatives from sociology as his social science consultants, first relying on Raymond Bowers, and later John Clausen. All three individuals played an important role in ensuring funds from the agency were directed towards sociological research during the 1950s and 1960s (Bloom 2000:17–9). In 1959, in response to requests for funds to study mental health in relation to social class, a Behavioural Science Study Section was established within the *NIMH* so that sociological research proposals could be reviewed separately from those of experimental psychology and psychiatry (Bloom 2000:19). Research training was given attention by the *NIMH* from 1958, with provision made for a significant budget for doctoral trainees (post-graduate candidates) in mental health, and 80 per cent of these funds went to sociology. These programmes were matched by similar funds from other federal agencies, and were a response to prevailing assessments about the looming shortage of PhDs in a context of rapid expansion in the university sector (Bloom 2000:20).

What this meant for the sociology of health and medicine was that ample funds were available during the 1950s and 1960s from private sources (such as *The Russell Sage Foundation*, the *Milbank Memorial Fund*, and the *Rockefeller Foundations*), but also from the *NIMH* and other federal agencies, to encourage interest in the field and support research and post-graduate training (Olesen 1974:7; Bloom 2000:17). For instance, Leo Simmons (a sociologist) and Harold Wolff (a medical doctor) were provided with funds from *The Russell Sage Foundation* to improve the use of social science research in medical practice, and establish a framework for inter-disciplinary collaboration (Cockerham 1983:1516). Private and public forms of funding provided many such opportunities for sociologists to engage in inter-disciplinary programmes within their universities, and these, for Bloom (2000:17), were critical to the formation of the speciality of medical sociology, more so than internal processes within the departments of its parent discipline. These events prompt some, such as Cockerham (1983:1514), to promote the view of early medical sociology as developing with a weak affiliation to its own parent discipline. However, one of the notable features of the 1950s and 1960s was the number of sociologists who took an interest in health and medicine but were employed within sociology departments. Very few sociologists during this period held secure employment positions within schools of health or medicine (Bird *et al.* 2000:2). As we shall see below, this situation provides a contrast with Britain, where there was little university-based sociology of health and medicine during the same period. Reflecting on this matter, Samuel Bloom states:

> Essentially, none of these individuals sought to join medical institutions; nor did medicine seek to recruit them as other than consulting scholars... throughout the entire period to this very day, they retained, with little or no thought to change, their prior status in the sociology departments of their universities
>
> (Samuel Bloom, unpublished paper of 1973, in Johnson 1975:229).

There were, during the 1950s, efforts to change this state of affairs. For example, the *Russell Sage Foundation* operated a scheme which placed social scientists in medical institutions as 'residents' (Olesen 1974:7; Bloom 2000:21–2). Such efforts were not broadly effective however, and this might have been partly the result of the known difficulties faced by sociologists who were interested in health and medicine in the 1950s and 1960s. These sociologists often faced challenges on two fronts: within sociology and from medicine. Their sociological colleagues often considered their field with 'disdain and suspicion', labelling it 'applied' and 'not theoretical', while health care providers and members of the medical profession were generally unfamiliar with sociological methods and concepts, and did not see a legitimate role for sociology in the evaluation of health care services. Moreover, many regarded sociologists as too radical in their political perspectives (Bird *et al.* 2000:1).

Nevertheless, with the assistance of the private foundations, the sociology of health and medicine finally started to take shape as an arena of social practice in its own right. Medical sociology began to appear in the sociology curriculum, and training in the field started in the 1940s and 1950s at the four major sociology departments: *Yale, Harvard, Columbia and Chicago* (Olesen 1974:7). Its 'neophyte' practitioners may have been tentative about their identity, unsure about the legitimacy of the new discipline and somewhat overwhelmed by the power of medicine, but they began to form networks and assist one another (Bloom 1990:4).

The process of institutionalisation for the intellectual field might be said to have finally begun in 1955 with the formation of the Committee on Medical Sociology, an *ad hoc* group within the *ASA*, organised by August (Sandy) Hollingshead, with Robert Straus as the secretary-treasurer (Olesen 1974:7; Bloom 1990:5), and funded by the *Russell Sage Foundation*. The origins of the Committee can be found in an even more informal group which had started meeting in 1954. This had been initiated by sociologists, but individuals from many disciplines were involved, including social workers, medical doctors, anthropologists and social psychologists (Bloom 2000:23). In 1962, the Committee eventually became the Medical Sociology Section of the *ASA*. It was the second section to be created within the *ASA*: social psychology was the first. (Even under the *ASA* the Section retained its multi-disciplinary character, and it wasn't until the 1970s that separate organisations began to be established to represent the various disciplines, see Bloom 2000:23). The Section continued to grow, and by 1965 it was one of the largest and more active sections of the *ASA*. During this period the Section obtained financial support for research, and later also for post-graduate and post-doctoral training, from an array of sponsors including the *Carnegie Foundation*, the *Milbank Memorial Fund* and the *Robert Wood Johnson Foundation*. Private foundations also gave funds to the universities to assist with the sociology of health and medicine. For instance, in 1952, the *Russell Sage Foundation* provided start-up funds to the sociology department at *Yale* to establish a post-graduate programme in medical sociology. This programme successfully obtained *Commonwealth Fund* support and began to take students in 1955. Ray Elling and Leonard Syme were among its first cohort of graduates (Bloom 2000:22).

A second indication of the institutionalisation of the field came with the establishment of the *Journal of Health and Social Behavior* (*JHSB*). This was first published in 1960 as the *Journal of Health and Human Behavior* (*JHHB*), and at this time operated as a private journal, started by E. Gartly Jaco as both editor and publisher (Bloom 1990:5). In 1966 it became one of the *ASA*'s official journals, and the first to come from a Section of the *ASA*. This occurred with support from the *Milbank Memorial Fund*, which agreed to underwrite any financial risks, and Elliot Freidson was selected as the first editor under the new arrangements (Bloom 2000:24–5). A third indication of the institutionalisation of the field came about in the late 1950s and 1960s with the publication of the first American textbooks for the sociology of health and medicine, including works by Norman Hawkins (1958), E. Gartly Jaco (1958), Howard Freeman and colleagues (1963), and Samuel Bloom (1963).

For William Cockerham (2005b), 1956–1970 was the 'golden age' for medical sociology, with a noticeable increase in sociologists taking an interest in matters of health and medicine. Structural-functionalism dominated both sociology and the sociology of health and medicine during the first part of this period, a theoretical template set in motion by the publication of Talcott Parsons' (1970) *The Social System*, in 1951. The book offered a general theory of society, and provided the discipline with a definitive statement about the nature of its subject and aims. (The 1951 text was a refinement of Parsons' previous 1937 work, *The Structure of Social Action*, which set out the methodological and meta-theoretical principles for the theory). Important for the sociology of health and medicine was one of Parsons' chapters in the 1951 text, which outlined a theory of 'the sick role'. It proposed illness to be a form of deviance appropriately managed and constrained within the social system (a theory taken directly from Durkheim's earlier work and combined with ideas from Lawrence Henderson and others). This statement about illness was a powerful symbol for the newly emerging speciality of medical sociology, for it distinguished its field from that of the professionalising arena of medicine of the 1920s and 1930s, and offered sociologists a new role: to examine 'sickness' rather than 'disease' (Parsons 1970, also 1968:372).

The dominance of structural-functionalism in sociology began to falter in the 1960s amidst growing unrest over conventional sociological explanations. In some quarters there was increasing disappointment with the prevailing emphasis on quantitative methods, for these did not appear capable of answering the critical questions about contemporary social life. This unease led to a revival of the older debates of the 1920s–1940s over 'soft' and 'hard' techniques and the strengths and failures of the case history or case study compared with statistical methods (Platt 1985, 1992). Debates in the 1940s concerning these issues had petered out with the rising domination of 'hard' techniques and quantitative methods in social research. In the 1950s and 1960s this second round of debate raised the possibility that 'applied' sociology might be a fundamentally different form of scientific work, and may even inhibit progress by attracting resources away from the discipline (Lazarsfeld and Reitz 1975; Bloom 2002:125). Another new element within these debates was the explicit connection made between methodology and ideology, for it was proposed that the sociologist, when taking on the social role of the applied researcher, was in danger of supporting the oppressive social 'system' (e.g. Mills 1956; Gouldner and Miller 1965).

This shifting landscape, characterised by dissent and restlessness but also a new vigour, is reflected in the publications of the era. Some were a continuation of the conservative, structural-functionalism of *The Structure of Social Action* and *The Social System*. This can be seen in Merton's study of medical education at *Cornell Medical College* (Merton *et al.* 1957), which demonstrated the process of professional socialisation. Others, however, reflected the emergence of radical alternatives within sociology. One of the new perspectives, which had an impact on both the parent discipline and the new speciality area of the sociology of health and medicine, was the labelling perspective. This focused on the way individuals and groups without power were isolated and oppressed, including those with mental illness (Sheff 1967). Other sociologists examined issues of class or ethnicity, such as Hollingshead and Redlich's (1958) *Social Class and Mental Illness*, and Snyder's (1958) *Alcohol and the Jews*. Goffman's (1961) *Asylums* also broke decidedly from structural-functionalism in its study of the extreme form of socialisation occurring in total institutions, as did Howard Becker's *Boys in White* (Becker *et al.* 1961). The latter, which was an undertaking by Everett Hughes with three of his former students (Howard Becker, Anselm Strauss and Blanche Geer), investigated the social basis of professional training in medicine. It was one of the first to use symbolic interactionism in studies of medicine, and provided the foundation for Glaser and Strauss' (1967) *The Discovery of Grounded Theory*.

These texts make the point that in this early period of the sociology of health and medicine in the United States, although there were sociologists who used medicine or illness as a means to test a range of theoretical propositions or establish new concepts (e.g. Robert Merton, Talcott Parsons and probably August Hollingshead), many others were interested in the field itself: the institutions of medicine and the social distribution of illness or disease. This view of the field may be an unpopular one, as conventionally it is argued that early sociologists only discussed health and illness as a means to demonstrate the application of 'core' concepts and theoretical frameworks (such as class, stratification, bureaucracy or social integration), to practical or contemporary problems (Susser and Watson 1971; Mechanic 1978; Grbich 1996; Idler 2001; Quah 2005). Nevertheless the evidence speaks largely for itself. The 1950s and 1960s were decades of rapidly increasing research interest in the sociology of health and medicine, and witnessed a considerable growth in published studies (Snyder 1958; Clausen 1959; Reader and Goss 1959; Freidson 1961; Faris 1964; Graham

1964; Mechanic 1967). The only 'blots on the horizon' were the low numbers of sociologists with secure employment in medical schools, and the rarity of undergraduate courses in this specialist field (Bird *et al.* 2000:2).

The 1970s in the United States

By the late 1960s and increasingly in the 1970s, the situation of sociologists interested in health and medicine began to change as it became possible to specialise in the field. Although there were some opportunities for specialisation emerging in medical sociology within the sociology departments (Pescosolido and Kronenfeld 1995:14), many sociologists moved to take up positions in medical schools. In part, this may have been encouraged by the large amounts of research money supplied by programmes such as the *NIMH*. Much of this research was inter-disciplinary, and this itself assisted sociologists to gain entry to medical schools where they could undertake studies of medicine and influence its curriculum (Johnson 1975:229–30). The funding structure also led to an emphasis in this early phase on mental health and the concerns of psychiatrists, as evidenced by the papers in the *JHSB* (Seale 2008:679). The field began to be seen as primarily an applied one, given that research monies were supplied in order to assist with a clinical or practical problem, or perhaps a policy issue, and not simply to address a conceptual matter. As Cockerham suggests, 'Funding agencies were not interested in theoretical work, but sponsored research that had some practical utility' (2005a:3).

Another factor which may have encouraged some sociologists to join the medical schools (and other disciplines in the universities), and sever their previously strong connection to mainstream sociology, was the poor treatment they received within sociology departments. In 1972, Geoffrey Gibson, secretary of the *ASA* Medical Sociology Section, described the situation this way:

> Increasingly in their research and in the dissemination of its results they are discovering more in common with health care researchers in economics, industrial engineering, geography, operations research, political science and management than with their colleagues in sociology. Department-based peer evaluation systems which have not heard of 'Inquiry, Health Services Research' and the 'American Journal of Public Health' or else count publications therein as inestimately less worthy than publication in the 'Journal of Health and Social Behaviour', the 'American Sociological Review' and the

'American Journal of Sociology', are either impelling young scholars into schools of public health or other multi-disciplinary settings or, more tragically, emasculating their growth by rewarding esoteric purist theorising and ignoring workmanlike multi-disciplinary health services research

(in Johnson 1975:230).

Despite these problems, the critical edge – which had emerged in sociology in the previous decade – continued to sharpen during the 1970s. Sociologists were more able to reflect on the problems in American society without fear of censure, and draw comparisons with other cultures without audiences assuming one was necessarily rejecting the American way of life. Moreover, unlike the previous generation, sociologists were less in need of reassurance and acceptance from conservative elements of society because they had become part of a new and much larger community of sociologists who shared their views (Lantz 1984:588–9).

A significant body of work began to accumulate during the 1970s, and the content of these sociological studies began to look quite different to the output of previous decades. Bird and colleagues (2000:5) suggest the 1960s and 1970s were decades of relatively strong economic growth and progressive politics, and with both government and community focused on ethnic and racial inequalities, an effort was made to improve access to health services for poorer groups within the population. This shift in concentration was assisted by changes at the organisational and institutional levels. For example, the Medical Sociology Section of the *ASA* received substantial funding in the 1970s from the *Carnegie Foundation* to build a programme of research on public policy and the health services. These efforts were driven by individuals such as David Mechanic, Sol Levine and Odin Anderson, and one of the aims was to overcome the narrow focus on the financing of services and address other aspects of the health system, its organisation and particularly the issue of preventative medicine. This change in emphasis for the Section returned the field to a 'close synchrony with social medicine' (Bloom 2000:26).

This re-orientation was reflected in the publications of the period. For instance, Mechanic and Levine's (1977) work on health services, Milton Roemer's (1976) volume on the world's health care systems, Andrew Twaddle's (1974) paper on health status and social stratification, Bonnie Bullough's (1972) study of the impact of poverty on access to family planning services and John McKinlay's (1975) study of migrants and their utilisation of health services. 'Iatrogenic medicine' became a prominent issue with the publication of *Limits to Medicine*, written by the European scholar Ivan Illich (1977). This concept directly challenged the Durkheimian and Parsonian thesis of the medical profession as a 'buffer' between the market and the patient, pointing to the processes of 'medicalisation' and the doctor as a cause of illness and distress. Studies of women's health also began to appear, with stinging critiques of the treatment of women by the medical profession and the health care services (Ehrenreich and English 1973; Scully and Bart 1973; Bagley 1976; Stark *et al.* 1979). These feminist studies were stimulated by the same social forces which led to the formation of the *Boston Women's Health Book Collective* (1973). The discipline and occupation of nursing, which had followed the pattern of medicine in adopting a 'scientific' approach to its roles in the first half of the twentieth century (Davis 1969, 1972), began to question its subordination to medicine and change its practices. This shift was reflected in a number of sociological studies (e.g. Ashley 1976; Reeder and Mauksch 1979).

Another, and rather important, interest which developed in the 1970s was 'the professions'. Although the years immediately after the war had seen the emergence of a critique of science (associated with the use of atomic weapons in Japan), by the 1970s this had expanded into a pervasive distrust of all forms of authority and expertise. There was a rising interest in alternative and traditional forms of medicine, in home births, and a growing critique of conventional medical practice. These views were reflected in the writings of sociologists and anthropologists of the period (Kleinman 1978; Baer 1981). Elliot Freidson's works (1970a, 1970b, 1975, 1978) on the medical profession took a central place, and Marxism became a significant and guiding perspective as the state struggled to gain control over spiralling health costs amidst an expanding and re-organising corporate, health care sector (Ehrenreich and Ehrenreich 1971; Johnson 1972; Navarro 1976; Relman 1980). For sociology, it was clearly a productive, critical, and diverse decade.

The 1980s in the United States

The period between 1970 and 1989 is considered by Cockerham (2005b) to be a time of 'maturity' for the sociology of health and medicine. He gives several reasons for this statement, one of which is that by this date the field had an independent literature and methodology, with a number of accessible textbooks, including his own *Medical Sociology* (first published in 1978), Andrew Twaddle and Richard Hessler's (1977) *A Sociology of Health*, and Peter Conrad and Rochelle Kern's (1981) *The*

Sociology of Health and Illness. Cockerham's (2005b) second reason is his optimism that the 'crisis' of potential subordination to medicine was over. The field certainly appeared to have broken free of its dependence on medicine, for in this decade Paul Starr published his Pulitzer Prize-winning book *The Social Transformation of American Medicine* (1983), damning the growth of corporate medicine in the United States and pointing to the consequences for professional autonomy in a new era of regulation.

Despite the virulence of this and other critiques of medicine, sociology had strengthened its foothold within medical institutions. Sociologists were represented on the staff of the majority of the 143 medical schools in the United States and Canada (Stokes *et al.* 1984), and the editor of the *Journal of the American Medical Association* wrote:

> The question should no longer be: Should the social sciences have a role in undergraduate medical education? Rather, it should be: How can we more effectively bring the lessons and insights of the relevant social and behavioural sciences to our students?
>
> (*JAMA* March 6th, 1981:955).

Such statements indicate the field had become well established (Bloom 1986:271). Sociologists were found within departments of psychiatry, social medicine, epidemiology, family medicine, community medicine and paediatrics, and to a lesser extent internal medicine, obstetrics and gynaecology, where they were less welcome (Hunt and Sobal 1990:319). Other evidence of the establishment of the field was the thriving Medical Sociology Section within the *ASA*, and the fact that almost every graduate department of sociology was offering a specialisation in the sociology of health and medicine by this date (Haney *et al.* 1983; Bloom 2000:27).

The 1980s, however, was a more politically conservative decade for the United States. Support for the social sciences had suffered a severe blow under the Nixon administration in the mid-1970s, with reduced spending on both research and professional training (Elinson 1985:269; Bloom 2000:20–1). Moreover, the decade of the 1980s began with a recession, severe cuts to the federal budget for welfare (but massive growth in military spending) and increasing unemployment under the Reagan administration. Some of the major sociology departments lost their post-graduate medical sociology programmes, and there was a decline in the number of medical sociology students being trained within sociology departments (though some found training in other departments, such as public health and preventative medicine, see Pescosolido and Kronenfeld 1995:15). The economy recovered around the middle of the decade, but these unstable years are remembered by many because of the stock market crash of 1987.

For Chloe Bird and colleagues (2000:5), the new social context shifted sociology from a focus on *inequality and access* to health care services towards a concentration on *effectiveness and efficiency*. Some sociologists resisted the general trend, focusing instead on the quality of life of specific population groups (e.g. Levine and Croog 1984). Others paid attention to the financial costs of care but turned this into a critique of the organisational structure of health care services. These sociologists pointed to the recent transformation of the health care sector, where corporations had come to purchase and control chains of hospitals, clinics, laboratories and insurance companies in a process of 'horizontal integration'. Legislative efforts to gain some semblance of control in this arena led to the establishment of the uniquely American phenomena of managed care and Health Maintenance Organisations, engendering many forceful sociological critiques (Relman 1980; Luft 1981; Starr 1983; Waitzkin 1983; Wolinsky and Marder 1985; Enthoven 1988; Melnick *et al.* 1989). Equally critical in its approach was the continuing work on the professions and professional autonomy (McKinlay and Arches 1985; Freidson 1986a, 1986b; Light and Levine 1988), as well as studies of inequality, such as Ray Elling's (1989) and Peter Conrad's (1988) concerns with workers' health and safety.

Alongside these developments were others also resisting the strictures of the neo-liberalist era: mainly by persisting with the sociological perspectives of the previous decade. Feminist works continued in strength (e.g. Reissman 1983; Olesen and Woods 1986; Martin 1987), as did studies on a variety of topics including Edward Yoxen's (1983) sociology of genes and genetics, Uta Gerhardt's (1989) focus on illness and the patient, and the investigation by Anthony and Patricia Walsh (1989) into the connection between love, self-esteem and multiple sclerosis. In addition to these diverse strands was an area of interest which had appeared in the closing years of the previous decade. These studies focused on health gradients and the social factors leading to various forms of stress. They were generally quantitative in methodology and addressed issues of concern to both sociologists and the agencies and institutions of medicine (e.g. Berkman and Breslow 1983; Hayes and Ross 1986; House *et al.* 1986; Link *et al.* 1986; Kaplan *et al.* 1987; Marmot *et al.* 1987; Liberatos *et al.* 1988).

The 1990s and beyond in the United States

The most recent two decades have seen a continuing growth of theoretical and empirical work in the sociology of health and medicine, and its accumulation has become widely apparent. This has, in itself, helped distinguish the field from other disciplines, such as public health, policy studies and health services research, and provided the field with a strong and unique identity. The sociology of health and medicine has developed into a well-established field, with most university departments offering courses in medical sociology. It is a common 'major' among American undergraduates, and continues to be one of the three largest sections of the *ASA* (Levine 1995:1; Bird *et al.* 2000:2).

During the 1990s and the first decade of the new millennium, the organisational and institutional context of health care services shifted dramatically. The growth of corporate medicine and the 'medical–industrial complex' – which had caught the attention of Starr, Relman, Waitzkin, Light and others in the 1980s – became a dominant and pervasive issue. Vast, and powerful, for-profit networks of hospitals, laboratories and medical centres developed as a feature of the health care system, and some of the literature reflects a concern with the rapidly rising costs of care (Chernew *et al.* 1998), a concerted effort to understand the phenomenon itself (Flood and Fennell 1995; Fox 1996; Leicht and Fennell 1997; Light 2000, 2001), the failure of the state to regulate or effectively manage the sector, and its effects on particular populations and the professions (Scott and Backman 1990; Frenk and Duran-Arenas 1993; Freidson 1994; Hafferty and Light 1995; Mechanic 1996).

Of course many other topics and subjects were explored over the same period, with some sociologists continuing with the interests of previous years, including medical technologies (Nelkin and Lindee 1996; Timmermans 1998), medicine as a profession (Buxton and Turner 1992), the sick role and the illness experience (Charmaz 1991), the social construction of illness and medical knowledge (Conrad and Leiter 2008), medicalisation (Conrad 1992), and gender and health (Lorber 1997). Of growing importance has been the field of 'sociological epidemiology', which made its first public appearances at the end of the 1970s. According to Bird *et al.* (2000:4), the field is concerned with the social patterning of illness in terms of gender and social class, and how these forms of inequality lead to exposure to a range of stressors (Link and Phelan 1995; Syme 1998; Ross and Mirowsky 1999).

These various interests and points of focus are provided here as indicative of the field during the most recent period. Despite the many commentaries on the state of the field we have come to know as the sociology of health and medicine, the literature does not provide an accurate assessment of its major characteristics, and details are known only about some areas, such as medical education (Badgley and Bloom 1973) or the use of statistics (Camic and Xie 1994). Indeed we have little information about the relative proportion of sociological research devoted to, for instance, health services analysis rather than medical knowledge, qualitative rather than quantitative methods, or Marxist versus Foucauldian theoretical frameworks.

There have been many astute and historically valuable reflections on the field, but neither those from the earlier period (Freeman and Reeder 1957; Straus 1957; Freeman *et al.* 1963; Waitzkin 1981; Wardwell 1982; Cockerham 1983; Freidson 1983; Mechanic 1983, 1989; Ruffini 1983, 1984), nor those published since the 1980s (Zola 1991; Pearlin 1992; Mechanic 1993; Bird *et al.* 2000; Cockerham 2005b), pay much attention to the institutional context (with the exception of Bloom 1986, 2000, 2002). Moreover, few provide a comprehensive review of the field, relying largely on personal experience and insight rather than systematically gathered empirical data (with the exception of Crane and Small 1992; Clair *et al.* 2007; Seale 2008). This means we have little indication about the dispersal of the various interests, perspectives or methodologies within the field. What level of interest is there in feminist perspectives among those studying the health services? Are sociologists employed in sociology departments more likely to use Marxist analysis than those in medical departments? Do female sociologists show a greater interest in the concept of social capital?

Such questions are addressed within the empirical study described in Chapters four and five. The study offers a systematic mapping of the field of the sociology of health and medicine in each of the three countries, as well as an analysis of the relationship between the use of sociological knowledge and institutional location. The next section, however, returns our focus to the institutionalisation of the discipline, this time in the United Kingdom.

The sociology of health and medicine in the United Kingdom

Our narrative begins in the United Kingdom in the opening decades of the twentieth century, when disciplinary boundaries were beginning to settle into their modern configurations. In a context dominated by a pervasive sense of national decline and dwindling 'vitality', fuelled by a perturbing level of infant mortality, low birth-rates (particularly among the middle and upper classes), industrial unrest and the near defeat in the Boer War (Moscucci 2005:1317–8); a plethora of intellectual and political claims were being made about how best to resolve the nation's problems, manage ill-health, and organise and administer industrial society as a whole (Warner 1992, 1995; Sturdy and Cooter 1998).

These claims coincided with a campaign by proponents of the new physiology (among other groups), for medical and social reform. Not entirely dissimilar to developments in the United States, efforts to transform medicine into a scientific discipline and build a profession were combined with the very public claim that military might and industrial production were dependent on a healthy population. Thus, even as early as 1921, national prosperity and industrial efficiency were being equated with health and illness (Warner 1992; Sturdy and Cooter 1998:447–8). The inclusion of science into these claims for resources and attention became the key to success, for proponents argued that the new laboratory and experimental sciences could best further the goals of the state and the corporate sector, and effectively manage the social and physiological body, through a specialised, politically and morally neutral, and hierarchically organised, array of technical experts. This process of transformation, completed by about 1930 in Britain, occurred despite significant defiance from many of its practitioners, for up until the First World War medicine was widely considered an 'art', the medical curriculum for the elite was based on a classical education with the aim of producing 'gentlemen', and there was strong resistance to 'science' and the new experimental method (Lawrence 1985). Eventually however, medicine was 'reformed', as it had been a decade earlier in the United States, and in both countries this involved the building of a new 'master' discipline based upon a combination of laboratory-based pathology, pharmacology, biochemistry, bacteriology and physiology (all of which only 'gained maturity' after the 1920s, see Stern 1927:22; Reader and Goss 1959:231). These various intellectual fields were eventually incorporated into a new and standardised curriculum for the medical schools, and the schools themselves increasingly coupled to the universities (Reid 1976). With the new interest from governments, philanthropists and the corporate sector in providing significant resources, the transformed discipline of medicine grew in strength, built its prestige and presented, for the first time, a public face of unity (Moscucci 2005:1318).

Although there had previously been a broad diversity of lay and scholarly perspectives on health and disease, these gave way to a new 'medical model'. In this model, well-being was reduced to a state of the individual, physiological body, and illness defined in new and strictly biological terms. The medical model, by definition, excluded collective, moral and political dimensions of well-being as causal factors in disease. Indeed the era was, according to Oakley (1991:166, 171), dominated by a narrow, eugenic model of health.

During the first four decades of the new century, academic sociology in Britain was largely confined to the *LSE*, and while some of the sociologists in London took a keen interest in matters of health, they did not continue to explore or extend the earlier sociological theories of health and medicine proposed by Engels, Marx, Durkheim and others (see Collyer 2010). Their sociology was instead built upon the framework of the new biology. For example, Alexander Carr-Saunders, at *Liverpool* from 1923 and the *LSE* from 1937 to 1955, was a biologist as well as a sociologist, and the focus of his research is encapsulated by the title of his major work: *The Population Problem* (also Carr-Saunders and Wilson 1964/1933). For Carr-Saunders, biological eugenics was a central piece of his theoretical analysis, and declining population quality was the result of high fertility among the 'inferior' races. In his view, the standard of living of the whole population was put at risk by those with an insufficient physical capacity to maintain industrial production. The perspective of Carr-Saunders was not unique among sociologists, and there was little to suggest that future sociologists might develop a critique of, and an alternative to, the medical model.

Academic sociology remained closely associated with the eugenics movement in Britain for the first three or four decades of the new century. The *Eugenic Education Society* held its first meeting in 1907 in the offices of the *Sociological Society* (Oakley 1991:167), and the societies had many members in common. For example, Richard Titmuss joined the *Eugenic Education Society* in 1937 and remained a member until just before his death in 1973 (Oakley 1991:169).

It is perhaps not entirely unexpected then to find that the institutional infrastructure, essential for the eventual development of an alternative to biological eugenics and the medical model of illness, was first established at some distance from academic sociology and the university system. This arena of intellectual and empirical activity was partially sociological, though not clearly differentiated from social policy or social administration (see Seale 2008:679). Such efforts were perhaps most apparent with regard to Benjamin Seebohm Rowntree, an industrialist, social reformer and self-described sociologist, who produced a number of works based on social surveys, including *Poverty, A Study of Town Life* (1901) and *Poverty and Progress* (1941). Others included Beatrice and Sidney Webb: Fabians, reformers and active in politics. Sidney Webb held an academic post for 15 years in public administration, and was also a member of parliament. Independently wealthy, the pair gathered data and wrote about many subjects, including eugenics, poverty, trade unionism and research methods (Webb and Webb 1910, 1916, 1968/1932). Their largely untheorised social surveys produced statistical evidence of the connections between illness, poor nutrition and poverty, and were carried out within the local municipalities and sometimes at the instigation of the *Medical Research Council* (*MRC*), an organisation set up in 1919. The work of other individuals such as Richard and Kathleen Titmuss, who investigated the association between social class and fertility, mortality, war and living conditions, also made major contributions to this field (Titmuss and Titmuss 1942; Titmuss 1943). Ironically, Richard Titmuss' interests in health and medicine, and his strategies to steer medicine away from its reliance on clinical models and measures, to integrate social factors into clinical education and examine health rather than merely disease, ended in 1950 when he moved to the *LSE* and took up the Chair of Social Administration. From this point his interests shifted towards the broader field of social welfare (Oakley 1991:185).

Mounting empirical evidence about the relationship between health and social organisation (Oakley 1991:188) assisted with the eventual replacement of eugenics with a new social model of health. Important also were the debates over eugenics that raged in the 1930s, for there was considerable concern about whether social or biological factors were responsible for illness, disability and infertility (Charles 1934; Pemberton 1934; Huxley 1936; Orr 1936). As an intellectual field, eugenics began to disintegrate from the mid-1930s when it was associated with Facism and Nazism. It was also difficult to sustain the idea of a genetic basis for joblessness in a context of continuing high levels of unemployment (Oakley 1991:176).

As a social model of illness began to take a place in the 'political vocabulary of health' in the early 1940s (Oakley 1991:172), and the hegemony of biological eugenics faltered, the social and institutional environment became more congenial to sociological efforts in the study of health, illness and medicine. An important element in this sequence of events, however, was the institutionalisation of social medicine in the 1940s. In 1943 the *Royal College of Physicians of London* urged all medical schools to establish departments of social and preventative medicine, and to integrate the teaching of social medicine with clinical studies (Pemberton 2002:343). The first department for Britain occurred with the granting of the Chair of Social Medicine at *Oxford* in 1943 to John Ryle, a consultant physician at Guy's Hospital. As Chair and also Director of the new *Institute of Social Medicine*, Ryle reported that the *Institute* was conducting statistical, radiographical, clinical, and also sociological work (Reid 1976). Ryle's position was that some groups within the population were at greater risk of illness as a consequence of the poor social conditions in which they lived. He called this *social* pathology (Pemberton 2002:343). Ryle also produced a book on social medicine, setting out the subject matter for the new discipline, distinguishing it clearly from public health in its focus on the environment rather than the individual, and claiming its subject matter extended beyond the field of communicable disease to a broad range of diseases (Ryle 1948; Oakley 1991:182–3). Not long after the establishment of Ryle's unit at *Oxford*, a similar department of social medicine was set up at *Birmingham University*, with Thomas McKeown in the chair (in 1945). Like the *Institute*, this too was funded by the *Nuffield Provincial Hospitals Trust*.

Other important institutional developments prior to 1950 included the formation of the *Committee for the Study of Social Medicine*. Members of this group included Titmuss, Ryle and the medical doctor Jerry Morris (Oakley 1991:183). Another was the establishment of a Social Medicine Research Unit at the Central Middlesex Hospital in 1948. The latter was funded by the *Medical Research Council*, with Morris as Director and Titmuss as Deputy (Oakley 1991:184). None of these early appointments were from individuals trained in public health, indicating that the universities were seeking to establish an alternative field, or at least a broader one, given that epidemiology at the time was focused on infectious fevers and had not yet expanded to study the distribution of non-infectious conditions (Pemberton 2002:343).

The formation of these organisational units (and the networks of scholars associated with them) were important in the *institutional* history of the sociology of health and medicine because they offered a forum for debate about the social aspects of illness, helped establish social networks among like-minded individuals and lent a much greater level of legitimacy to the field. They were also critical mechanisms for the fostering of empirical research into the social factors associated with illness in the 1940s. This was because, in addition to their role in medical education, staff in these units were usually involved in medical social surveys, and began to expand the conventional epidemiological approach to investigate non-infectious diseases in the population (Pemberton 2002:343). Despite this, the social medicine units cannot be seen as providing a direct *intellectual* link with the development of the sociology of health and medicine in Britain because, according to Oakley (1991), they represented divergent approaches to their subject matter. For Oakley (1991:185), the social medicine of the 1940s was a pragmatic programme of endeavour, and while it was not based upon a distinctive theoretical framework, its ideological affinity was with medicine, and its epidemiological emphasis clearly distinguished from sociology. These differences would eventually widen as sociology became a more coherent discipline, severed its ties with biology and eugenics, and lost its pursuit of a scientific methodology. At this stage however, the two fields had a tense and somewhat unstable relationship, with only two significant points of compatibility. The first was their shared assumption about scientific method as the most appropriate means to explain human behaviour. The second was the humanitarianism of sociology at this time, which appealed to proponents of social medicine in their need to find social and political solutions to social problems (Reid 1976).

The institutionalisation of social medicine prior to 1950 therefore provided a context within which sociologists and others could broadcast the connection between disease and 'social factors' in the British context, and offered material evidence that this connection was finally being taken seriously by decision-makers: even if the term 'social' was used in a broad and rather anomalous manner. There was other evidence also, for similar ideas were reflected in the Goodenough Report (Ministry of Health 1944), which made a number of recommendations concerning the introduction of sociology and other social sciences into medical education in Britain. Other recommendations of the committee included the re-orientation of medical schools towards education rather than vocational training, their integration into the university system, the development of post-graduate education and the tying of funding to a policy of accepting women students (Rivett 1986). Each of these would have an impact on the eventual formation of a sociology of health and medicine.

The 1950s and 1960s

At the end of the war, although Britain had recently celebrated a victory over Germany, its infrastructure was in ruins, the population was significantly depleted and it was still a place of ration books and identity cards. Over the next few years, and initially under the direction of a Labour government, there was a rapid shift in focus from the war and the military to a programme of reconstruction, re-building the towns, closing down industries no longer required in a time of peace, repairing the housing stock, planning new industries and building essential services. One of the more significant events of this era of renewal was the creation of the *National Health Service* (*NHS*) of 1948, which nationalised all hospitals, voluntary and council, and placed all health care services within a state-funded, regional framework. The creation of the *NHS* reflected the collectivist norms of the war years, which continued in Britain into the 1960s, and are possibly still in evidence today. These sentiments helped to maintain the commitment of both Conservative and Labour governments to the funding and provision of social services (Jefferys 1986:48). The extensive expansion of state services occurred in the midst of two decades of significant economic growth, though less so in the 1960s than the 1950s. The level of employment was very high, and the demand for labour was such that older workers were encouraged to remain in the workforce. This, and the high wages, also brought young people and married women into the paid economy, at least on a part-time basis. The greater material prosperity and the altered position of young people and married women can be understood as at least partly responsible for the subsequent shift in 'generational and male–female relationships in and outside the family' (Jefferys 1986:48).

The expansion of state interest in the *public* provision of services, and in health and medicine in particular, *should* have provided significant opportunities for sociologists. However, in contrast to the United States, with its relatively large population of sociologists, there were very few academic, university-based sociologists in Britain in the 1950s (Jackson 1975:19). The more prestigious of the universities, *Cambridge* and *Oxford*, did not have sociology departments; few university-based sociologists showed an interest in health services or health-related behaviour (Jefferys 1997:124); and only a 'handful' of sociologists were employed in medical establishments through the 1950s and 1960s (Illsley 1975:65; Jefferys 1991:16).

One reason for this situation might be found in the funding context for medical research. Since the 1930s and the formation of scientific medicine, the profession had become well established and powerful. Along with this came an exclusion of the social sciences: even public health and infant welfare were firmly under the control of medicine (Jefferys 1997:121). As medicine strengthened its alliance with the laboratory sciences, and sociology distanced itself from biological eugenics, the social sciences were increasingly perceived as contrary to the clinical discipline of medicine, and considerable boundary-work became necessary to build a new bridge between the two.

By the beginning of the 1950s, medical research in Britain had become the almost exclusive domain of doctors from the leading university teaching hospitals and the Royal Colleges. Unlike the United States, where sociologists had by this time begun to establish viable connections with private and public foundations and agencies, health research in Britain was conducted by subordinate staff (such as medical statisticians and epidemiologists) under the direction of medical doctors, and its focus was on laboratory medicine, particularly new fields such as genetics and bio-chemistry. Much of the funding for medical research came from the *MRC*. This body, still in operation, instigates its own research, responds to requests from government departments and provides funding for research to outside bodies or individuals from universities and hospitals. In the 1950s, most decisions about research funding from the *MRC* were made by medically qualified scientists from the teaching hospitals, with sociologists having little representation on the decision-making bodies (Illsley 1975:64; Reid 1976). Despite the growing awareness among policy-makers of the need to provide less expensive, and therefore non-clinical solutions to the constantly expanding demands for health and other social services (Jefferys 1986:50), sociologists had little in the way of a recognised role in the health system. They were considered irrelevant to developments such as genetics, and other disciplines (such as epidemiology and public health) had stronger claims to be 'interpreters of societal influences to the medical profession'. This left to sociology the arena of social and preventative medicine (Illsley 1975:64–5), a low-status field which continued to be resisted by medicine.

The social sciences, then, were not welcomed into the medical curriculum in the 1950s and 1960s. Although there had been some expansion for the social sciences (Oakley 1991:186), there was little employment for sociologists within medical departments in either decade. For the few sociologists who *were* given work in medicine, it was often temporary with little security. Moreover they found themselves treated as subordinate staff, with promotion barred for anyone without medical qualifications (Jefferys 1997:127). One of the factors behind this was the restriction on funding for medical education (Rivett 1986). Another was the early association between sociology and social medicine, for it meant sociology was still considered one of the disciplines of medicine, able to apply some of the methods of mainstream sociology but few of its concepts. Social medicine itself continued to be active during the 1950s, with several members of the *Socialist Medical Association* creating the *Society for Social Medicine* in 1956 (Pemberton 2002:342). The MRC funded some of its activities, including a conference on the Social Sciences and Medical Research in 1957, and another on Social Classification in 1959 (Oakley 1991:186).

The implications for the infant stirrings of a sociology of health and medicine in Britain were that its first notable institutional context was in the departments and units of *social* medicine, which played host to a few sociologists, rather than the departments of sociology or the departments of medicine (Pemberton 2002:344). For instance, McKeown's Department of Social Medicine at *Birmingham* encouraged the employment of social scientists and their participation in social research (Jefferys 1997:124). Sociologists were also made welcome at meetings of the *Society for Social Medicine*, as were statisticians, for it was open to anyone who held an academic or research post in social medicine or related subject (Pemberton 2002:344). (Margot Jefferys, a sociologist who joined the public health department of the *London School of Health and Tropical Hygiene* in 1952, was a regular participant). Added to this was the fact that the 1950s and 1960s were generally decades of broad inter-disciplinary and multi-disciplinary mixing across the social sciences and across the boundaries of the university sector, and it was in these circumstances that the roots of the sociology of health and medicine (as a specialised field within the British discipline, with its own networks and journals) first began to be laid down.

An indication of the permeability of the disciplinary boundaries of the period is given by the events of the 1953 *BSA* conference, in which one-third of the papers concerned matters of health or medicine, but five of the seven presenters were medical doctors (Illsley 1975:65; Reid 1976; Stacey and Homans 1978:281). The heterogeneous nature of these groupings was evident also in the early membership of the *BSA*, which included many individuals who were not sociologists. This was not just because there were few sociologists in the 1950s, but because many of the individuals interested in this field called themselves 'social scientists', which Jefferys (1997:125) regards as a peculiarly British academic group made up of individuals with an initial education in disciplines such as economic history, economics or political science. The boundaries between sociology and the other social sciences were consequently highly permeable at this point, and sociology was often used as a general term or synonymous with the social sciences. Important also was the lack of restriction on who could become a member of the *BSA*. This changed over time, but rather slowly. In 1951, 75 per cent of its members were employed outside the universities. By 1964, this had fallen to about 50 per cent (Platt 2002:186).

The growing number of individuals with a shared interest in the sociology of health and medicine eventually led, in 1956, to the holding of the first professional meeting for this nascent cluster, and, in 1969, to the founding of a Medical Sociology Group of the *British Sociological Association*. This was one of very few special groups forming within the *BSA* in the 1960s, for many sociologists were busy attending to the establishment of new sociology departments. New study groups became more common over the next few years, including one on political economy, another on socialist development, and a women's caucus was formed in 1974 (Platt 2002:186–9). Other signs of the growing field included the publication of the first British textbook, by Mervyn Susser and William Watson in 1962 (primarily directed at medical students). Such developments had their disappointments also. For example, the Oxford-based Pergamon Press began publication of a new journal *Social Science and Medicine* (*SS&M*) in 1967, but, perhaps because of the greater interest in medical sociology in the United States, it was to be published from the company's New York offices.

Commentators on early British sociology usually consider the 1950s and 1960s a period when the sociology of health and medicine reflected and pursued the issues and problems defined by medicine and other non-sociologists, notably physicians and government agencies, rather than those of the discipline of sociology (Straus 1957; Johnson 1975:229; Reid 1976; Stacey and Homans 1978; Scambler 2005:3; Cockerham 2005b; Seale 2008). The products of this period are usually referred to as a 'sociology *in* medicine', rather than a 'sociology *of* medicine', for only the latter subordinates medical values, perspectives and problems to sociological principles and concerns. It is difficult to shake off the rather negative image of the 1950s and 1960s as a 'dark' period prior to the development of a 'real' 'sociology *of* medicine'. Ann Murcott (2001) is one of the few to suggest an alternative account, pointing to the inventiveness of these individuals in pursuing new opportunities and their capacity to produce sociological work that could be understood (and funded) by a variety of audiences. It should also be noted that the 1960s was the decade in which the 'medical model', as it later came to be called, first came under scrutiny and criticism (Jefferys 1986:52).

These were therefore important decades, and not least because, along with the general expansion of the social sciences, sociology began to find institutional homes beyond the *LSE* and London (Halsey 2004:98). In the 1960s, medical sociology became a component of several existing research centres, including the *Nuffield Centre for Health Services Research* at *Leeds*, and the *Health Services Research Units* at *Canterbury* and *St Thomas' Hospital Medical School*. Three new research centres dedicated to medical sociology were also established at *Aberdeen, Bedford College* at the *University of London*, and the *University College of Swansea*, though none have continued to function in their original form.[1]

The growing band of sociologists and social scientists interested in pursuing the new sociology of health and medicine included Margot Jeffery (originally an economic historian) in the Department of Public Health at the *London School of Hygiene and Tropical Medicine*; Raymond Illsley, the first Director of the *Medical Sociology Research Unit* at *Aberdeen*; Tilda Goldberg, a psychiatric social worker from the Social Medicine Unit at the *Central Middlesex Hospital* who investigated psychosomatic illness (Goldberg 1958), as well as the relationship between social class and mental health; George Brown, a social anthropologist at the *Maudsley Institute of Psychiatry*, who undertook studies in psychiatric medicine, the social basis of mental illness, and eventually the relationship between class and depression (Brown 1959; Brown and Harris 1978); Ann Cartwright, a statistician who later founded the *Institute for Social Studies in Medical Care* (in 1970); Fred Martin, a social psychologist from the *LSE* who lectured in the Department of Social Medicine from 1956; Joe Loudon, a social anthropologist at *Maudsley*; Derek Allcorn, a social anthropologist from the Social Medicine Unit at the *Central Middlesex Hospital*; and Barbara Wootton (1959) from *Bedford College*, who studied the impact of psychiatric ways of thinking on attitudes towards mental health and illness, and the relations between social pathology and class, family characteristics, and physical health.

The 1970s in the United Kingdom

In the 1970s, despite the oil production crisis, there was significant new government funding of medicine, leading to a general expansion and the creation of several new chairs (Rivett 1986). The recommendations of the *Royal Commission on Medical Education*, the 'Todd Report' (1968) – to introduce the social sciences into undergraduate medical education in an effort to convert training into a system of education – took some time to be implemented. Although sociology had hardly made an appearance in the curriculum of medical schools, nursing colleges or health visitor training schools at the beginning of the decade (Illsley 1975:65), by 1977, 28 of the 34 British medical schools had introduced sociology, while 31 were teaching psychology (Field 1988:294). Sociology, as a subject for the curriculum, had made an appearance, but it was primarily offered by individuals – some of them sociologists – employed outside the schools of medicine. This had been the effect of one of the recommendations of the *Todd Report*, that is, for sociological and psychological contributions to medical education to be made by academics from mainstream sociology or psychology departments, not those working in medical faculties (Jefferys 1997:129). This recommendation had taken into account the negative experience of non-medical staff within departments of medicine – and perhaps also the disdain rendered by sociologists to their sociological colleagues who showed an interest in working with medicine – and was an attempt to ensure sociologists and psychologists remained attached to their discipline (Jefferys 1997:129, 131). The result was that most medical sociologists in Britain were located in sociology departments rather than within medicine, though opportunities for employment within medical schools (and not just departments of social or community or public health medicine) grew to a small degree during the 1970s (Reid 1976; Jefferys 1997:129). By this decade it was also becoming apparent that other fields such as social work, nursing and health visiting were professionalising and taking on a greater research role. Sociology was becoming important as a theoretical framework for their studies and sociologists were provided with new arenas for health-related interactions as well as new opportunities for the teaching of medical sociology (Reid 1976).

The same decade was one of growth for sociology. The women's movement began to have an effect on the discipline, as women represented 35 per cent of the higher degrees in sociology and took 21 per cent of the new positions in the university system. By 1973, women constituted 26 per cent of the membership of the *BSA* (Platt 2002:188), and in 1974/5 held 22 per cent of the positions in British sociology departments (though only ten per cent of these were at the professorial level, see Roberts and Woodward 1981:538). This improvement in the position of women occurred within the context of a dramatic increase in the size of the university sector. The impact of the growing prominence of women in the discipline, plus the general politicisation of the population, brought (controversial) changes to the running of the *BSA* conferences. For example, conference subsidies ensured broader attendance, child-care was provided, a larger number of papers and speakers included, and a more democratic process of selecting topics, speakers and papers introduced (Platt 2002:189). Within the *BSA* organisation itself, an income-related scale of fees was created in 1976 to make the association more accessible to all sociologists, a book club began to offer sociology books at lower prices, and the *BSA* took over the publication of the journal *Sociology* (Platt 2002:191).

Changes came also for medical sociology. The women's movement encouraged sociological studies in issues such as human reproduction and childbirth (Oakley 1975, 1976; Comaroff 1977; Hart 1977); contraception, abortion, and illegitimacy (Horobin 1973; MacIntyre 1973; Cartwright 1975); as well as the role and status of women in the health services, particularly with regard to nurses and midwives (Donnison 1977; Elston 1977). Raymond Illsley (1975:65–7) wrote that the field of medical sociology was by this time predominantly occupied by sociologists from university teaching departments, had been accepted into the sociological mainstream as one of its specialities and made solid contributions to sociological theory. Although it had initially been treated with derision by mainstream sociologists, the sociology of health and medicine had finally adopted the same set of methodological and theoretical underpinnings as its parent. For Illsley (1975), this process had been assisted by the 'flood' of publications from the United States, for sociologists in the speciality field were at last able to engage in the same form of 'non-involved criticism, discussion and synthesis' as their other sociological colleagues.

The main forms of funding for sociologists of health and medicine in the mid-1970s were the *Department of Health and Social Security* (which had the primary responsibility for running the *NHS*) and the *MRC* (a body set up to fund research). Both were state agencies, supporting four or five research units dedicated to research in the sociology of health and medicine (Illsley 1975:65). From the 1960s it became evident that the strong medical orientation of the *MRC* had produced a gap in the research system, for the growing demand for evaluation and research on the health services was not being met (Illsley 1975:66). At the same time, the *Social Science Research Council* was averse to funding proposals concerned with medicine, and hence medical sociology research proposals were constantly rejected by both bodies (Reid 1976). The *Department of Health* sought a partial solution by commissioning research on, and evaluations of, the health services. This led to tension between the two organisations, the removal of some of the autonomy of the *MRC* with respect to 25 per cent of its budget and the creation of a Health Service Research and Development unit within the *Department of Health*

(Illsley 1975:66). One of the consequences for the sociology of health and medicine was that research with an obvious benefit to medicine or the administration of the health services would be funded, while the study of, for example, cross-cultural differences in health behaviour, or the doctor–patient relationship in the seventeenth century, would not.

This context had a number of effects on medical sociologists. One was a greater involvement in project work with members of other disciplines. On the positive side this meant an increase in access to medical sites and medical data, as well as opportunities for a wider role in the health system. On the less positive side it meant working in projects where the research objectives and methods were pre-determined and framed by medical scientists according to their own models and career needs, thus favouring non-threatening methods (such as surveys rather than observation) and theories (such as interactionism or interpretivism) (Illsley 1975:66). Greater access to medicine and the health system was rarely, therefore, on one's own terms. This situation was exacerbated by the persistence of a 'liberal reformist ideology', a set of beliefs about the intrinsic value of health and the progressive improvement of health services. This ideology had led to the creation of the *NHS* and ensured that even sociologists were committed to 'making the health services work' (Reid 1976).

Despite these factors, previous concerns about the lack of independence of sociologists of health and medicine from the institutions of medicine seemed to have largely disappeared by 1975. Illsley (1975:67) suggested that gains had been made in sociology's capacity to formulate its own research programmes, and where once sociologists were permitted to participate in medicine from outside the field, they had more recently been 'promoted to observer status within medicine'. To some degree, invitations to observe medicine came from health administrators rather than clinicians, for the first group tended to regard sociology 'as a counter-balancing force to the strength of medicine itself'. This in itself prompted a new concern among sociologists about the potential for becoming agents of the civil servants and the state (Illsley 1975:67). After all, sociologists were now involved in evaluating the operation of the health services but were not given the opportunity to take part in the decision-making processes at the top, where policy was made regarding the shape of the *NHS* (Illsley 1975:67).

By the mid-1970s there were clear signs that a new speciality of the sociology of health and medicine had taken an institutional form in Britain. In 1976 the annual conference of the *BSA* was devoted to the sociology of health and medicine, leading to the publication of two volumes of papers (Dingwall 1977; Stacey *et al.* 1977), and signalling an acceptance within the sociological mainstream. By this time also, the Medical Sociology Study Group had become the largest and most organised section, holding its own annual conference (Reid 1976; Stacey and Homans 1978:281). More medical sociology textbooks appeared, such as Cox and Mead's (1975) *A Sociology of Medical Practice*; David Tuckett's (1976) edited collection, *An Introduction to Medical Sociology*; Tuckett and Kaufert's (1978) edited collection, *Basic Readings in Medical Sociology*; Jones and Jones' (1975) *Sociology in Medicine*; and Robinson's (1973) *Patients, Practitioners, and Medical Care*. At this time, such texts relied heavily on material from the United States (Field 1988:296).

Members of the new field also formed their own journal in 1978, the *Sociology of Health and Illness* (*SHI*), to provide a forum for qualitative studies of health and medicine (Seale 2008:680). It offered its first edition in 1979. In contrast to the journal *Sociology*, which is owned by the *BSA*, the *SHI* is owned by a charitable foundation, and there is no formal, legal association between the study group and the journal. The *Foundation for the Sociology of Health and Illness* was created in December 1999 after concerns about tax liabilities.[2] The journal is the only asset of the *Foundation*, and the charity currently provides funds to support editorial process as well as students, conferences, workshops, and seeding grants for research activities. The *Foundation* has no legal ties with either the *BSA* or the *BSA* Medical Sociology Group, but the three bodies collaborate in activities such as the *Sociology of Health and Illness* Book Prize.

In the 1960s and 1970s, British sociologists of health and medicine began to turn away from their previous focus on epidemiological studies and take greater note of sociological theory. In a search for theory, British sociologists initially found the American works of Parsons of some interest, but later the works of Elliot Freidson (1970a, 1970b, 1975) took on a greater importance, perhaps because these offered an alternative to the consensus model as well as an independent view of medicine (Bury 1986:139; Seale 2008:680). Althusserian Marxism and ethnomethodology also became important in British sociology (Platt 2002:186), along with many other schools. The field was described as 'one of great activity, but little theoretical or methodological unity' (Stacey and Homans 1978:281).

Davies (2003:175) lists a number of social scientists working on health and medicine during the 1970s in the United Kingdom, including David Towell from the *Fulbourn Hospital* (and later the *King's Fund*), who examined the psychiatric care setting (Towell and Harries 1979); Wieland and

Leigh (1971) and Revans (1972) from the *King's Fund*; and McLachlan (1977) at the *Nuffield Provincial Hospitals Trust*. Many of their studies were 'administrative' rather than 'academic' in focus (Davies 2003:175). An important historical work published in this decade was Thomas McKeown's (1979) *The Role of Medicine*, which challenged the claims of medicine and the medical profession as responsible for the major health improvements of the modern era. Also influential was Nick Jewson's (1976) paper on medical cosmology, which reflected the rising influence of the sociology of knowledge on the field (also see Wolff 1970; Waddington 1973; Scull 1975; Skultans 1975; Atkinson 1977; Hughes 1977; Posner 1977).

Another growing area of sociological research, as noted by Cockerham (1983:1520), was the analysis of clinical work employing symbolic interactionist and ethnomethodological perspectives. These ethnographic studies offered rich, descriptive accounts of social practices and the relationships between patients and practitioners: perspectives which were not present in American sociology of the same period. Examples include the works of Paul Atkinson (1977, 1981); Gerry Stimson and Barbara Webb (1975); Michael Wadsworth and David Robinson (1976); Alan Davis and Gordon Horobin (1977); and Robert Dingwall (1977, Dingwall *et al.* 1977). Other sociologists of health and medicine from the 1970s include Margaret Stacey (1976), Margot Jefferys (1973, Phil Strong (1977), Ray Jobling (1977), Jean Comaroff (1976, 1977), Lesley Doyal (1979) and Sally McIntyre (McIntyre and Oldman 1977).

The 1980s in the United Kingdom

The new decade opened with the publication of the 'Black Report', a report from an expert committee examining health inequalities and chaired by Sir Douglas Black. The report had been commissioned by the *Department of Health and Social Security* in March 1977 by David Ennals, Labour Secretary of State. Although ready for publication in early 1979, it was not immediately made public due to the election of a new Conservative Government in May of that year. The report offered evidence of an improvement in the health of the population since the introduction of the *NHS*, but also of ongoing inequality in mortality rates according to social class. This provoked a flurry of political and policy activity in many other countries, in the *World Health Organisation* and the *Office for Economic Co-Operation and Development*. It also led to debate and empirical investigation into health inequalities among sociologists of health and medicine in Britain (Williams 1984; Blane 1985; Calnan and Johnson 1985; Boulton *et al.* 1986; Bloor *et al.* 1987). It had little positive impact on the new British government.

Overall, the 1980s were not very positive years for sociology in Britain, as the Thatcher Conservative government continually denigrated the discipline's central issues and concerns (Iphofen and Poland 1997:44). University funding from the state – its primary source of funds – was severely cut in the late 1970s and again in the 1980s, a reduction of about 13 per cent between 1981 and 1984. These budget decreases were more severe in the humanities and social sciences than elsewhere, so that senior members of staff were encouraged to take early retirement and members of the workforce were subjected to widespread redundancies (Platt 2002:190). Threats were also made to abolish the *Social Science Research Council*, though this was effectively salvaged through the political action of social scientists and the *BSA*. A number of very public attacks were made on sociology, notably from conservative sociologists Julius Gould (in 1977) and David Marsland (in 1988), indicating serious ideological divisions within the discipline (Platt 2002:190).

The number of posts for sociologists in the medical schools did not grow as rapidly as they had in the latter part of the 1970s, but there was an increase in the number of medical sociologists employed outside the sociology departments as several new positions were created. The period was, according to David Field (1988:296), one of consolidation rather than growth, marred somewhat by the employment of casuals and non-sociologists (in some medical schools) to service the teaching of the discipline. With regard to the field's relative presence within these schools, it still had a lower profile than psychology. Sociology's lack of power within medicine was also evident in the restriction of its role to teaching delivery, for few sociologists were invited to be part of significant committees or the admissions processes (Field 1988:297).

Sociologists continued to face problems where they were employed in the medical schools. Isolated from the focal concerns of their own discipline, it became difficult to resist the definitions and perspectives of their medical colleagues. They also suffered from a lack of career prospects, 'because they have no clear sponsor to vouch for their worth and to push for their promotion in the relevant university bodies' (Field 1988:299). Speaking of this situation, Horobin (1985:95) says:

> Medical sociologists...inhabit the interstices between the citadel of medicine and the suburb of sociology. In many cases this is reinforced by the institutional arrangements under which medical sociology is practised, for relatively few are firmly based in departments of

sociology and those located in medical departments are seldom given full accreditation by their medical colleagues. So medical sociology is still searching for an identity...

Boundary disputes with other disciplines were also in evidence in the 1980s. Sociologists were continuing to put up with various 'intruders' into its field, most of whom were without sociological training or even actively practising sociology. Gordon Horobin (1985:96) argued that like sociology in general, the sociology of health and medicine was defensive rather than aggressive in Britain, and 'too beset by self-doubt to make any really committed assaults on the neighbouring tribes'. At the same time however, he regarded it as essentially 'healthy' for the sociology of health and medicine to have been forced, as it was during the 1970s and 1980s, to engage in 'practical' work. The separation of the field from academic sociology and its 'uneasy symbiosis with medicine' had led to a considerable proportion of its output being interesting and meaningful. Horobin suggested he was 'content to let a thousand flowers bloom even though [he] would personally water only some of them' (1985:104).

On a more positive note, the textbooks of the 1980s reversed the position of the 1970s, and for the first time included British rather than American material (Field 1988:296). Several British medical sociology textbooks appeared, raising the profile of the field (especially within medicine), as well as providing valuable resources for teaching. These included David Armstrong's (1980) *An Outline of Sociology Applied to Medicine*; Patrick and Scambler's (1982) edited collection *Sociology as Applied to Medicine* (specifically written for medical students and the medical curriculum); Scambler's (1987) *Sociological Theory and Medical Sociology*; and Margaret Stacey's (1988) feminist analysis of the field *The Sociology of Health and Healing*.

From the 1980s, sociologists of health and medicine in the United Kingdom began to show an interest in the theoretical ideas from continental Europe (Seale 2008:680), and there appeared a number of debates about social constructionism in the journal *SHI* (e.g. Nicolson and McLaughlin 1987). For example Mike Bury (1986:139) argued that Freidson's relativist approach to disease was problematic, resting on a distinction between illness as a social phenomenon and disease as a bio-physical state independent of human knowledge. To resolve the impasse, Bury (1986:139–40) suggests British sociologists turned to the Marxian-influenced critical theory of the Frankfurt school, and to Foucault (1970, 1977). For William Cockerham (1983:1520), this small movement towards theoretical development in the sociology of health and medicine first became apparent in the 1970s, and he found it contrary to the past emphasis on producing work with a practical application. Cockerham points to the work of Robert Dingwall (1976) and George Brown (Brown *et al.* 1968; Brown and Harris 1978) as examples of this more theoretical strand of development in the field.

The sociology of knowledge approach to the sociology of health and medicine, evident in the previous decade, continued to develop in the 1980s. Some of the works of the period had a strong historical focus, for instance Lawrence (1985), Comaroff (1982), Cooter (1982), and Wright and Treacher (1982). Others seemed to gain inspiration from the works of Michel Foucault, for instance Armstrong (1982, 1987), and Bryan Turner (1995/1987), the British sociologist who left for Australia in the early 1980s.

According to Davies (2003:177), in the late 1980s and during the 1990s, sociology tended to examine health from either a 'micro' or a 'macro' perspective, leaving the middle ground, 'where policy and organisational processes tend to be concentrated', to others such as health policy analysts or political scientists. Health policy thus strengthened as a field from the end of the 1980s, and this meant, says Davies (2003:178), sociologists were more likely to investigate the boundaries between health workers, such as between nurses and doctors (Cartwright and Anderson 1981; Hughes 1988) than broader organisational practices, and this trend has continued (e.g. Daykin and Clarke 2000). This observation is supported by the interests of the sociologists of health and medicine during the 1980s, for it includes Stacey's (1980) investigation of an assessment centre for children with disabilities; David Hughes' (1988) exploration of nurse–doctor interaction; a study by Hughes *et al.* (1987) on teenagers with mental disabilities; and Rawlings' (1989) examination of the symbolic significance of hygiene. Despite this area of weakness, the sociology of health and medicine is generally thought, by the 1980s, to have established a 'sociology *of* medicine', with the sociological perspective finally prioritised ahead of medicine (Cockerham 1983:1519).

The 1990s and beyond in the United Kingdom

By the late 1980s, many researchers and policy analysts began to predict serious shortfalls of labour throughout the health professions, particularly in medicine and nursing. Efforts were made to increase cost-effectiveness in the health services as well as in education and training, and the reform of the medical curriculum became increasingly urgent. The Thatcher-led Conservative government's response to the former was to introduce, in 1990, an internal market into the *NHS*, which split the purchase of health care services (GP fundholders) from the provision of services (*NHS Trusts*), ostensibly to promote competition between providers (i.e. hospitals) within the *NHS* and enhance efficiency. Opportunities for privately provided health care services were also encouraged by the state. The new Labour government scrapped the internal market when it came to power in 1997, and its reforms limited competition and emphasised co-operation. This (and no doubt the significant increase in resources for health services) raised the general level of satisfaction with the *NHS* (Propper *et al.* 2003:28). Nevertheless, a second round of reforms in 2002 included a greater capacity for patients to select a private source of care (outside the *NHS*), and for private services to compete with public ones. The cost-effectiveness of these various reforms has been the subject of considerable debate, with some researchers suggesting the privatisation of health services and the involvement of private financing arrangements to extend the *NHS* have been the more expensive options and left a burden of debt for future generations to service (Rowland *et al.* 2001). Concerns have also been raised about the issue of equity: a key social value endorsed in the 1948 establishment of the *NHS*. Others have argued that chronic under-funding, the introduction of private forms of health care and private–public financing schemes may have harmed the ability of the service to respond effectively to the needs of many social groups (Pollock 1993, 2000; Pollock *et al.* 1997; Gaffney *et al.* 1999a, 1999b; Calnan *et al.* 2001; Cant and Calnan 2008; Harley *et al.* 2011; Hughes *et al.* 2011; Pollock and Price 2011).

The 1990s were the beginning of a set of dramatic changes for sociology. The period began with a continuation of the Conservative government's assault on the social sciences and sociology. In contrast, the Labour victory of 1997 brought with it a new policy of multi-disciplinarity for the health field, particularly in public health. Since the formation of community medicine in the 1970s, training, and all senior career paths, had been closed to non-medical professionals, and public health effectively equated with public health medicine (Evans 2003:961). The Labour government's emphasis on multi-disciplinarity for this field and its opening of a small number of senior management posts to non-medical experts in public health have encouraged new roles to develop (particularly for those with epidemiological skills), and led to a limited (though valuable) alteration in the traditional medical hierarchy (Evans 2003:964–5). It is not clear whether the new Conservative government of 2010 will seek to expand or reverse this process of multi-disciplinarity in the health field.

Moreover, although still recovering from a decade of assault by the Conservative government, the discipline has finally been able to acknowledge the success of its efforts – in train since at least the 1950s – to influence the medical curriculum and raise the educational levels of lower-status health care professionals (such as midwifery and nursing) (Cooke 1993; Iphofen and Poland 1997:44). As Margot Jefferys (1991:15) states:

> Today, all UK medical and dental students are expected to have some rudimentary knowledge of sociology and its actual and potential contribution to the theory and practice of modern medicine. They are also introduced to the principles of epidemiology and medical statistics, and their role in medical research and practice. Scarce resources of time and staff still restrict the contribution which both disciplines can ideally make to the education of medical practitioners, but few teachers are now prepared to deny their intrinsic value.

By the 1990s, *if there had been* a previously narrow set of concerns within the sociology of health and medicine in Britain, the field had changed considerably. In 1995, Bryan Turner wrote about the new developments of mainstream sociology (including the sociology of the body, the sociology of risk and theories of globalisation), as having been introduced into the sociology of health and medicine, bringing about a new meeting between the sub-field and its parent. In agreement with this viewpoint is Celia Davies (2003:179), who suggests that recent British medical sociology – or at least that reflected in the journal *SHI* – shows the strong influence of Foucauldian and post-modernist analysis, and a pre-dominance of concepts such as 'embodiment, identity, self, narrative, biography, history and risk'. For Graham Scambler (2005), evidence of this stronger interest in social theory can be found in the number of new journals established during the period, including the multi-disciplinary journal *Health*, which started in 1997, the *Body and Society* in 1995, *Health, Risk and Society* in 2000, and *Social Theory and Health* in 2003.

The extent of interest in health and the body in British sociology is also demonstrated by the devotion of the annual *BSA* conference to these topics in 1990 and 1998 respectively. Other topics of interest to sociologists since 1990 have included the illness experience, particularly chronic illness (Bury 1991; Kelly and Field 1996; Lawton 1998, 2003; Williams 2000; Taylor and Bury 2007), and 'emotional labour' (Straus *et al.* 1982). Lawton's (2003:33) review of the field found very little emphasis on health and the healthy body, suggesting most studies focus on illness and the diseased body (with Monaghan's 2001 study of body-building as an exception). Seale's (2008:679) analysis of the publications of the period indicates that social inequalities associated with social class did not hold a high level of interest, although there were a few exceptions, including Wilkinson's (1996) *Unhealthy Lifestyles*, and Blaxter's (1990) *Health and Lifestyles*.

In the 1990s, many sociologists sought to investigate the health care services and the *NHS*. Some have been mentioned above with regard to the introduction of private health and private–public financing schemes. Others focused more firmly on the social processes and practices within the health services, for instance Jon Gabe, Michael Calnan and Mike Bury (1991); Nicky Britten (1991); Phil Strong and Jane Robinson (1990); Judith Green and David Armstrong (1993); Mike Dent (1990); Paul Atkinson (1995); and David Hughes and Lesley Griffiths (1999). Others continued the trend of examining various aspects of illness, including James Nazroo (1998), Mike Kelly and David Field (1996), and Julia Lawton (1998). Sarah Nettleton (1995) and Ellen Annandale (1998) produced new textbooks for medical sociology.

With regard to the methods and methodologies in use by sociologists of health and medicine in Britain, Seale (2008:680) suggests most sociological work by this time had become qualitative. There are, however, branches of sociology where quantitative policy-work is conducted, where 'atheoretical' work can be found, and where a social problems approach is taken which draws on sociological theory but seeks to address political and policy issues. The smaller field of British quantitative work published over the decades in *SHI* has been investigated by David Blane (2003) and Bechhofer (1996). Here it was found that about 72 per cent of papers were qualitative or not empirical, and 28 per cent quantitative in the period 1992–1994, and that this hadn't changed a great deal from 1981, when the relative proportions were 80–20 per cent. Bechhofer (1996:586) tells us this represents only a 'modest shift toward the quantitative group'. Blane's (2003) study draws strongly from Bechhofer's analysis, and also examines papers published in the journal. It is quite difficult to judge, from either analysis, how large the quantitative field might be, as the authors do not distinguish between the papers according to nationality, and as a result include sociologists from other countries (such as Jake Najman from Australia, Irene Wennemo of Sweden, Espen Dahl of Norway and Ichirō Kawachi of the United States). Nor do the reviews distinguish between sociologists and individuals from other disciplinary fields. Although some, such as Nick Jewson (1976) and James Nazroo (1998), have sociological qualifications and/or identify themselves as sociologists, the inclusion of others raises questions about disciplinary boundaries, for also mentioned are scholars Doreen Massey (a geographer), Richard Wilkinson (an epidemiologist) and Peter Goldblatt (a statistician). It appears reasonable to conclude, therefore, that most sociologists of health and medicine in Britain favour a qualitative approach, and that this is reflective of British sociology as a whole.

Qualitative studies of health and medicine, based on the interactionist paradigm, first became popular:

> ... in mental illness research where the slipperiness of diagnostic concepts was most apparent and where the status of the dominant profession – psychiatry – was somewhat uncertain. The spread of the interactionist perspective to the analysis of somatic illnesses and the agencies dealing with them was quite rapid once sociologists allowed themselves to think of the social meanings without its biophysical character. Early scepticism of soft data and soft methods on the part of grant givers was replaced by low key approval when research began to document the processes by which agencies or specialities create clients. 'Need' could then be seen to be a political as much as a descriptive concept, a very useful notion when resistance to demands for further resources is the order of the day
>
> (Horobin 1985:101–2).

The continuation of an emphasis on the qualitative approach in British sociology may have been prompted by quite different factors. For Clive Seale (2008:680), the primarily qualitative, theoretical approach resulted from the assaults on the discipline of the 1980s, turning sociologists away from the political, policy context.

There have been a few other reviews of British efforts in the sociology of health and medicine, and interest has been shown in the sociological workforce. Thus we have some information about the research interests of this group, and about the characteristics of sociologists. For example, in a recent review of the discipline of sociology as a whole (Holmwood and Scott 2010:24), it was pointed out that the academic cohort is still disproportionately male, with 92–94 per cent white nationals, and considerable gender differences in attainment. Where international sociologists are employed, these are also generally white (and from the European Union, North America or Australia).

Hence there is very little racial or ethnic diversity among staff, with little sign of any shift in the trend.

The sociology of knowledge indicates the likelihood that these and other social characteristics of the sociological workforce have consequences for the kind of medical sociology conducted in Britain. Until the publication of this volume, little has been known about the field in relation to its institutional context. In Chapters four and five, an empirical study is described and its findings presented on a range of matters, including the extent to which sociologists working in medical departments use quantitative rather than qualitative methods. For the present however, it is time to turn to an examination of the processes of institutionalisation in the Australian context.

The sociology of health and medicine in Australia

The early twentieth century

In the previous chapter it was pointed out that although there was a dearth of independent departments of sociology in Australia prior to the 1950s, there were sociological works and courses of teaching. These took place within other university disciplines, within the classes of the *Workers' Educational Association*, and also outside the university system. Some of the individuals engaged in this research and the teaching of sociology had interests in health and well-being, including Meredith Atkinson, Clarence Northcote, Herbert Heaton, and John Gunn. Some had post-graduate qualifications, usually from Britain and rarely from sociology, as Australia had no capacity to award sociology PhDs at this time and Britain had few sociologists it could spare for its former colony. Indeed the first sociology PhD awarded in Australia was to Robert Pike, and this wasn't until 1965 (Willis 2005). Fortunately, during the pre-departmental period, a number of the new arrivals had previously been introduced to sociological theories or methods, and this experience, particularly in social surveys, assisted with the building of sociological expertise within the country.

Australia in the first half of the twentieth century was a curious mixture of progressive social and political reform and conservative parochialism. In July of 1900, Queen Victoria gave her assent to a bill before the British Parliament for the six Australian colonies to form a federation. Federation came into operation as of the first of January 1901, providing the country with a constitution, its own parliament (though it was yet to have its own building), a Governor-General (Lord Hopetoun), a Prime Minister (Edward Barton, appointed by Hopetoun), and no actual government or political parties. In 1902 women were given the vote at the federal level, forcing the laggard states to introduce women's suffrage. The world's first Labor government appeared in Australia in 1904 (though it was not to last long in its first incarnation, losing office after only four months). The same year also saw the creation of the world's first Court of Conciliation and Arbitration. In 1907 pensions for the aged were introduced, and in 1908 the High Court – established in 1903 – ruled on the matter of wages, leading to a response from the Court of Arbitration to bring in the 'basic wage', a law which remained in place for almost a century. These historic developments were combined with others of a far less progressive nature. For example, the political preference in the country swayed towards protectionism rather than free-trade, the Immigration Bill introduced to the Commonwealth Parliament in 1901 was designed to ensure a 'White Australia', the social and living conditions of the indigenous peoples were appalling, the maternity allowance introduced in 1912 was available only for white Australians, and loyalty to the Empire (Britain meant 'home' to most of the country's white population) essentially over-shadowed any early glimmerings of nationalism.

During the first half of the twentieth century, Australian's experienced two major wars (1914–18 and 1939–45) and a depression (1929–33). This meant the economic fortunes of the country were continually shifting, with widespread social and financial hardship. In Australia, as in Britain, concerns were continually raised about the falling birth rate and high maternal mortality, and in the 1930s it was estimated that approximately 40 per cent of Australian children were malnourished. The government pursued a policy of 'populate or perish', and in an effort to improve the health of the nation, built its research capacity by expanding the *Federal Health Council* and transforming it into the *National Health and Medical Research Council (NHMRC)* in 1937. The new body was given a new research function to investigate matters of public health, and it also became an advisory body for government. In this expansion, members of the medical profession were included for the first time, indicating something about their growing strength.

There was also mounting concern about the lack of widely accessible health services. Under the constitution, the Commonwealth was responsible only for quarantine-related health matters, while State governments were required to provide health services. The extent to which such services were adequately funded and accessible to the population varied greatly. Religious and secular charities provided care for some of the population, those with employment were able to join Friendly Societies (and exchange voluntary contributions for health care services), wealthier individuals paid doctors and hospitals on a fee-for-service basis, while members of the defence forces were able to attend government services. Assistance with health care costs for the general population was generally inadequate, with patients often having to make some contribution towards the cost of services and there was widespread means-testing to attend public or community-based hospitals. A federal *Department of Health* was established in 1921, but even the holding of two Royal Commissions during the 1920s (to investigate the means to improve the co-ordination of State and Commonwealth services and reduce the cost of health care) had led to little progress in the creation of a national health system.

Several efforts towards a national system were made. The first, in 1928 by Earl Page (a surgeon, business owner and Treasurer), was thwarted by the Friendly Societies (voluntary insurance schemes), employer and doctors' groups. Plans for the further reform of health and welfare services were shelved as economic conditions worsened. The second was in 1938 by Richard Gardiner Casey. Casey was a Treasurer in the Lyons government, and he proposed *The National Health and Pensions Insurance Bill* as a means to provide sickness benefits, pensions and medical benefits. This would be funded from contributions of two per cent from the wages of the workers, and differed from the 1928 proposal because it offered treatment and medicines which would be free (at the point of service) for the insured. The plan was opposed by employers, workers, charities, the medical profession and even the Curtain-led Labor Party. The latter, in opposition, argued that health services should be free and not drawn from wages. Australian doctors were represented by the *British Medical Association (BMA)* at this time, and the government was offered support for its programmes only on the basis that all medical services would continue to involve a cash payment. Agreement was initially reached between the *BMA* and the government with regard to issues such as remuneration and conditions of service, but Casey's plan met further opposition in the parliament and although eventually passed into law, was not enacted in the face of the looming war in Europe.

A third effort was made, on this occasion by the Labor government in the 1940s (in power from 1941 to December 1949). By this period there was widespread debate about the need for some form of national insurance, but fearful the government would attempt to bring in a system akin to the British *NHS*, Australian doctors campaigned to protect their financial interests. When the government brought in the 1944 *Pharmaceutical Benefits Act*, aiming to provide essential medicines free of charge, the doctors joined forces with the United Australia Party (a forerunner of the Liberal-Country Party), and fiercely resisted all proposals. The doctors took the matter to the High Court, and this ruled against the Commonwealth, finding it did not have the power to legislate on medicines or other health services, and ruling the legislation invalid. This prompted a referendum in 1946 to enable an extension of Commonwealth powers. The referendum was successful, but the doctors had also won: for they had effectively limited government from taking any actions which might involve 'civil conscription'. This meant the government would be unable to force doctors to work in a public dental or health care system.

The Labor government went ahead with a more limited national health programme, began negotiating with the states for free access for public patients in public hospitals in return for some Commonwealth subsidies, and brought in the 1947 *Pharmaceutical Benefits Act* and 1948 *National Health Service Act*. The *Pharmaceutical Benefits Act*, like its 1944 forerunner, aimed to provide a selection of free medicines upon presentation of a government-issued prescription form. This effort was also challenged by the coalition of doctors and other interested parties, who took the matter to the High Court on the basis that the requirement to use an official form amounted to civil conscription. With the Act ruled invalid, the Labor government passed new legislation to give patients free medicines only where the practitioner 'chose' to use the official form. Without the requirement to use the prescription forms, doctors acted *en masse* to thwart the intentions of government and the will of the people, and refused to use the forms. This meant patients continued to have to pay full price for medicines. It wasn't until the Labor Party lost power in 1949 that the fear of nationalisation diminished. From this period doctors began to use the free medicine scheme (Dewdney 1989:73).

The first five decades of the century thus saw very little progress in the improvement of the population's health or in the creation of a more accessible health care system. Yet these years also witnessed the emergence of a small but growing band of experts, who, from the 1940s and 50s, began to undertake social surveys of all areas of social life, including the incidence of disease and poverty in the aftermath of war, as well as urbanisation, industrialisation and migration. Most of the surveys were untheorised and fairly rudimentary with regard to method (Ancich *et al.* 1969:49), but nevertheless provided a foundation for future work and reflected the rather late formation of an interested, reformist, intellectual, middle class: previously absent in the country. Social surveys appeared mostly in Melbourne, Adelaide and Sydney, and included studies by the educationalist W.F. Connell, the social psychologist Oscar Oeser, and the many research studies of the *Brotherhood of St Lawrence*. The *Brotherhood* was something of an anomaly in a country with no true history of non-religious philanthropy, very few large companies, and an entrenched propensity to turn to government for assistance. In this environment it was a significant player, filling a niche where there were few academic sociologists and even fewer sociology departments. By the late 1960s the *Brotherhood's* role diminished as it shifted its focus from research to services. By this time however, 'there were other researchers, including members of the newly founded departments of sociology at *Monash* and *La Trobe*, who were better able to take up the broader social research agenda' (Davison 2003:158).

The 1950s and early 1960s

Although the 1950s brought increasing economic growth and full employment to the country, no progress was made in the 1950s and 60s with regard to the implementation of a national health service in Australia. With the newly forged Liberal Party in power from December 1949 (in coalition with the Country Party), and Robert Menzies at the helm of this conservative government, a fourth attempt was made to create a health scheme. This one occurred in 1953 when Earle Page (from the Country Party), this time as Health Minister, put forward a government-subsidised, voluntary scheme (*The National Health Act*), shifting the balance back towards an emphasis on individual contributions. Patients paid into a registered medical insurance fund, and this fund acted as an agent of the government, paying an agreed upon amount for the doctor's service. In Page's new scheme, access to the subsidy was dependent on the capacity to purchase private health insurance, and this left a large proportion of the population uninsured (de Voe and Short 2003:348).

Somewhat greater progress was made in other health-related areas, such as the monitoring and testing of pharmaceuticals. Efforts to improve the population's access to medicines had thrown the spotlight on the quality of drugs, and, with the Commonwealth becoming a significant purchaser of drugs by the 1950s, their cost also became an issue. Prior to the 1950s the testing of pharmaceuticals was conducted at the *Universities of Sydney* and *Melbourne*, but after the passing of the *Therapeutic Substances Act* in 1957, the *National Biological Standards Laboratory* was set up at the *Australian National University*. This new facility enabled the creation of a national, uniform system of biological standards and labelling for drugs. An *Institute of Social Medicine* was planned for the *ANU* (Rowse 2002:173), more effort was made to take a role in the *World Health Organisation*, and closer relations were fostered within the Asian region through the establishment of the Colombo Plan (a programme which sponsored many thousands of students, including in the health professions, to study at Australian tertiary institutions).

The poor treatment of Australian soldiers by the British in the First World War, and Britain's lack of regard for Australia's own defence from Japanese invasion during the Second World War (Ward 1968:156–7), coupled with the arrival of new consumables and cultural products (e.g. the car, the movies), turned the loyalties of the general population increasingly away from Britain towards America. Within the universities however, the ties to the 'home country' were more resilient, and the institutional establishment of sociology in Australia closely parallels many aspects of the British case. Chairs and departments of sociology began to be formed from 1950, but there were very few until the later 1960s. The relatively late start for the discipline of sociology within the university sector is often explained as a result of ideology (Bryson 2005; Richmond 2005:58–9). As was the case in the United States and Britain, the 1950s and 60s in Australia were difficult for intellectuals on the political Left, as there was a widespread fear of communism: particularly from the 'Catholic Right'. Peter Worsley, for example, as an anthropology student, was prevented from doing fieldwork in New Guinea in 1952 by the Australian government due to his 'political affiliations'. Numerous other intellectuals were denied appointments or promotions for this reason (Rowse 2002:257). The Communist Party was banned in 1950 with the passing of the *Communist Dissolution Bill*, which also barred communists from employment within the Commonwealth government. The legislation was overturned by the High Court in 1951 (Ward 1968:165).

Until the broad establishment of sociology departments, sociological perspectives on health and medicine, like other sociological investigations, were generally produced by scholars with qualifications from other disciplines, working in other departments of the universities, and sometimes even by individuals outside the university system. Consequently the specialist field's beginnings can be found in an interdisciplinary mix of social psychology, history, demography, anthropology, social work, social psychiatry, social epidemiology, public health and medicine.

Many of the individuals involved in its earliest days were health/ medical practitioners who frequently attended sociological gatherings and displayed an enthusiasm for investigating the social aspects of illness. One of these was Jerzy Krupinski, a medical doctor and epidemiologist, employed at the *Mental Health Research Institute*, a unit established in 1956 by the *Victorian Health Department* to monitor the state's psychiatric services. Krupinski identified one of his interests as 'medical sociology' in his application for membership to the *Sociological Association of Australia and New Zealand (SAANZ)*, and was an active member of the association. His studies were concerned with the mapping of social class and the ethnic characteristics of psychiatric patients. A second practitioner who attended the early sociological meetings was Alan Stoller. Stoller was a government psychiatrist from the *Mental Health Authority* in Melbourne, and interested in similar issues but also the phenomenon of transsexualism. The pair collaborated on a number of projects (Krupinski and Stoller 1968, 1971, 1974). Another was Neville Yeomans, a biologist, psychiatrist, psychologist, and barrister. Unlike Stoller and Krupinski, Yeomans also had some sociological qualifications. In certain respects, Yeomans was the New South Wales (NSW) equivalent of Krupinski, being the founding director of Fraser House (a community-based psychiatric unit set up in 1959 by the *NSW Health Department*). Yeomans pioneered action-research among the mentally ill, working on the principle that the re-building of a patient's social network would reduce their mental distress and help them back to 'functionality'. His work incorporated sociological theory, including the philosophical ideas of Karl Marx (Yeomans 1965; Clark and Yeomans 1969; also Spencer 2006). In the 1960s Yeomans set up the *Clinical Sociology Research Study Group*, and in 1967 this radical psychiatrist led a tour group of sociologists from the annual *SAANZ* conference to see Fraser House at the *North Ryde Psychiatric Hospital* (Richmond 2005:60). Individuals such as Krupinski and Yeomans were important in this early period, for they gave the infant sociology a 'shelter' within the medical sphere when it did not have a secure place elsewhere.

Specialisation was not a feature of sociological work in these decades, as the community of university-based sociologists was too small (the membership of *SAANZ* was less than 150 in 1965, see Frank Jones 1973:1), and most sociologists who published on health also wrote on other topics. An early sociologist, Athol Congalton, was typical in this respect. Congalton, originally from New Zealand, was the Professor of Sociology for many years at the *University of New South Wales*. He became known for his work on social status and stratification (Congalton 1969), but also for investigations into nursing (Congalton 1963) and undergraduate texts on health sociology (Congalton and Najman 1971; Congalton 1976). The career of John Western offers a second example of the extent to which scholars of the period moved easily between disciplines and rarely specialised on one topic. Western completed his *Social Studies Diploma* in 1954 and collected a Masters degree in psychology at *Melbourne*. He completed a PhD in sociology in 1962 at *Columbia* before returning to Australia, and early publications range from student attitudes (Anderson and Western 1967), to policing (Wilson and Western 1972), military conscription (Western and Wilson 1968), but also health and medicine (Western 1976; Najman *et al.* 1981).

In the 1960s the appearance of several new scholarly journals indicated an intensification of interest in sociology. In 1961 came the *Australian Journal of Social Issues*, and in 1965 the *Australian and New Zealand Journal of Sociology*. Foreign sociology journals also began to be made available in Australia, such as the American publication, the *Journal of Health and Social Behavior (JHSB)* (published from 1960), and the British journal, *Sociology* (from 1967). A review of health-related journal publications by Australian sociologists of the period indicates the prevalence of topics such as alcohol abuse, health and welfare services, policy, and social class, with something of a lesser focus on Aboriginal health, fertility trends, mental illness and the problems of the migrant population. Most papers were untheorised, but where sociological theory was in evidence, the dominant theoretical paradigm was functionalism, with a small component of feminist and interactionist perspectives also apparent. Quantitative methods were the primary methodological approach.

The late 1960s and 1970s

By 1965 the Australian economy was second only to Japan with regard to the strength of its economy, with a vigorous manufacturing sector and a healthy and still growing export trade in both primary and secondary industries. The arts began to be patronised, emerging artists and performers began to make a career within Australia rather than necessarily leaving for foreign shores, the local publishing industry began to grow – despite strong competition from overseas – and a more sophisticated, urbanised culture became evident (Ward 1968:169–70). An intensification of the discipline began in the late 1960s with the general expansion of the university system. Boosted by a still increasing population and a continuing flow of European migrants, the university sector saw a growth in student numbers, in new universities, and in new sociology departments. Amidst the rise of student movements, the university sector also experienced an influx of mature students. This heightened the awareness of social issues and students began to place demands on the staff of sociology departments to address social problems and offer, in addition to the 'core' courses (on method and theory), a set of 'electives' on specialist areas (Scott 1979:5–8).

Several associations were formed during this period. One of these was a Medical Sociology Section of *SAANZ* in 1967 (*ANZJS* 1967:149; Richmond 2005:60–63). It was the first of the speciality sections, followed in 1970 by a Sociology Teachers' Section and in 1976 a Women's Section. The Medical Sociology Section was organised by Katy Richmond – the first convenor of the group – and developed from the work she and Rosemary Otto were conducting on psychiatrists and psychiatric hospitals at Larundel, a mental hospital 800 metres from Richmond's office at *La Trobe* (Richmond 2010). Under the convenorship of Richmond, and assisted by Otto, informal meetings were held monthly in inner-city Melbourne. One of the participants was Herbert Bower, a psychiatrist who is widely remembered for the sensitive support provided to transgender people. In 1975, along with Trudy Kennedy and William Walters, Bower developed the Gender Dysphoria Clinic, first at the *Queen Victoria Hospital* and later at the *Monash Medical Centre*. Although Bower eventually became convinced of a genetic basis to gender dysphoria, he was a fierce advocate for social justice for his patients, and took a keen interest in sociological thought (Collyer 1993; see also Bower 1960, 1964, 1972, 1986). Some of the 30-odd participants of the Medical Sociology Section were *SAANZ* members, and the group attracted some interest from 'health oriented social scientists and doctors around Melbourne', because 'sociology was then the flavour of the month, and there were few other outlets for medical researchers with a sociological bent to gather and talk' (Richmond 2010). The Melbourne-based group operated during the late 1960s and until the early 1970s (Richmond 2005:60–63).

The first formal national meeting of the *SAANZ* Medical Section was opened by Sol Encel, the Chair of Sociology at the *University of New South Wales*. At this meeting, the speakers were all specialists in medicine or public health rather than academic sociologists, including John Cawte, a psychiatrist (*ANZJS* 1967:152). *SAANZ* had been formed in 1963, only a few years prior to the Medical Section, and so this was the first of the speciality areas to emerge. Despite a subsequent change of name to the Health Sociology Section, it has remained the largest, attracting a significant proportion of the papers at each annual conference.[3]

Another relevant association was the *Australian and New Zealand Society for Epidemiology and Research in Community Health* (*ANZSERCH*), formed in 1970 by Basil Hetzel, Professor of Social and Preventative Medicine at *Monash*.[4] Hetzel's interest in the social aspects of medicine and health lent a much needed legitimacy to the growing sub-field. A number of lecturers and researchers working with Hetzel in the Department of Social and Preventative Medicine were members of the Melbourne-based Sociology Group convened by Richmond, and attended the monthly meetings (Richmond 2010). *ANZSERCH* eventually became the *Australian Public Health Association*, but in its earliest manifestation was an important forum for sociologists to meet other sociologists but also epidemiologists, public health specialists, medical practitioners, and a very small band of health economists who had no other place to meet (Deeble 2004:1).

Some of the early attendees of the *ANZSERCH* meetings included Neville Hicks (public health), John Deeble (economics), Thelma Hunter (political science), Jane Shoebridge (nursing and sociology) and Evan Willis (medical sociology). These meetings provided a forum for the inter-disciplinary group, for the sociologists of health, like the small epidemiological-public health community and the health economists, were struggling to find an institutional niche. *ANZSERCH* was both evidence of a mutual interest and a vehicle for furthering these interests, and it gave impetus to several new disciplines during this formative period. In the first few years, the group focused on matters of medical concern, but from about 1973, the emphasis shifted and papers increasingly reflected a more sociological interest in the political and social dimensions of health (Hicks 1976:1). Participants were encouraged to offer sociological and historical insights and 'avoid treating community health within a traditional medical paradigm' (Hicks 1976:2). Debates and papers given at the various gatherings focused on the problems of the medical paradigm, on strategies to combat the 'intellectual imperialism of the medical perspective', the growth of a social movement to establish a multi-disciplinary approach to community health in Australia, and acknowledged *ANZSERCH's* role in such efforts (Donahue 1976; Line 1976). Despite this level of interest, insufficient papers were offered to justify a separate section on social epidemiology, and it was noted by Neville Hicks (1976:2) that the majority took, as a given, the institutional structures, practices and assumptions of medicine.

There were other indications of the strengthening of the sociology of health as a specialist field. One was the increasing number of members listing their 'area of special interest' in the association's public membership directory as 'medical sociology', and the proportional increase in this group over the decade (*SAANZ* 1970; Scott 1979:21). A second was the rise in university courses on health sociology, one of the earliest taught by Athol Congalton at *New South Wales* (see Willis 1982:145), and another in the Department of Anthropology at *Western Australia* (*ANZJS* 1965b:136). These new courses occurred at a time when sociology itself began to have a greater presence in the university system, for the discipline was introduced as a 'major' in the 1960s (i.e. as a continuous course of study throughout the undergraduate degree programme) in at least four universities, and in another seven during the 1970s (Scott 1979:3).

A third indication of the rising interest in the field can be found in the number of health-related papers presented at conferences. At *Monash* in 1965, several papers were of a health or medical nature, including one from Alan Stoller and Jerzy Krupinski (*ANZJS* 1965b:133). With the formation of the Medical Section of *SAANZ* in 1967, the quantity of papers at subsequent conferences increased significantly (*ANZJS* 1967:152; 1970:70). Papers presented at the 1969 conference offer an insight into the topics of interest of the period. In the Medical Sociology Section, Basil Hetzel gave the opening address, and presentations were given by Alan Stoller on the social characteristics of patients with schizophrenia; Frederick Ehrlich (a surgeon from the *NSW State Psychiatric Services*) offered a paper on disability; Jerzy Krupinski, a paper on deserted mothers; Julius Roth (a visitor from *California*), a paper on the natural health movement; G. Graves, a paper from her study of attitudes towards mental health; Barry Maley (a student of anthropology at the *ANU*), a paper on social stress; and John Brehaut (from the Department of Anthropology and Sociology at *Monash*), a paper on hospital organisation (*ANZJS* 1970:70; *SAANZ* 1970).

It may be suggested that a 'sociology *of* medicine' emerged in Australia during the 1970s, somewhat later than its occurrence in the United States. Prior to the 1970s, the sociology of health and medicine in Australia, as in Britain and Germany, appears to have been predominantly applied and mainly concerned with problems identified by non-sociologists, notably doctors and government agencies. Increasingly however, Australian sociologists began to offer an alternative view. This new 'sociology *of* medicine' had made a debut in the 1960s, as evidenced in the work of sociologists such as Athol Congalton (1963),

Neville Yeomans (1966), Margaret Sargent (1968), and Robert Pike (1963). Egged on by a group of Left-wing economists and progressive individuals in nursing, psychiatry, and community health; the infant field began to build a critique of medicine and the health care system. By the 1970s the 'trickle' of books had become a fast-running creek if not quite a flood, and several new health sociology books were published and became invaluable for teaching in sociology, nursing, and other areas of health and medicine. Some of these publications were very critical of medicine, seeing it as failing to provide equal access and appropriate forms of treatment for all social groups (Sargent 1973; Bates 1977; Brownlea 1977). Medicine was shown to be characterised by vested interests and a lack of professional accountability, and the health care system unable to attend to the needs of patients and protect their fundamental rights (Hetzel 1974; Boreham *et al.* 1976; McEwan 1977; Ward 1979). Such texts offered perhaps some of the first distinctly sociological perspectives on health and medicine from Australian authors, as opposed to the many books on the *social aspects of health* written by public health specialists, epidemiologists, economists, and practitioners (Sax 1972; Scotton 1974, 1977; Diesendorf 1976; Moss and Piggott 1976; Hicks 1977; Legge 1977).

The strengthening of the field and the development of a distinctive 'sociology *of* medicine' in Australia, coincided with a number of political and social changes. By the end of the 1960s there was a widespread view among political and social reformers and within the academic community that the provision of health and welfare services was inadequate (Hunter 1963; Sax 1967; Whitlam 1968; Scotton 1969). Health expenditures were rising and nearly 17 per cent of Australians were not covered by health insurance. This meant, under the Menzies-Page health system, the existence of a large group of Australians who were not entitled to public health care services but also without the means to purchase health services. In 1968 the Coalition government formed a *Committee of Inquiry into Health Insurance* (the Nimmo Committee). This examined the problems of health insurance, and made a number of recommendations about reducing the complexity of the scheme. Although some minor changes were made in subsequent health legislation under the Gorton government, it took a number of years of debate in the media and the parliament about the difficulties of accessing services and the costs of 'high technology medicine' – and a change of government – before the situation was substantially changed.

Neville Hicks (1976:1) argues that the election of the Whitlam Labor government in 1972, after 23 years of rule by the Liberal-Country

Party, brought a new priority to social welfare and health services. The Whitlam government also took on organised medicine, legislated for the introduction of universal medical insurance (Medibank), and made a variety of incursions into the established institutions:

> Funds were made available for several new forms of health service, a few of them well out on the fringes of medicine. Ear-marked grants were provided in nine universities to establish departments with names like 'Community Medicine' in medical faculties which would have [otherwise] taken decades to shift recurrent funds away from traditional clinical departments. (There were already three or four departments of this kind where people like Gordon and Hetzel had been trying to achieve a change in emphasis for several years)...The fruits of those changes are yet to be harvested but...their growth has begun
>
> (Hicks 1976:1).

These changes in the political and social context were reflected in the more critical *stance* of the sociology publications of the 1970s, but it took somewhat longer for these publications to show any change in the subjects under examination. Thus a brief review of the publications of the 1960s and 1970s shows little substantive difference with regard to the topics of interest. The focus on alcoholism, deviance, and the health system continued (Hunter 1963; Saint 1963; Cawte 1964; Krupinski and Stoller 1968; Sargent 1968; Maxwell 1975; McGrath 1977; Bates 1979; Durrington *et al.* 1979; Whitlock 1979), though a few more studies appeared on the subjects of class and professionalisation, particularly towards the end of the period (Pike 1963; Western 1963; Duff 1973; Darby 1977; Egger 1978; Glasner 1979; Willis 1979). However, there were some differences between the theoretical perspectives of the two periods, for papers became more *sociological* in orientation rather than simply focusing on the *social* aspects of illness or the health system; and there was a shift in the theoretical frameworks themselves, for functionalism was on the wane and Marxist, Weberian, Durkheimian, interactionist and feminist perspectives on the rise (Betts 1976; Burton 1977; Homer 1977; Wild 1977; Storz 1978; Swain and Harrison 1979). Quantitative methods were still in the ascendance (e.g. Najman 1979).

Important in the development of health and medical sociology during this period was its close association with sociology departments. In the British case, medical sociology was initially established inside departments of social medicine, and disciplinary boundaries reduced the extent to which the sociologists could engage with the theories and concepts of mainstream sociology. In contrast, Australian health sociology began in the same way as general sociology: in an inter-disciplinary context. When general sociologists were given an institu-tional perch in sociology departments, so were the sociologists of health and medicine. There *were* Australian sociologists who found positions within nursing, public health and medicine, but they either maintained their links with the discipline, or took on a new disciplinary identity. No significant sociological *groups* were established outside the new soci-ology departments. Thus the speciality of health sociology formed in conjunction with the broader discipline, and groups claiming a socio-logical identity gathered within, or closely attached to, the faculties of arts and the social sciences.

Looking back from a distance of many decades, the emergence of the sociology of health and medicine might be seen as a coherent, progres-sive movement. At the time however, there were many groups acting in relative isolation, responding to local problems, or at least, to what appeared to be a local problem. In Adelaide for instance, some of the same individuals who had expressed their concerns about medicine at the *ANZSERCH* meeting of 1976 successfully set up an education unit as a joint venture between the *University of Adelaide* and the *South Australian Institute of Technology* to produce a multi-disciplinary, and team-work approach to the education and training of health and medi-cal workers (Moss and Piggott 1976:209). Individuals working on these initiatives were aware of similar ventures elsewhere (at *McMaster Uni-versity* in Canada, the *Montefiore Hospital* of New York, and the *Royal Prince Alfred Hospital* in Sydney) (Moss and Piggott 1976:210). Within such initiatives, 'health' and 'health care' become boundary objects, enabling diverse groups to communicate across intellectual fields and build a commonality of purpose. In these cases, the production of intel-lectual knowledge is subordinated to other purposes, such as designing courses of study to ensure medical students develop skills in commu-nication and teamwork. Nevertheless, these inter-disciplinary ventures were critical to the vitality of the new speciality field of the sociology of health and medicine, for they forced both observers and participants to clarify and define the nature of sociological knowledge and practice.

The 1980s

Another shift occurred in the 1980s as a result of changes within the university sector itself. The dramatic increase in tertiary sector students to 330,000 by 1980, coupled with the construction of many new universities, the transfer of nursing education into the university system, and a major restructuring of the system eradicating the differences between institutes, colleges and universities, meant the creation of additional sociology departments and many more possibilities for service teaching in areas such as nursing, education and social work.

Books and journal articles also began to appear in Australia by sociologists who were, for the first time, able to build a career within the speciality area of health sociology. One of the more notable of these was Jackob Najman. Najman completed his PhD in 1978 with Athol Congalton, and took up an interest in health and health services, particularly with regard to migrant health. In subsequent decades, Najman has essentially kept to the field of health and social epidemiology (Najman 1979; Najman *et al.* 1981, 1983; Lupton and Najman 1995). A second prominent sociologist of health and medicine is Evan Willis. Willis was born in New Zealand but arrived in Australia in the late 1970s to pursue doctoral studies. This sociologist produced a significant treatise on the division of labour in medicine (Willis 1983), and subsequently followed an almost exclusive interest in the health sector (Willis 1979, 1988, 1994, 1998; Daly *et al.* 1987, 1992). The field was given a further boost when Bryan Turner, a sociologist from the United Kingdom, took up the Chair of Sociology at *Flinders University* in South Australia, and in 1984 produced *The Body and Society*, followed in 1987 by *Medical Power and Social Knowledge*. These works, like Willis' 1983 *Medical Dominance*, helped to invigorate the field and encourage theorising in the sociology of health and medicine. Other significant books published in the 1980s include a study of Aboriginal health called *Health Business*, authored by Pam Nathan and Dick Leichleitner Japanangka; *Sociology and the Nurse* by Frank Lopez; *Health Systems and Public Scrutiny* by Erica Bates; *Where It Hurts* by Cherry Russell and Toni Schofield; *Healers and Alternative Medicine* by Gary Easthope; *Health Care and Public Policy* by George Palmer and Stephanie Short; and the textbook, *Sociology of Health and Illness* by Gillian Lupton and Jake Najman.

The publications of the 1980s reflect a continuing concern with fertility, contraception, and reproduction (Callan 1980; Montague 1980; Mugford and Lally 1980; Betts 1980, 1981; Caldwell 1984; Neuendorff 1986; de Lepervanche 1989; Klein 1989). They also indicate an intensification of interest in medicalisation, professionalisation, and medical dominance (Gibson and Boreham 1981; Gibson 1985; Wilson and Gorring 1985; Turner 1986b), in capitalism (Braithwaite 1984), social movements (Osborne 1984), and inequalities such as disabilities

(Rubinstein 1982; Rees and Emerson 1983; Sutton and Beran 1983). Relative to the previous decade, far less interest was shown in alcohol and drug abuse, migration, race and ethnicity, religion and deviance. New issues emerged towards the end of the decade, with a small sprinkling of papers beginning to appear on AIDS (Ross 1988) and the new reproductive technologies (Albury 1989; Sullivan 1989). In general, few of the papers were fully theorised, but among the small group which were theoretically framed, functionalism had disappeared entirely while Marxism and Feminism continued to gain in strength (Rubenstein 1982; Baker 1983; Casswell and Smythe 1983; Hopkins 1984; Hatty 1987; James 1987; Alcorso 1989). Weberian, Durkheimian, interactionist and constructionist perspectives were still in evidence (Willis 1983, 1988; George 1984; Hopkins 1989). Empirical papers were generally quantitative (Betts 1981; Najman *et al.* 1983; Ryan and Dent 1984; Neil and Jones 1988; Minichiello 1989), but there was considerable excitement in the sociological community over the development of Lyn and Tom Richards' (1981) new software for the analysis of qualitative data; and Yolande Wadsworth's (1984) manual for qualitative evaluation research. For the first time, there was a sufficiency of Australian materials for research and textbooks for teaching the sociology of health and medicine. Overall, the decade was one of growth and consolidation for the discipline.

The 1990s

The sociology of health and medicine was a significant intellectual field by the 1990s. Sociologists were able to specialise, and the field offered a viable career path through sociology. The majority of members of the Health Sociology Section of *TASA* were now women, reflecting in large part the influx of women graduates into the university sector. Over the previous decade the Section had developed a constitution, formed state branches, appointed convenors for each branch, and begun to hold regular meetings to recruit 'early career' sociologists into the field. Membership continued to reflect a diversity of disciplines, including members from the health professions, but now had a strong 'core' of academic sociologists. A major development of the Health Section was the creation of its own academic journal in 1991, the *Annual Review of Health Social Science* (which became the *Health Sociology Review* from 2001). Initially edited by Jeanne Daly and Allan Kellehear from the Department of Sociology at *La Trobe* (with Evan Willis joining the team in 1992), the editorship thereafter changed hands fairly frequently.[5] In the 1990s, the journal provided sociologists with a much needed, local outlet for their work. The support of members of the Health Section was crucial to the success of the publication, as these individuals were, and continue to be, major constituents of the journal's community of peer reviewers, contributors, and subscribers. Other indications of the strength of the field in the 1990s were the many textbooks published for the teaching of undergraduates (Willis 1994; Cheek *et al.* 1996; Daly 1996; Grbich 1996; Petersen and Waddell 1998); as well as a variety of other books on health sociology (Daniel 1990; Kellehear 1990; Turner 1992; Lupton 1994; Petersen and Bunton 1997).

Sociological theory was rejuvenated during the 1990s by the return of several expatriates, the appointment of foreign sociologists, and visits to the sociological 'metropole' of Britain and France. The new theories of risk, post-structuralism, embodiment, of Bourdieu and Foucault, appeared in Australian publications (Turner 1992; Lupton 1993, 1994; Petersen and Bunton 1997; Petersen 1998). Somewhat surprisingly, existing theoretical frameworks did not suffer. While many journal publications in the sociology of health and medicine had previously been untheorised, the 1990s witnessed a heightening of theory. Thus feminist, interactionist, and constructionist theories were employed by more sociologists (Broom 1995; Collyer 1996a; Guillemin 1996; Hunt 1996; Lane 1996; Reiger 1999; Zadoroznyj 1999), at the same time as the new theories came into vogue. Also of continuing interest was Marxian analysis, which represented a sociological response to the many incidences of privatisation within the Australian health care sector (Collyer 1997a, 1998; Collyer and White 1997; White and Collyer 1997, 1998).

Fragmentation was a second characteristic of this period. The growth of cultural studies on many university campuses – a multi-disciplinary rather than inter-disciplinary arena for research and teaching – was symptomatic of this new phenomenon but at the same time a driving factor in the proliferation of speciality areas. The creation of a *Centre for the Body and Society* at *Deakin*, headed by Bryan Turner, was also a relevant development. New journals, new thematic groups, specialist conferences, and new departments, all began to draw sociologists away from activities within a general sociological 'core' towards sites of innovation: Leisure Studies, Queer Studies, Gender Studies, Criminology, Socio-Legal Studies, Masculinity and Society, and so on. This new concern with 'culture' rather than 'structure' saw a dramatic fall in sociological interest in social class for the first time, but also a decline in sociological concern with ethnicity, race, and religion. It brought with it a new concentration on sexuality and masculinity (Connell and Dowsett 1993; Kippax *et al.* 1993; Dowsett 1996), and science and technology (Martin

1991; Wajcman 1991; Hepburn 1992; Collyer 1994, 1996a; Martin and Richards 1995; Willis 1998).

The 'cultural turn' was associated also with the switch from quantitative to qualitative analysis, for the enthusiasm for qualitative methods had emerged and become the dominant form in a very short period. This radical shift cannot be fully explained without reference to gender. Prior to the 1990s, Australian health sociology and the parent discipline were comprised primarily of men. This was reversed in the space of a decade as women drew on the support of the Health Section and the Women's Section of *TASA*, and became vocal proponents for health sociology, feminism, and qualitative methodologies (Richards and Richards 1981; Wadsworth 1984, 1991; Daly 1996; Grbich 1999; Kirkman 1999; Richards 2005). In the process, the much smaller group of quantitative sociologists (who were primarily men) were overwhelmed. The discipline was radically and irrevocably re-oriented.

A new phenomenon which emerged in this period was an interest in sociology *itself*. Although attention had been paid to the examination of sociology during previous decades, particularly with regard to issues of professionalisation and the permeability of the borders of the discipline (Bottomley 1974; Cock *et al.* 1979; Zubrzycki 1979; Willis 1982), the 1990s brought new debates on sociology. Reflections appeared in the sociological journals, at conferences, in monographs, and government reports (Baldock 1994; Western 1998), stimulating debate about the future of the discipline. The sociology of health and medicine was not unaffected, and reflections on this area of sociology also intensified (Turner 1990; Willis 1991; Daly 1998). The period was consequently one of renewal and self-reflection in Australian sociology, and indicated a new maturity for both sociology and the sociology of health and medicine.

The contemporary period

Recent years in Australian sociology have been characterised by consolidation rather than radical change, for health sociology has continued as one of the more significant areas of teaching and research (Marshall *et al.* 2009:24). It has also been a period of internationalisation. Although Australia has long been a country of immigrants, with many of its health sociologists born overseas (Jake Najman, Evan Willis, Dorothy Broom, Margaret Sargent, Kevin White, Bryan Turner, Alec Pemberton, Charles Waddell, Fran Collyer); there has been increasing pressure in recent years for sociologists to engage more directly with global intellectual networks and publish in the 'core' European or American journals. The response from sociologists of health has been an increasing level of international collaboration for sociological research and publication, a rise in the number of foreign visitors in Australian sociology departments, a greater representation of Australian sociologists at international conferences, a weightier presence of international publishing houses in the Australian market, and an influx of foreign authors seeking to publish in the Australian-based journal *Health Sociology Review* (*HSR*). This internationalisation process has reduced the amount of time between the development of new theories or concepts in Britain, Europe or America, and their uptake in the Australian context. It has also increased the sharing of ideas between Australian health sociologists and those of Britain and the United States. All three countries, for instance, now demonstrate an increasing concern with the concepts of globalisation, internationalisation and social capital; while sociologists in Britain and Australia have paid increasing attention to Bourdieu (Seale 2008:692).

The field continues to draw its major theoretical perspectives from Europe and the United Kingdom. Deborah Lupton (2005:430–1) sees Australian medical sociology as characterised by two dominant perspectives. The first of these is the political economy perspective, dominant since the 1970s, and examining the major social categories of class, age, gender and ethnicity (Diesendorf 1976; Willis 1983; Broom 1991; Reid and Trompf 1991; Germov 1995; Collyer 1997a; George and Davis 1998; Collyer and White 2001; Palmer and Short 2010). The second, and now more common strand, is the post-structuralist perspective. This has a social constructionist orientation, is often based on Foucault, and became apparent from the late 1980s (Lawler 1991; Petersen and Waddell 1998; Pringle 1998). As we shall see in Chapter five, our Content Analysis of publications confirms this view of two dominant perspectives, though it also points to the presence of a broader spectrum of theory in the Australian context.

These various theoretical traditions are currently being employed to guide empirical work reflecting Australian concerns and issues. An interest in reproductive issues has been maintained, with a focus on the new fertility technologies (Gilding 2006; Dempsey 2008), and the new genetic technologies generally (Leontini 2006). A revitalisation of interest has occurred regarding ethnicity, race, and Indigenous health (Saggers and Gray 2001; Pyett *et al.* 2008), sparked by the controversial Commonwealth government intervention in the Northern Territory. Fewer papers now address the topics of sexuality, though this is likely to indicate the emergence of new specialist journals rather than an overall fall in research interest. Finally, we are also seeing a healthy number of locally produced health sociology textbooks (White 2002; Gray 2005; Willis and Elmer 2007; Willis *et al.* 2009), as well as a range of research studies exploring theories of consumerism, the health care system, death and the body (Kellehear 2000; Henderson and Petersen 2002; Stanton *et al.* 2005; Collyer 2007; Petersen 2007).

The United States, the United Kingdom and Australia compared

The above analysis indicates the development of three relatively unique, historical trajectories for the sociology of health and medicine across three countries. In the United States, the sociology of health and medicine developed from the 1950s as a distinct speciality of sociology in conjunction with demands from government and the institutions of medicine, and greatly stimulated by the provision of both public and private resources. In that country, the sociology of health and medicine was established within the shelter of its parent discipline, with its early practitioners (of the 1950s and 1960s) employed primarily within departments of sociology rather than those of medicine. The 'sociology *in* medicine' was the first field to be developed. It began to blossom from the 1950s, as money began to pour into medical education and sociologists made the most of the opportunity to influence the medical curriculum and engage in inter-disciplinary research. By the 1970s, sociologists were able to specialise in health and medicine, to find employment in the medical schools, and apply for funding to undertake inter-disciplinary work. Finally shaking free of the repressive effects of 'McCarthyism', sociologists sharpened their critical approach and a 'sociology *of* medicine' emerged during the decade. Taking into account these various events and processes, it is apparent that the *institutionalisation* of the speciality was completed during the 1960s, a period which saw the establishment of its own journal, the production of American textbooks, and a formal *ASA* Section. This means the institutionalisation of the specialist field of the sociology of health and medicine occurred several decades after the completion of the same process within its parent discipline.

In the United Kingdom, by way of contrast, empirical, sociological research had traditionally been conducted outside the university sector, and the discipline of sociology initially dominated by biological eugenics. This very different foundation for sociological endeavour discouraged the emergence of a new speciality field within the sociology departments themselves. Thus when medical sociology first began to take shape, it appeared at some distance from the departments of sociology, and was spurred on by the activities of individuals employed within departments of social medicine and public health. These social and intellectual networks stretched across an inter-disciplinary field, with individuals coming from medicine, psychiatry, public health, and social medicine as well as sociology and anthropology. A 'sociology *in* medicine' emerged in the first instance, becoming evident from the 1950s, followed by the solid establishment of a 'sociology *of* medicine' by the 1970s. The process of institutionalisation for the speciality began in 1956, with a series of professional meetings organised by an inter-disciplinary mix of experts. A milestone was reached in 1969 with the formation of a Medical Sociology Group of the *BSA*, and the process of institutionalisation completed in the 1970s with the production of student textbooks, substantial in-roads into the medical curriculum, and the creation of a speciality academic journal. In that country, the institutionalisation of the speciality field took about a decade longer than it had in the parent discipline, and though its foundational phase occurred outside the departments of sociology, it was substantially integrated into the discipline during the 1970s.

The Australian case differs from both the British and American models. In Australia, there has always been a close association between the development of the discipline of sociology and the specialist field of the sociology of health and medicine. Specialisation within the discipline remained rare in the 1960s and 1970s, and became a possibility only from the 1980s, when sociology as a whole expanded. The secure institutional, intellectual, and theoretical connections between the subfield and the parent discipline in the contemporary era have been the result of three historic factors. One, the common, inter-disciplinary history of 'mainstream' and health sociology. Two, the small size of the sociological community, which has encouraged the inclination towards generalisation rather than specialisation and inhibited the formation of organised groups outside the sociology departments or the national professional association. And three, the tendency for many sociologists of health to be provided with employment within the social sciences rather than in departments of medicine or social medicine. As a consequence, contemporary research in the sociology of health and medicine in Australia is an arena which shares the theoretical and methodological concerns of the discipline of sociology, and is similarly broad-ranging in its choice of subject matter. On the other hand, the inter-disciplinarity

of the *collegial networks* within the sociology of health and medicine
has continued into the current period, even though this feature has
largely disappeared within the parent field. With regard to the institutionalisation of the specialist field, this began with the development
of the Medical Sociology Section of *SAANZ* in 1967, and proceeded
rapidly as demand for speciality courses for undergraduate teaching
grew during the 1970s and brought with them a rash of Australian textbooks. Although a 'sociology *in* medicine' was evident during the 1960s,
a 'sociology *of* medicine' did not begin to flourish until the 1970s,
indicating a very brief and intense period of institutionalisation. This
means institutionalisation was completed in the 1980s when it finally
became possible, and profitable, to forge a career in the speciality field.
In Australia, as in Britain, the sociology of health and medicine took an
institutional form about a decade after its parent discipline.

Thus we can see that the timing of the institutionalisation processes
differ somewhat from one country to the next, with the speciality taking an institutional form in the United States during the 1960s, in the
United Kingdom in the 1970s, and in Australia during the 1980s. With
regard to the processes themselves, the three countries shared many similarities in their patterns of development, even though some aspects
of these trajectories have been quite unique. One of the shared features was the general expansion of the university system during the
post-war period accompanied by a significant boost in state funding.
A second was the re-orientation from the 'training' of doctors and health
workers to their 'education', producing new opportunities for undergraduate teaching in both the social sciences and in medicine. A third
was the new emphasis on research. Although researchers had always
been available to the state as well as private interests, this function
was systematically developed from the post-war period and became a
significant component of the university budget. Individual and institutional strategies to pursue research funding encouraged – or perhaps
more accurately, forced – interaction and collaboration between the
disciplines, including those of sociology and medicine.

There are many other factors which shaped the historical development of the sociology of health and medicine, some shared, others
unique to each country, and some continue to shape the content and
form of the discipline in the current context. These need to be explored
if we are to understand the contemporary field, and this requires a focus
on the nature of disciplines themselves. For this we turn to the next
chapter.

3
Disciplines, Professions and Specialities

Disciplinary 'specialities' are conventionally regarded as mere divisions of larger, formal bodies of knowledge. Defined by a specific set of problems and objects of study, they are assumed to emerge in a rational process of cognitive division. Ronald Akers (1992:4), for example, distinguishes between disciplines (bodies of knowledge with their own perspectives) and specialities (areas of study) on this basis. In this chapter we re-consider the idea of disciplinary specialities, suggesting that they, like their parents, should be theorised primarily as sites of social action and structural forms. Extending this new understanding of disciplines into an investigation of disciplinary specialties means paying close attention to the *social* relationships between the parent and its speciality. This has been an arena of particular neglect in the social science literature. Here we take the opportunity to examine the forms of differentiation existing within and between all intellectual fields – no matter how large or small – and regard these as the product of social action and structure. This means taking note of the competitive as well as collaborative social arrangements which constitute the field, but most importantly, building a focus on the 'fracture lines' of academia, for every struggle over resources, prestige or territory within one field tends to reverberate through its neighbours. Only in this way can a full understanding of disciplines and specialities be produced, because these are, in a fundamental sense, produced and reproduced through their relationships with other intellectual fields: that is, by their *border* relations.

A number of factors shape these border relations. One of these, briefly discussed in the first chapter, is professionalisation. Professionalisation has long been a subject of research interest to sociologists, but it has also been one of the few research topics adopted by sociologists to reflect on their own practices and social roles. Self-consciously reflecting on the discipline as a profession has allowed sociologists to consider the discipline as having an *organisational* presence to support its members, provide services, and encourage communication between sociologists and the broader public. Yet this has also been a fraught exercise, for not all sociologists have been comfortable with the notion of sociology as a profession. While some of the features of professions may be welcome – perhaps its capacity to represent the discipline in the public arena, provide it with a public identity, and defend its reputation and standards – others have been more controversial. In particular, the social control function of the professions has brought discord, for our own sociological theories of the professions have linked all claims to expert knowledge with political and market power, prestige and social inequality. Comfortable with offering a critique of other professions, sociologists have been less keen on self-analysis and have often resisted strategies to further the discipline's professional status.

This matter is of relevance at this point because although sociology has been regarded as both a discipline and a profession, the *relation between* its disciplinarity and its professional status has not been at the forefront of social theorising. Ironically, this is in large part the result of specialisation within sociology, for historically, some sociologists have explored disciplines while others have separately studied the professions. Moreover, those investigating disciplines have regarded them primarily as intellectual fields and formal bodies of knowledge concerned with specific subjects and organised around particular methodologies or approaches; while those engaged in studying the professions have, since the 1970s, focused on these as mechanisms of social control and fundamentally about power, that is, as special occupations with the capacity to control their own work and the labour of others. More recent theoretical development has bridged the divide between power and knowledge, enabling their inter-play to be given greater attention. These newer ways of thinking about the social world need to be introduced into the investigation of the history of sociology and its specialities.

This chapter will suggest it is sociology's twin status as both a profession *and* a discipline which is the key to understanding the nature of the field and its specialities. The professionalisation of sociology has been particularly evident in the capacity of sociologists to bargain in the broader marketplace, but its full effects are dependent on the processes of disciplinarity. This is because professionalisation is mostly 'blind' to the particularities of our knowledge base and the subtleties of status positions between sociologists. It is the forces of disciplinarity – albeit girded by the profession – which give us our relative positions within the sociological community and the universities. We have seen the academic professions theorised as entities which employ professionalisation processes to ensure they are granted, and continue to be granted, the right to occupy space within the university system and teach specific areas of knowledge. The academic professions thus engage with formal knowledge, and as members of a profession, sociologists are 'institutional vehicles' for its production and transmission (Freidson 1986a:688). Disciplines, on the other hand, are central to the construction and exchange of *scholarly* rather than merely *practical* knowledge. As such, disciplines are not just discrete territories of intellectual endeavour, but domains of social relations and social structures that produce the rules of interaction and competition between sociologists, and hence indirectly give rise to a *specific* knowledge base, a set of cultural and social practices, and, significantly, an hierarchical ordering of tasks, roles and status positions. Thus it is the relationship between its disciplinarity and professional status which provides sociology with its character and capacity to operate in the social sphere.

This third chapter draws from the theoretical framework developed in the first chapter and the historical material presented in Chapter two to examine the processes through which disciplines and speciality fields form and alter over time. Where the second chapter provided an historical view of the *institutionalisation* of the specialist field of the sociology of health and medicine, this focuses on its disciplinarity and the way this interacts with, and is shaped by its professional status. The Section 'Sociology and its specialities' offers an introduction to the concept of specialities, and explains what is meant by the external and internal relationships of an intellectual field. The subsequent section reflects on the processes through which the *external* disciplinary boundaries of the sociology of health and medicine have been constructed and maintained. This is followed by discussion on the management of *internal* disputes and the maintenance of a disciplinary hierarchy.

Sociology and its specialities

Disciplinary specialities became an issue in the 1950s and 1960s, particularly in the United States, when the diversity of interests within sociology became evident and were constructed as a 'problem' by its leadership (e.g. Merton *et al.* 1959; Naegele 1965a; Shils 1965; Warner 1976). Yet the status of sociology's specialities have still to be adequately theorised and investigated. One of the problems with specialities is the lack of clarity over what they are. In some countries criminology, for example, is identified as a discipline but elsewhere thought of as a speciality of sociology. This problem also occurs with disciplines to some extent. Medicine, for instance, despite its lack of a discrete 'object of study', is regarded in certain countries as a discipline but elsewhere as a complex of disciplines or even as having no disciplinary status at all. This problem with nomenclature echoes Thomas Gieryn's (1983) rather controversial finding that science is 'no single thing', for it can be represented in a variety of ways and be historically and contextually flexible. If the same logic is applied to disciplines and specialities, we might find their identities and labels equally dependent on social context.

In the discussions below, specialities and disciplines will be distinguished primarily by the configuration of their boundary relations at any particular historic moment. Where there is a rigid or relatively impermeable boundary between two arenas of social action, these can be regarded as distinct disciplines (e.g. mathematics and geography). Where the boundary is readily permeable, the probability is greater that the two areas are specialities of one discipline (e.g. political sociology and the sociology of work), or a speciality and its parent (chemistry and bio-chemistry). This is because specialities generally enjoy a more co-operative set of boundary relations with a relevant discipline, and share its social identity and external boundaries.

Specialities may provide advantages in status and resources for both the individual and the discipline. For individuals, specialities offer an informal social context within which ideas can be considered and exchanged more rapidly than through the more extended disciplinary community. Specialisation also provides a formal sphere of social action wherein individuals can more easily compete for status, for the more limited arena allows them greater visibility and recognition while rendering large literatures more manageable (Ben-David and Collins 1966; Hackett 2005). Membership of a speciality may also confer particular advantages, depending on the nature of the speciality and the context. For instance, it seems that specialists in the American context have higher incomes (Leahey 2007). For the discipline there are also certain advantages and disadvantages to specialities. A discipline's specialities may result in the extension – or annexation – of territory, and can weaken or strengthen its presence in the university system and the wider public sphere.

The nature of disciplines and specialities can be analysed using the concept of external and internal boundaries. These boundaries are socio-temporal-historical constructions, sensitive to geography, with both local and global dimensions. They are formed largely through various forms of boundary-work, sustained over extended periods. Where this boundary-work is directed outwards at other disciplines, at the state, university management, or broadly at 'the public', it can be regarded as an *external* form of boundary-work, for it usually involves action to reinforce or extend the discipline's perimeters. As such, the boundaries of sociology might be regarded as largely constituted by their 'external' relationships with other intellectual fields, for these are constantly under negotiation and re-alignment. Alternatively, *internal* boundary-work is generally about governance, for disciplines can be regulatory systems and maintain order and 'discipline' within their own borders. The difference between internal and external boundary-work is essentially an analytic distinction, for in practice both forms are closely entwined.[1] The distinction is employed below to provide greater clarity in the investigation of this complex set of processes. As we shall see, both *internal* and *external* forms of boundary-work have been fundamental to the development of the speciality field of the sociology of health and medicine, and continue to give it shape in the contemporary context.

External boundary-actions: Economics, medicine, psychiatry and epidemiology

During the early decades of the twentieth century, several new intellectual fields were in the process of formation, including biology (Pauly 1984), the new physiology, medicine, psychology (Good 2000), and also economics (Fourcade-Gourinchas 2001). This social and disciplinary turmoil was the back-drop to the institutionalisation of sociology and its specialities, and continued to have an impact during its major professionalisation period (from the 1930s through to the 1950s). Often referred to as the *sociological project*, this professionalisation process involved the manipulation of the discipline's boundaries, a reformulation of its intellectual territory, and the establishment of a new strategic direction for the field. Led by Robert Merton, Talcott Parsons, and other members of the sociological elite in the United States, its effects were soon to reverberate through both Britain and Australia.

A powerful symbol for the re-formulated discipline of sociology was the publication of Talcott Parsons' text, *The Structure of Social Action* in 1937. For Charles Camic (1987:434), this text was not a decisive break with existing trends but a deliberate action to bring into sociology a methodological approach employed by one of the more successful disciplines of the period: neo-classical economics. Parsons' choice of the conservative, *neo-classical*, rather than *institutional* form of economics reflected not only a set of political preferences, but his professional concerns. Parsons took an active role in the debates between the two forms of economics, and was aware that institutional economics was premised on an holistic model of the social sciences in which sociology could play its part; while in contrast, neo-classical economics argued that no discipline could explain all aspects of reality and thus its role should be to focus on one aspect (Camic 1987:429). This meant a selection between two methodologies: (1) the institutional form in which sociology would be unlikely to have a unique role, and may even be dispensed with by one of the other social sciences or (2) the neo-classical one, which would focus on aspects of reality and 'turn over [the non-economic elements to the] sociologist' (Parsons 1968:141; Camic 1987:429). For Camic, *The Structure of Social Action* held significance for sociology because its publication was an explicit strategy aimed at the professionalisation of the discipline. The adoption of the methodological schema of neo-classical economics was a means to increase the status of sociology, and at the same time ward off the encroachment of economics, which Parsons perceived to be a very real threat (Camic 1987:429).

With the professionalisation project underway, sociologists looked nervously over their borders towards the discipline of economics, but could not fail to be also aware of the now-dominant presence of medicine. Although this is obviously the more crucial border relationship for the sociology of health and medicine, its importance for mainstream sociology has rarely been acknowledged. The association between sociology and medicine has varied considerably over time, and from one country to the next. Nevertheless the historical processes which initially established the broad structure of this boundary have been remarkably similar in all three locations. In the 1920s in America, and a little later in the other two countries, social groups began to organise for the professionalisation of medical education and practice, adopting the new experimental laboratory methods as a means to build a new public image for medicine as a scientific *discipline*, introducing new practices of standardisation for its curriculum, attending to its processes of credentialism, and creating new measures to control the behaviour of its members. By the 1940s, many forms of 'undesirable' social conduct had been subjected to medical explanation and intervention, and medical authority and control had been extended throughout the political, moral, and cultural domains. Medicine had become a powerful institution with its own associations, schools and journals, and was well resourced by both the state and the corporate sector. It had also been successfully presented as a coherent *discipline*, its diverse practices and knowledges cobbled together into an hierarchically organised mega-field with various surgical and clinical fields at the apex, and others (such as nursing and public health) on its lower margins. In this process, the institution of medicine successfully claimed sole expertise over well-being, re-defining health as the absence of disease, and narrowing its focus to physical manifestations of biological dysfunction.

These developments could not fail to impact on sociology and the other disciplines. Sociology in the nineteenth century and the early decades of the twentieth century had incorporated physical, psychological *and* social phenomena in its explanations of well-being, suffering and inequality. This broader vision is evident, for instance, in the works of Albion Small (1923:404), who argued sociology could only advance upon a foundation of knowledge about the physical and psychical basis of social behaviour. As a model for sociology, it continued to appear in texts of the 1930s and 1940s (e.g. Ogburn and Nimkoff 1964/1947). This meant the border between the two territories – medicine and sociology – was highly permeable and their lack of differentiation led to frequent disputes. A defining moment in the relations between sociology and medicine was the production of a second text by Parsons – *The Social System* – in 1951. In this re-working of his previous book, he offered a definition of health and disease which radically departed from that of medicine, but in the same movement endorsed medicine's authority. 'Illness', Parsons announced, was partly 'organic' or 'biological' and partly 'social'. On the one hand, 'sickness' was an adopted social role, but on the other, disease was fundamentally a physiological 'fact' (Parsons 1970, also 1968:372). In this dualistic theory of ill-health, Parsons claimed a niche for sociology which (temporarily at least) resolved the border dispute with medicine. While early twentieth-century sociology often mixed (what we would now see as) biological, sociological and psychological factors, and indeed did so deliberately, the new approach to sociology declared the investigation and treatment of 'disease' as within medicine's territory; while sociology's role was to examine how social facts (such as norms and roles) might contribute to (i.e. influence the severity or distribution of) ill-health. In taking this position, Parsons handed the embodied, suffering individual to the more powerful discipline of medicine and retained for sociology only those aspects of illness which had become problematic for medicine. In dropping its claims as an authority on the nature and causes of health and disease, sociology avoided direct competition with medicine and reduced the friction between the fields. The new boundaries of sociology were defined according to what was 'not medicine', and its new province became 'the social'.

The pronouncement of sociology's unique role re-oriented its disciplinary boundary with medicine and produced a new intellectual division of labour around the phenomenon of illness and the health care system. Although this boundary-activity may have appeared a strategic 'master stroke' to observers of the 1950s, the historic separation of disciplinary knowledges within this sphere of action has continued to plague both disciplines. The symbolic, discursive boundary rapidly solidified into a social boundary and eventually led to the construction of an institutional frontier, barring entry for sociologists to departments of medicine in Britain, Australia and the United States. It placed sociology in a defensive position, requiring continuous struggle to establish its credentials and convince others of the value of including 'the social' aspects of health and healing in teaching, research and practice. At the same time, this social boundary has led to the theoretical impoverishment of medicine, for, as noted by Levine (1987:2), that discipline has never answered the intellectual challenges posed by sociology, and remains essentially unreflexive about its own role and perspectives.

The exclusion of sociology from the institutions of medicine has never been complete, for there have always been some sociologically trained individuals employed in its departments or interested in collaborative projects. However these sociologists often find themselves in a subordinate position. Margot Jefferys offers an illustration of the effect of this subordination on sociologists from her own experience of Britain in the mid-1960s. Where joint papers were submitted to medical journals, she found the editors insistent on re-arranging the order of authorship to ensure those with medical qualifications were placed first (Jefferys 1997:127). This privileging of the medically qualified is an example of medicine patrolling its borders. In this case, the response from the authors was to threaten the withdrawal of their paper. This is an example of sociology patrolling *its* borders. Sociologists working in departments of medicine in those decades were at considerable disadvantage relative to their sociological colleagues in sociology departments, but also compared with their medically qualified colleagues. As Jefferys (1997:127–8) describes, the sociologists were regularly denied both promotion and job tenure, and many had little choice but to return to sociology or other social science departments.

In subsequent decades, the borders between sociology and medicine have continued to be relatively impermeable, but sociologists have occasionally been successful at influencing the medical curriculum and medical practice. This has usually been with the assistance of medical 'insiders'. Bloom (1990:2) talks of key medical practitioners who were influential in the establishment of social medicine in the United States: individuals such as Rudolf Virchow, Henry Sigerist, Lawrence Henderson, Leon Eisenberg and George Reader. These 'insiders' engaged in boundary-work to convince others to take into account the 'social' aspects of illness and include sociological perspectives, theories, concepts or methods in intellectual work and the medical curriculum. They also lent some of their authority to assist sociologists to gain access to the broader public and political discourses of health. In Australia, medically qualified individuals such as Basil Hetzel and Fred Ehrlich performed similar roles, as did John Ryle and Jerry Morris in the British context.

The role of 'insiders' has also been important in establishing legitimacy for the developing speciality of medical sociology, heightening its respectability and improving its relations with medicine. From the perspective of the medical establishment, sociologists were:

> ... rank outsiders in the medical world. Their claims to knowledge of use to medical practitioners could be disputed and were disturbing. They had to find patrons from within the academic branches of the profession if they were to gain a foothold in institutions dominated by the medically qualified
>
> (Jefferys 1991:16).

Such 'patrons' were sometimes found in the central disciplines of medicine, as we have argued; but more often in the marginalised disciplines of psychiatry, epidemiology, public health, community health, community medicine, nursing and midwifery, and even at times in general practice. In all three countries, the boundary-action of 'insiders' had the effect of inserting sociology into the territory of medicine. Over time, their actions helped shift the status of sociologists working in the medical faculties from *assistants*, where they were providing useful skills in survey analysis and interviewing, to *colleagues*, with expert knowledge of human behaviour. This change was made possible because these disciplines offered sociologists 'shelter' within their departments, and 'sheltering', like 'mentoring', is a constructive form of boundary-work which is often decisive in the institutionalisation of disciplines.

The disciplines which mentored the sociology of health and medicine often had one element in common: they were low in both status and power (Field 1988:298). Psychiatry played a particularly important mentoring role for the sociology of health and medicine in the 1950s and 1960s in all three countries under consideration. By engaging in intellectual debate and research work with sociologists, psychiatrists sought to counter allegations that their discipline was capable of treating only 'pseudo' medical conditions, that its disciplinary status was questionable, and its knowledge basis unscientific. As Jeffery's notes, the assistance given to sociology was not an altruistic act on the part of psychiatry, but a strategy to use sociology to overcome the discipline's own problems. In Britain at that time, psychiatry's crisis of legitimacy and lack of authority within the medical hierarchy made it difficult to attract sufficient student enrolments relative to the more prestigious areas of surgery and general medicine (Jefferys 1991:17). Collaboration with sociology offered psychiatry a set of discourses to explain the nature of mental illness and the possibility of bolstering its academic standing.

In the Australian context, the sociology of health and medicine was also given assistance by psychiatry: indeed psychiatry was the first of the disciplines to act as a mentor for the new speciality field. In this country, collaboration between psychiatry and sociology was driven by the need for the construction of a 'public' and an audience, rather than a problem with student numbers *per se*. If psychiatry was to provide itself with a unique and viable intellectual field, it had to engage in academic and public debate. Yet Australia of the 1950s and 1960s had a very small intellectual and academic community, and there were few opportunities for public gatherings or outlets for publication. Thus almost all forms of public debate were by necessity inter-disciplinary. Several psychiatrists, including Alan Stoller, Neville Yeomans, Jerzy Krupinski and Herbert Bower, took a prominent role in shaping the intellectual networks from which medical sociology eventually emerged. The consequences of such collaboration were beneficial to both disciplines: opportunities for joint research provided psychiatry with a set of outlets for its work and a capacity to contribute to public debates, while sociology was given access to hospitals and clinics and the possibility for influencing the medical curriculum. Even at this time however, the greater prestige and power of medicine shaped this interaction, for the psychiatrists' clinical and research interests dominated the emerging field of health sociology until the later 1970s.

Psychiatry performed a similar role in the United States, where it was also the first medical discipline to build an alliance with sociology. Although psychiatry began to establish itself in the medical schools during the 1930s, it initially excluded the social or behavioural sciences from its curricula (Bloom 2002:112–4). By the 1950s psychiatry began to open its curricula to sociology and enter into collaborative research. Eventually an effective partnership developed between the two disciplines, evidenced by joint projects such as the investigation of the link between social class and mental illness undertaken by Hollingshead (a sociologist) and Redlich (a psychiatrist) (Hollingshead and Redlich 1958). Under the auspices of the *National Institute of Mental Health* (*NIMH*), a number of inter-disciplinary projects were initiated. In these psychiatry was a willing partner, in part at least because it was undergoing its own struggle for professional status within the hierarchy of medicine at that time (Badgley and Bloom 1973; Cockerham 1983:1516).

Other fields within the disciplinary hierarchy of medicine also assisted in the processes of institutionalisation of the sociology of health and medicine in all three countries. These included public health, epidemiology, social medicine, community medicine, midwifery and nursing, and most have maintained important border relationships with sociology.[2] The histories of these disciplines are as complex as those of sociology's own past, and because *their* intellectual territories have not been constant over time, their many borders within medicine, as well as the borders they share with sociology, have constantly been re-aligned and re-forged. There is insufficient space in this volume to do justice to sociology's relations with them all – or the significant national differences between them – and hence only a few comments can be made in this chapter about some of the more important of these.

One of the more salient is their changing, and changeable, nature. A notable example would be psychiatry, for although this discipline provided an important impetus for sociology during the 1950s and 1960s in Australia, Britain, and the United States, the relationship soured as the anti-psychiatry movement, first evident from the late 1960s, grew in strength and threatened the close alliance. By the 1970s, psychiatrists began to reduce their level of interest in the social aspects of mental illness and turned to biological mechanisms for causal explanations and pharmaceutical solutions for clinical problems. Sociologists became increasingly critical of psychiatric practice, particularly the widespread use of tranquilliser drugs as a means of social control over women (Foucault 1965; Cooper 1967; Szasz 1971). The relationship between psychiatry and sociology has strengthened a little in more recent years in association with de-institutionalisation (Cook and Wright 1995), and sociologists have once again found employment in departments of psychiatry. However their presence in these departments is more common in the United States than in Britain or Australia, and not as prevalent as it is in public health (Bloom 2005:83).

A second significant aspect of these border relationships is the extent to which they are the product of national, and sometimes even regional or institutional factors, and thus vary from one context to the next. The cases of public health and epidemiology are good examples of this. Both are multi-disciplinary intellectual fields, with public health often combining epidemiology, biostatistics and health services research, and sometimes also occupational health and other social sciences. Epidemiology, which initially focused on the management of infectious diseases, appears to have divided since the late 1960s into social and clinical branches, with the latter primarily undertaken by medically qualified personnel. In Britain, clinical epidemiology has been known as community medicine, and is focused on the evaluation of clinical interventions (Jefferys 1986:54–9). Social epidemiologists, on the other hand, have training in the social sciences and medical statistics and, like public health advocates, take an interest in preventative health, education, health systems analysis and policy (Jefferys 1991:19).

Unfortunately the distinction between 'social' and 'clinical' epidemiology is not consistently used in the literature, nor in practice, and variations in the labelling of the disciplines between countries, and indeed often within countries, make it difficult in a study such as this to clarify the border relations and distinguish the medical from the non-medical disciplines. For instance (and as shall be revealed in Chapters four and five), the relationship between epidemiology and sociology appears more co-operative in the United States, where epidemiological skills are taught within the institutional space of sociology in some universities (and may be given the name of *social* or *sociological* epidemiology); and where medical sociologists may have training in several fields, including social psychology, social stratification and biostatistics (Pearlin 1992:2). Thus, in the United States, boundary-action has resulted in a process of disciplinary 'capture', where sociology has extended its border into neighbouring sites such as social epidemiology and social psychology, and re-fashioned these as specialities of sociology. In Britain and Australia in contrast, where post-graduate work is research, rather than training-focused, and under-graduate degrees are relatively more discipline-based, departments of sociology generally do not provide students with epidemiological skills, nor offer courses in psychology, indicating a more adversarial relationship between the fields, less permeable borders, and indeed the continuation of distinct disciplines. Some evidence of these national differences can be found in the student textbooks, for the inclusion of epidemiological material in British sociology textbooks for medical students has been regarded as a sign of the undue influence of medicine (cf. Reid 1976); whereas student publications in the United States consistently contain sections on epidemiology (as well as psychology), indicating closer ties between these disciplines (e.g. Bird *et al.* 2000).

A third important dimension of the relationships between disciplines concerns the process through which they are constituted. It is common for these relationships to be discussed as if their similarities and differences were essentially cognitive, theoretical or methodological. For instance, social epidemiology and medical sociology are said to differ with regard to their key concerns, perspectives, and theoretical and conceptual approaches (Spruit and Kromhout 1987:586; Bird *et al.* 2000:2–3; Syme 2000); psychiatry and sociology to share a common concern with human behaviour (Bloom 2005); epidemiology and social medicine to be differentiated on the basis of intellectual objectives, underlying beliefs and motivations (Jefferys 1997:131); medical sociology and medical anthropology to vary in concepts, methods and topics (Olesen 1974:8); and medical sociology and psychology to have contrasting theoretical underpinnings (Umberson *et al.* 2000). The historical investigation of the sociology of health and medicine, undertaken in this chapter from a sociology of knowledge approach, shows another dimension to disciplinary boundaries. This is the extent to which these are essentially created when individuals, groups and institutions employ disciplinary similarities and differences – symbolic distinctions – as tools in the academic, policy, and public marketplace to negotiate and compete for resources. In the process, relationships between disciplines are reformed and manipulated.

The manipulation of the boundaries of science has been one of the more notable examples of such boundary-work, for several new intellectual fields were brought forth in the early part of the twentieth century – including medicine, psychology and biology – as a result of effective strategies to adopt a 'scientific approach' and incorporate some of the methods of the new laboratory sciences. Even sociology has re-shaped its territory and formed closer alliances with science at various times in its history. Yet the borders with science have been only one of many sites of boundary-action, for the manipulation of boundaries is a consistent feature of disciplines. It features in the adoption of a 'holistic' perspective by the *discipline* of nursing for instance: in this case serving to differentiate its knowledge base from the central disciplines of medicine (and psychology), and build alliances with sociology and other social sciences. 'Holism' is also used as a symbolic resource for nursing as a *profession*, for it legitimates the presence of nursing practice within the hierarchy of medicine, and is utilised by the representative bodies of nursing to indicate occupational control over a discrete body of specialised knowledge and obtain or formalise jurisdictional support from the state.

These symbolic distinctions are often discussed as 'tensions' and 'contradictions' within the intellectual fields of disciplines. Epidemiology, for example, is argued to contain within itself a:

> ...tension between an approach oriented toward biology and the study of mechanisms, and an approach oriented to populations and their interactions with the environment. This tension initially took the form of an opposition between microbiology and statistics, and more recently between molecular biology and public health...the tension is still present and is in fact essential for the success of the discipline
>
> (Parodi *et al.* 2006:358).

Such tensions or divisions are also present within many of the sub-disciplines of medicine. In psychology and psychiatry, for instance, there is a *social* as well as a more *clinical* or biological form of the discipline. These tensions and points of potential fragmentation provide disciplines with a formal collection of symbolic resources. In the case of the 'mega-discipline' of medicine, these symbolic resources enable it to claim or dispute ownership over its less central disciplines. At the same time, they provide the various sub-fields with some independent capacity to sever or build essential alliances in the struggle for resources within the hierarchical arrangements of medicine. As a conglomerate, medicine is able to use this flexibility to advantage in the public sphere and manipulate its external border relationships.

Sociology too is part of a conglomerate – the social sciences – but this arrangement does not provide it with the level of protection experienced by those in the medical hierarchy. Unlike medicine, which has engaged in sustained professional action to organise its disciplinary structure, the social sciences have failed to generate a cohesive public image and do not enjoy broader support for their role. Evidence of this is widespread. In the Australian case, by way of example, medicine's official representative in the nation state is the Chief Medical Officer. The occupant of this position is the principal medical adviser to the Minister and the key Commonwealth government department of health (the Department of

Health and Ageing). It guarantees the institution of medicine a strategic role in the development of health policy and the administration of programmes. The natural sciences have an equivalent representative: the Chief Scientist, the occupant of which advises government on matters of relevance and heads the *Prime Minister's Science, Engineering and Innovation Council*. The social sciences are without official representation and fare poorly with regard to policy influence and public resources.[3]

Possibly the only positive consequence of not being part of a disciplinary conglomerate is the greater independence experienced by sociology and its kindred disciplines (e.g. anthropology) in the construction of their boundaries. Without an overall mantle, the social science disciplines are capable of more diversity in these relationships and the configuration of their disciplinary landscapes. Focusing on sociology, we can see that this intellectual field covers a broad and heterogeneous territory rife with tensions and divisions which are rarely commensurate. This diversity – which is relatively greater in sociology than in many other disciplines – provides sociology with a 'discursive repertoire', which is constructed by disciplinary actors over extended periods and forms a central part of its public image. A critical element of a discipline's repertoire is its 'tensions' and 'contradictions'. Indeed the deployment of these aspects of sociology's discursive repertoire enables its members to vary the presentation of the discipline in order to forge alliances or create distinction and distance, engage in scholarly exchanges in the academic and policy arenas about the nature of social problems, and put forward claims about the discipline's capacity to offer solutions. Some elements of sociology's highly flexible repertoire (which will be familiar to readers) include the contrasts between its qualitative and quantitative methodologies; its interactionist, conflict and consensus theoretical frameworks; and its realist, constructivist, and interpretivist epistemologies. These have all been successfully employed in academic as well as public arenas to further disciplinary and professional objectives.

A final dimension of disciplines and their border relations which must be discussed at this point is the way the disciplinary fields are themselves structured by broader societal relations of power. These influence the outcomes of rhetorical conflicts between disciplines and the formation and maintenance of border alliances. As a consequence – and despite the concerted boundary-activity of individual knowledge workers – the disciplines can be swept up in radical movements which restrain disciplinary activity, reduce access to resources, or imperil previously acquired status positions. An example can be found in the pervasive antithesis to communism from the 1930s until the 1970s in both Australia and the United States. This retarded the full realisation of the sociology of health and medicine in both countries, for sociological perspectives in the health arena were often perceived as proposals for 'socialised medicine'. In the United Kingdom in contrast, where a similar collectivist ethos led to the establishment of departments of social medicine and the *NHS* in the 1940s, the institutionalisation of the sociology of health and medicine was less effected by a general aversion to communism, but instead stalled by the disruptions of war and subsequently, in a period of national re-construction, by the promotion of multi-disciplinary health research as a pragmatic solution to immediate social and policy problems.

More recent examples can also be given which show how the discipline has changed in response to broader social processes and shifts in the socio-economic context. If we look to the 1970s, for instance, we find the sociology of health and medicine as an established field in the United States, and on its way to disciplinary respectability in Australia and the United Kingdom. During the 1980s a new set of intellectual claims regarding the problem of illness was put forward from the discipline of economics. The sociological framework – which proposed illness to be a product of material conditions and structural inequalities – was forcefully pushed aside by more conservative and individualistic perspectives. In its stead was a revival of the notion of illness as a problem of individual risk-taking and irresponsibility, and the promotion of a set of market-based solutions based around the building of (allegedly) more effective and efficient *private* health care services. This shifted the previous emphasis on improving equality and accessibility towards an imperative to investigate and reduce the cost of health care services.

This radical alteration of the disciplinary landscape can be seen, in part at least, as a result of changes in the sphere of government from the 1980s: by the election of neo-liberal conservative political regimes, state responses to declining economic conditions, and pressing military conflicts (the Falklands, Afghanistan, the Gulf War). The re-orientation of the policy context severely impacted on the relative capacity of the disciplines of social science to contribute to health policy. Fewer resources and opportunities were available for the sociology of health and medicine at the same time as orthodox economics and the fields of management and business improved their fortunes. In a sense, this has been a 're-run' of the 1940s and 1950s, when the discursive association between the sociology of health and medicine and 'social' medicine inhibited the growth of the discipline, and it became difficult for sociologists to engage in broader political discourses concerning health and health care. In the more recent era, the synergy between neoliberalist discourses (or economic rationalism in the Australian context) and market interests has silenced sociological voices and led even the government of the United Kingdom to adopt pro-market policies and encourage its citizens to purchase private health insurance and utilise private services (Harley *et al.* 2011).

The concept of neo-liberalism captures those aspects of the *symbolic* world where 'individuals and groups struggle over and come to agree upon definitions of reality' (Lamont and Molnár 2002:168). It fails to fully address those elements of the *social* world that pattern and structure social action and which have contributed to the recent subjection of the academy to the vicissitudes of the capitalist market and its 'norms of profitability and instrumental efficiency' (Kurasawa 2002:335). In the three countries under consideration here, the strengthening influence of the discipline of economics in the determination of health policy, and the sharp decline in interest in collective and state solutions to health care services, reflects not just a discursive shift, but an alteration in the relative power of the market vis-à-vis the state. In the new era of transnational corporate power, the disciplinary landscape has generally been opened to the brutal effects of the structures of class and capital. These new pressures on disciplines have been various, and include imperatives to collaborate with political and economic players, produce research of policy or industrial 'relevance' rather than for the consumption of one's peers, engage in multi-disciplinary research teams, and publish in a limited range of high-status outlets.

The concept of 'academic capitalism', introduced in the first chapter, embraces these elements of the social world and the re-shaping of the disciplinary landscape amidst the growing ascendancy of market forces. Yet even the advancement of academic capitalism has not impacted equally on all disciplines. As previously argued, disciplines have their own sets of rules and intellectual power relations (Bourdieu 1969), and the capacity to differentially 'translate' the pressures for the instrumentalisation of knowledge coming from the political and economic fields (Albert 2003:149). Some, such as the applied branches of the natural sciences and engineering, appear to have succumbed more readily to the processes of academic capitalism (Slaughter and Leslie 1997; Rhoades and Slaughter 1998). The academic culture of the humanities and social sciences, on the other hand, appears to have more effectively resisted such pressures. Sociology has been protected by two of its significant features: (1) its fragmentation into numerous sub-fields, which makes it difficult for one form of legitimation to be imposed across the whole discipline and (2), the tendency for large numbers of sociologists to engage in 'dual production' (i.e. research produced for peers as well as political or economic actors) (Albert 2003:178).

The resistance of the discipline of sociology to the processes of academic capitalism has brought with it certain penalties in terms of resources and access to the political and economic arenas. The extent to which the speciality of the sociology of health and medicine has suffered the same fate as its parent discipline has yet to be fully assessed. Given the greater *instrumentalisation* of the applied sciences, including medicine, and the relatively greater dependency of the sociology of health and medicine on *medicine*, there is some potential for the specialty to display more of these characteristics than its parent. Moreover, because the discipline's boundary relationship with the nation state and the market sector varies somewhat between Australia, the United Kingdom and the United States, it is also likely that sociologists would be differentially capable of marshalling the necessary resources to protect their discipline – and specialist fields – from these political and economic forces.

More research is needed to fully investigate the impact of academic capitalism on the sociology of health and medicine, and the other specialist areas of sociology. However, some of the consequences of these political and economic transformations for the specialist field have been examined in the study described in Chapter four. Differences between the three countries are also discussed in some detail in subsequent chapters.

Internal boundary-actions: Maintaining discipline within the ranks

In the section above on external boundary-actions, we examined some of the processes through which speciality fields or sub-disciplines – such as the sociology of health and medicine – are produced through their 'external' relations with other fields. In this section it is appropriate to examine the 'internal' boundary-work of the discipline, for these forms of social action also contribute to its terrain. While external boundary-action is largely directed towards other disciplines and institutions, the state and the market, internal boundary-action focuses on the sphere of action *within* the discipline. In practice of course, both processes often occur together. For instance, internal boundary-work may be a response to threats posed by other disciplines or changes in the funding decisions of the state, and these may in turn impact on, or even re-fashion the external border relationships. Nevertheless examining the boundary-work *within* the discipline provides a focus on the processes through which rules and norms are fashioned and social order maintained.

One of the more notable acts of internal governance in sociology occurred during the middle years of the twentieth century. It took place in the United States, where the discipline was strongest and the number of sociologists and sociology departments was rapidly increasing. The situation was provoked by the proliferation of a diverse range of specialities within the discipline, for this created some uncertainty about the relationship between the sub-fields and its parent and the capacity of specialities to contribute to general sociology (Reader and Goss 1959; Selznick 1959:117–8; Simpson and Yinger 1959). For some members of the sociological community in particular, the diversity of interests was regarded as something of a challenge to the new and still-fragile unity of the sociological project (Naegele 1965a:24; Shils 1965:1406).

The potential for disruption in the field was resolved by leading figures putting forth a series of 'official' statements. These distinguished between various forms of sociological practice, with some forms re-named as *specialities:* that is, fields of endeavour peripheral to the sociological *core* and concerned only with the application and testing of classical sociological theory. Other areas of sociological practice were declared to belong to the *core* of sociology: a sphere of intellectual concern formed from timeless, universal and enduring human concerns, with continuing validity, viability, and relevance, basic to human experience, and remaining problematic and insolvable (Naegele 1965a:26; Parsons 1965:31; Shils 1965:1412, 1447; Nisbet 1967:7, 318; Warner 1976:11). The problems investigated within the specialities were claimed to be quite different. Distinct from the unit ideas of the classical period, these were the product of the *new* social concerns of the twentieth-century urban context (Merton *et al.* 1959:xxxiii).

These pronouncements had ramifications for all sociologists. Work within the specialities was henceforth to be of lesser value than that within the 'core', for the former was useful only for demonstrating the application of sociological theory. Indeed the specialities were declared peripheral to sociology itself, for they focused on phenomenon which was not, by definition, to be found in any systematic form within the classic, canonical texts. The specialities each had *their own history* (Merton 1959:xxx, xxxiii), and likewise *their own precursors* and founders (Lipset 1959). They were the result of *new* problems and concerns, *new* offerings, not previously examined sociologically (Simpson and Yinger 1959:399), and as such, their subjects were *not of sociological interest in themselves* (Reader and Goss 1959:232; Merton 1971:802).

These programmatic statements about the nature of specialities within the discipline may have assisted efforts towards professionalisation by proffering a view of the field as unified and coherent; but they offered an inaccurate view of the discipline's past. The portrayal of the classic, canonical texts as 'lacking' in concern for the problems of illness or practices of healing was to become a widespread view within the discipline. Even today, in Britain, the United States and Australia, sociologists are regularly (mis)informed. They are told of the neglect of the classical theorists for the subject of illness (Cockerham 2005a:11); that Durkheim's work on suicide was not an interest 'in health or suicide *per se*' (Scambler 2005:1); and that past theorists only discussed illness as a means to demonstrate how *core* concepts and theoretical frameworks (such as class, bureaucracy, or social integration) could be *applied* to practical problems (Mechanic 1978:326; Grbich 1996; Idler 2001:171–2; Quah 2005:24). Just as insistent is the message about the 'late development' of the speciality field, for it is repeatedly stated that 'the earliest texts' on the sociology of illness were from individuals such as Blackwell and Warbasse (Scambler 2005:1), and Parsons' book was the 'pivotal event' when, for 'the first time a major sociological theorist included an analysis of the function of medicine in his view of society' (Idler 1979:723; Petersdorf and Feinstein 1980; Turner 1987:6–7; Armstrong 2000:25; Cockerham 2005a:5).

With very few exceptions (perhaps Foucault 1980:151; Levine 1995:1), this has become the official view of the discipline. Recent work by the author (Collyer 2010) has indicated the falsity of this 'history', revealing Comte, Engels, Marx, Mills, Weber, Durkheim, and many other classical founders to have taken an active and public role in debating theories of disease causation and offering assessments of medical education and healing practices. Yet the twentieth-century processes of professionalisation and medicalisation ensured these efforts were 'written out of history'. The 'official' view has had a profound and lasting effect on sociology.

It was the sociology of health and medicine which was to bear the full brunt of these pronouncements about the nature of the specialities. In constructing a distinction between the discipline's 'core' and its 'periphery', specialities soon came to be regarded as intrinsically less worthy than other areas of sociology, and commonly charged with being 'atheoretical' and 'applied'. Indeed their apparent 'paucity' of theory was asserted in reviews and assessments as early as the 1950s, for some of the first to take heed of the 'official' statements were sociologists interested in the emerging field of health and medicine. The issue was stirred by Robert Straus in 1957 with his articulation of a difference between the 'sociology *of* medicine' and the 'sociology *in* medicine', with the former examining sociological problems and the latter based on medical definitions of a problem. The allegations and criticisms mounted, with the speciality said to have no theoretical content of its own, to import its theory from mainstream sociology, to fail to add to the conceptual 'stock of knowledge' of the sociological core, and to make insufficient use of theoretical constructs (Freeman and Reeder 1957:77; Olesen 1974:6; Johnson 1975; Figlio 1987:95; Light 1992:911, 913–4; Gray and O'Leary 2000:260).

Few of these criticisms can be fully substantiated, and yet such claims have become part of a mythology or doctrine, obscuring the speciality field's substantial contributions to the discipline. Close attention to the historical record will show, for instance, that medical sociology has attracted funding into the discipline from the better-resourced faculties of medicine, and its inclusion in the medical curriculum has promoted the discipline as a whole, raising its profile and increasing its impact on policy. And despite protestations to the contrary, the sociology of health and medicine *has* developed its own theory and exported this into other areas of sociology. Chief among these would be theories of the medical profession, providing a theoretical framework for the study of all professions (Bird *et al.* 2000:3), but also the theorising of normality and 'deviance', which Durkheim (1951) developed in his studies of suicide, and was later expanded by Parsons (1970) to indicate illness as a form of aberrant social behaviour with positive benefits for the social system. There are many other examples of theories and concepts developed within the speciality and later incorporated into mainstream sociology, including the concept of *cultural lag*, which derived from studies of medical care (from Ogburn 1922); *grounded theory*, a methodological innovation emerging from studies of dying patients (from Glaser and Strauss 1967, 1968); and an argument might also be made for the wholesale exportation of post-structuralism and Foucauldian analysis from the specialist field, beginning with Foucault's (1973) *Birth of the Clinic*.

In addition to the production of theories which have later been taken up in the sociological 'core', the investigation of medicine and health has broadened sociological knowledge of the state, the market, organisations and institutions (Light 1992:914), and assisted with the formation of key sociological paradigms which grapple with social control, regulation, order and organisation (Gerhardt 1989). Medical sociology has also modified 'core' theories to explain illness behaviour and patient–doctor interaction; developed new concepts such as *medicalisation* and *bio-graphical disruption* (see Bury 1982); chartered new theoretical and methodological territory in comparative health-systems analysis; and methodologically clarified the causal relationship between inequality and the distribution of illness.

Yet within the sociological community, the level of awareness about the many theoretical and methodological contributions of the speciality field is extremely low. The constant repetition of claims about the speciality's 'atheoretical' status has produced a set of beliefs among sociologists which serves to maintain the distinction between *core* and *periphery*. Rather than search for evidence of such contributions, the tendency for each new generation of sociologists is to assume the speciality has been a net *importer* rather than *exporter* of theories, concepts and methodologies. This discursive regime, set in motion at mid-century and adopted as standard fare in almost every sociology text-book, ensures the continuance of an inaccurate view of sociology's past and of its knowledge base.

The primary function of this discourse of 'failure' and 'poor performance' appears to be the maintenance of order within the ranks of the sociological community. This order is unmistakably hierarchical. Despite a pervasive ideology of camaraderie and democracy, all sociologists are 'not born equal'. In addition to the usual structuring by gender, sexuality, class and ethnicity, an additional hierarchical feature is a grading according to the disciplinary canon. Here we find a set of prescriptions about the relative value of all sociological tasks, roles and ideas, and work is ranked according to its proximity to the 'core' rather than merit (or its potential for contributing to other realms such as policy, public well-being or student education). The result is a hierarchical system with sociologists engaged in the 'core' (i.e. generalists) placed above those working in the specialities; the privileging of *academic* sociologists relative to those in industry, government or the community; and the valuing of theoreticians above the methodologists and 'applied' sociologists. Surprisingly, this hierarchical arrangement has not been of central concern to sociologists, though it has occasionally been noted:

> Those who teach 'theory' enjoy high status in academic departments, while those who are actually engaged in theory building have the highest status of all. It is mainly from those who aspire to these exalted positions that the cry that there is not enough theory in medical sociology comes
>
> (Horobin 1985:103).

The hierarchical order of the discipline, which sets out the relative status positions and defines what constitutes theory and theory-building, is largely maintained and reproduced through the internal boundary-actions of its members. A recent Australian example of *internal boundary-action* directed at maintaining this hierarchical ordering involved the health sociology journal, the *Health Sociology Review* (HSR). This journal was initially created in 1991 by members of the Health Sociology Section of *The Australian Sociological Association* (TASA). During its first decade it was financially dependent on the support of the hosting university. With the editorship moving constantly from one institution to the next, some editors were more successful than others in obtaining resources for the editorial process. Rarely 'breaking even' financially, TASA was eventually lobbied by health sociologist Stephanie Short and some other Health Section members, and for a few years the association provided a small sum to assist with the cost of its production.

By the year 2000, the journal was adopted by *TASA*, and its name changed to the *HSR* in 2001. The executive of the association – an elected group of sociologists representing the membership plus the editor of the *Journal of Sociology* (JoS) (but not the editor of *HSR*) – was divided over its new responsibility to produce *HSR* under its auspices. Some saw the journal as presenting unwelcome competition with its 'flagship', *JoS*. Ownership of *HSR* was given to a local publisher, *eContent Management*, as a means to resolve the dispute, and thus legal ownership of *HSR* no longer resided with the Health Section or the association. Despite the change of legal ownership, *HSR* continued to be regarded by Health Section members as their own, who credited it with both symbolic and social value. The association's subsequent refusal to support, or even acknowledge *HSR*, prompted health sociologists to take internal boundary-action and lobby the executive to provide support for the journal on the same basis as *JoS*. Although it took several years, lobbying eventually resulted in some financial support for the editorial process and an acknowledgement of the value of the journal to Australian sociology. It was not until December 2009 however (and a complete change in the membership of the executive), that the association's constitution was altered to include *HSR* as one of its official journals and its editors given equal representation on the executive.

The dispute over *HSR* is an illustration of how disciplines – as sites of social action – respond to challenges to the disciplinary order. The growing interest in, and rising status of health sociology, was clearly perceived by some members of the sociological community as a threat to other areas of the sociological field. The resultant boundary-action by the executive to give *HSR* to a commercial publisher, remove it from the association's arena of responsibility, and seek to encourage members to return to the mainstream journal as an outlet for their work; can be seen as having the effect of restricting and de-valuing the knowledge products of health sociologists, entrenching established distinctions between 'core' and 'applied' areas of the discipline, and emphasising differences in the relative status of members of the community. Boundary-action on the part of some sections of the sociological community challenged these efforts and eventually achieved greater parity for the speciality.

A situation not unlike the one faced by *HSR* in Australia arose in the United States in the 1960s. E. Gartly Jaco had created the *Journal of Health and Human Behavior* in 1960, but by 1962 found the role of both editor and publisher difficult to maintain (Bloom 1990:5). Jaco approached the *American Sociological Association (ASA)* for support, and requested the association to take it as an official journal. The Publication Committee of the *ASA* did not respond warmly to this invitation, suggesting there might not be a sufficiently large readership for a new specialist journal and this would make it difficult for the association to support it financially:

> The Publication Committee worried about opening the door to specialised journals...They also did not seem to like the idea of medical sociologists as a professional group...The atmosphere became heated...In the end, approval was granted (grudgingly), but only with the commitment of the Milbank grant to pay any deficit that might be incurred [and] a trial period of three years during which a minimum number of subscribers would have to be enlisted
>
> (Bloom 1990:5–6).

Medical sociology has since become the largest speciality of sociology in the United States, but internal disputes continue to be a feature of the discipline. For instance Pescosolido and Kronenfeld (1995:8) write about the conflict between members of the Medical Sociology Section and the *ASA* in the 1980s, where members of the speciality considered themselves to be under-represented, particularly within the discipline's general journals.

The struggles of *JHHB* and *HSR* are examples of internal boundary-work which provoke friction within the discipline and challenge its order. Neither case resulted in an overall re-arrangement of the hierarchical arrangement between the specialities and 'mainstream' sociology;

but in reaching a more suitable, institutional accommodation, the speciality gained some resources and recognition.

These processes show us three things about the relationship between specialities and the parent discipline. First, that discursive, symbolic statements from authoritative figures can lead to the construction of social boundaries composed of a system of internal stratification and inequality, with differential treatment, status and resources.

Secondly, that all members of the discipline are complicit in the production of its hierarchical order. Although the original statements about distinctions between the discipline's 'core' and its 'specialities' were produced by sociologists of 'the mainstream', in more recent periods, the acceptance of such distinctions has been widespread, and commentary has come primarily from sociologists in the specialities. This suggests the successful completion of a process of internalisation, where sociologists have adopted the rules and principles of the intellectual field (Bourdieu 1984:66), even where they may be contrary to their own interests.

A third lesson which can be drawn from these illustrations regards the process of specialisation and how this might be connected to the hierarchical order of the discipline. One view is that as specialities have become a common phenomenon, this has itself reduced the hierarchical order. Albert (2003), for instance, argues the increasing heterogeneity within the discipline and the proliferation of specialities has meant a multiplicity of organisational principles, for each speciality has its own set of standards and distinctive configurations of power. This he suggests, brings less consensus over standards, and multiple criteria for measuring the quality of knowledge output, making it difficult to evaluate researchers 'according to a common scale' (Albert 2003:171; also Collins 1986; Stinchcombe 1994). The cases of *JHHB* and *HSR* do not support this view. Instead they provide examples of where specialisation might be used to create or entrench the hierarchical order of the discipline rather than flatten its structure. It is possible of course, that some national sociologies are more resilient to internal challenge than others, given their diverse external relations with government and industry (particularly the publication industry). In Australia, for example, there is little opportunity for a discipline to independently alter its firmly entrenched, internal relationships with its specialities and radically reform its social order. One of the reasons for this is the dominating presence of the state in the university sector, which allows disciplines very little independence to negotiate their own disciplinary boundaries. This is well illustrated in the current evaluation process (the *Excellence in Research for Australia* or *ERA*), which, like the *RAE/REF* in the United Kingdom, forces compliance from the universities in return for government funding.

The *ERA* replaces the previous *Research Quality Framework* (*RQF*), and unlike the former, is not a metrics-based system. The *RQF* reinforced the *external* hierarchy of the disciplines, for its metrics-based system favoured the natural sciences with their much higher citation rates. Fierce lobbying from the university sector about the flawed nature of citation analysis for the humanities and social sciences, accompanied by a change of government, led to the development of this new evaluation system (Steele *et al.* 2006:281; Genoni and Haddow 2009:3). The *ERA* in contrast is a discipline-specific system and does not allow for comparisons between the disciplines. One of its more significant measures of 'performance' is the value of the publication output of academics, and this is measured in several ways including the application of peer review to assess and rank the journals in which the papers appear (ARC 2010). This aspect of the system mimics the *European Reference Index for the Humanities* (*ERIH*), which aims to give funding bodies an exact measure of research quality.

In Australia, the ranking of journals has been highly contentious, for it has a bias towards English-language journals; under-estimates the importance of journals in emerging fields (Macintyre 2009); gives greater weight to for-profit at the expense of open-access journals (Atkinson 2010:4); and privileges international journals from Western Europe and North America, thus discriminating against scholars of local and Australian subjects (Genoni and Haddow 2009; Atkinson 2010). Moreover, despite some exceptions (e.g. *Social Science and Medicine, SS&M*), there is a tendency within the system to rate generalist journals (such as *JoS*, the *British Journal of Sociology*, the *Annual Review of Sociology*) more highly than specialist journals (e.g. *HSR, Sociology of Health and Illness* (*SHI*), the *Sociology of Law, Teaching Sociology, Sociology of Sport Journal, Journal of Historical Sociology*).

In this way, the rank order of the journals in the Australian case mirrors the social order within the disciplines, favouring some groups (English-language speakers, sociologists working in established fields, theoreticians and generalists) at the expense of others (more innovative sociologists, those with first languages other than English, sociologists working in the specialities). An examination of the ranking process indicates why the *ERA* reinforces the internal disciplinary hierarchy, and in effect, pre-determines the outcome of the exercise. The initial ranking exercise took place in 2008 and the subsequent list was released in 2009. (It is currently in a second process of revision for the 2012 evaluation).[4]

The ranking process differed widely between the disciplines (Genoni and Haddow 2009), but essentially relied on committees drawn from disciplinary peak bodies and the learned academies. In the ranking process, journals were allocated to one of four categories in a manner which ostensibly took into account such information as their acceptance/rejection rates, the academic status and international standing of the individuals on their editorial boards, and the seniority and international standing of the contributors. The resultant rankings indicate that these criteria could not have been followed, for many journals do not publish this information, and information about the contributors or board members was not sought from the editors. Moreover, journals rating highly on these indices have not been ranked in the top positions. Given that the 'logic' of the process remains unclear, it is difficult to draw any conclusions from these rankings regarding the relative 'quality' of the journals (Genoni and Haddow 2009:9; Genoni *et al.* 2009:13; Atkinson 2010:6). The general response to the *ERA* ranking of journals has been negative. Like the *ERIH*, it is thought to produce 'defective' data, for it confuses internationality with quality, and assumes all papers within a journal are of equal quality, whereas:

> Great research might be published anywhere and in any language. Truly ground-breaking work may be more likely to appear from marginal, dissident or unexpected sources, rather than from a well-established and entrenched mainstream. Our journals are various, heterogeneous and distinct. Some are aimed at a broad, general and international readership, others are more specialised in their content and implied audience. Their scope and readership say nothing about the quality of their intellectual content
>
> (Editorial, *History of the Human Sciences* 2010, 22(1):2).

Little information has been published about the ranking process with regard to either the *ERA* or the *ERIH*, but it is not difficult to understand why the relative ranking of the journals privileges the generalist journals. When we examine the committees involved in the *ERA* consultation process, it is apparent these were not fully representative of the discipline but composed of sociologists of high status within the discipline *and* primarily generalists. Thus few had any familiarity with the speciality journals, their major debates, or the leading figures in the various speciality fields. In combination with prevailing disciplinary discourse about the allegedly poor performance and 'applied' nature of the specialities, the committees produced a ranking of journals reflecting the disciplinary order. The ranking of the discipline's journals is therefore another example of internal boundary-action. Although it is a response to external events (for the process is imposed on the discipline by the state), the exercise provides actors within the discipline with the means to enforce the disciplinary order and ensure its specialities remain in their place.

These examples have emphasised the processes through which the external and internal boundaries of the discipline are produced through a complex process of boundary-action. They have also shown the divisions between, and within the intellectual fields as historically contingent, formed in distinct national contexts, and shaped by the particularities of that arena. We have seen these boundaries develop in response to challenges from other disciplines and the broader environment (including changes instigated within the universities, the state and the market), as well as from internal disciplinary processes. These boundaries not only differentiate one intellectual field from another and thus organise the social relationships between the disciplines but also impose an internal hierarchical structure on the discipline itself. Questions remain about the extent to which these boundaries are similar in the three countries under consideration, and how they impact on the production of sociological knowledge. Such issues will be addressed further in the chapters ahead.

4
The Study and Its Methods

Recent decades have seen an increasing number of sociological papers reflecting upon the field of the sociology of health and medicine. As might be expected, the greater proportion of the literature assessing the field's progress and predicting its future trends is from the United States (e.g. Freeman and Reeder 1957; Straus 1957; Wardwell 1982; Cockerham 1983, 2005b; Bloom 1986, 2002; Mechanic 1989, 1993; Zola 1991; Pearlin 1992; Gaziano 1996; Waitzkin 1998; Clair *et al.* 2007; Evans 2009). The United Kingdom also provides a significant set of assessments, though on a lesser scale (Johnson 1975; Stacey and Homans 1978; Jefferys 1991; Blane 2003; Scambler 2005; Seale 2008), and there is a proportionally smaller offering from Australia (Ward 1979; Willis 1982, 1991; Manderson 1998; Willis and Broom 2004; Collyer 2011b).

These contributions are of considerable value to the discipline, pointing to gaps in our knowledge, new topics we should address, or alerting us to the need to increase our critical stance, consider an alternative viewpoint or more fully theorise our subjects. There are a number of ways our reflections on the field might be improved, and become even more useful to practitioners in the discipline. One approach might be to take greater note of the necessity, in an increasingly global world, for scholarly observations to be more carefully *situated*. Many local, regional, or national sociologies are presented *as if they were* entirely self-contained bodies of knowledge and arenas of social practice. Even a local form of sociology must be provided with a social context and described *in situ*, that is, enmeshed within a set of relationships with other sociologies, disciplines and institutions. The general trend however, has been otherwise, for there are only a handful of studies providing cross-national comparisons (Cockerham 1983, 2005b; Waitzkin 1998; Seale

167

2008) or positioning the sociology of health and medicine firmly within its socio-political context (Johnson 1975; Mechanic 1993).

A second suggestion is for more rigorous, empirical investigations to be conducted. Although a number of studies of the field have been published – some of them very insightful – few draw on systematically collected data. There are a handful of exceptions (Crane and Small 1992:198; Willis and Broom 2004; Clair *et al.* 2007; Seale 2008), but most are commentaries and reviews, setting out the key issues, shortcomings, or shifts in perspective over time, and drawing primarily upon the personal experiences and reflections of individual sociologists (Murcott 1977; Stacey and Homans 1978; Ward 1979; Freidson 1983; Cook and Wright 1995; Lawton 2003).

A third recommendation is to engage in more comparative, global studies of the field. Much of the current literature concentrates on a brief period in history, a university department, an intellectual school or aspect of sociology. As a result we have only a fragmented view of the domain of the sociology of health and medicine, and know very little about practices and experiences in other corners of the world.

A fourth suggestion is to undertake studies which take greater note of the institutional or organisational context in which the sociology of health and medicine is practised. The greater proportion of existing studies focus on the substantive content of sociological knowledge and its theoretical progress and tend not to reflect on its context. This leads to difficulties in explaining paradigmatic, methodological or theoretical shifts over time, or even variations in development from one country or region to another. It also encourages the (very problematic) view of sociology as independent of its social structure and not located in a specific historical period, geographical environment or cultural milieu. As a result, studies of the sociology of health and medicine often proffer 'a view from nowhere', failing to consider the impact on our work of the organisations and institutions we work within and how even these are shaped by the broader policy and market contexts.

These issues and omissions have become more obvious over the recent decade, and when taken together, suggest a more rigorous and inclusive study of the discipline is well overdue. The current volume is a contribution towards this important project. It has a number of aims. One, to provide an *empirical* study of the sociology of health and medicine *in situ*, taking an 'evidence-based' approach that goes beyond personal reflection and anecdote, and systematically gathers data on the trends and topography of the field. Two, to undertake a *comparative* approach, situating sociology within specific socio-temporal locations and examining the differences and similarities across several countries. Three, to offer a study that pays attention to *institutional context*, emphasising the connections between formal bodies of knowledge and the political, organisational and institutional settings in which that knowledge is produced. And four, to fully *theorise* this account of the field, applying the sociology of knowledge approach to explain the nature of the sub-discipline and its processes of change and growth.

This chapter describes the many questions underpinning this research; a discussion of the research design and the selected methods, and explains how choices were made to focus on three countries. It offers a justification for the inclusion of the key journals as sources of empirical data, and explains the sampling strategy employed in the Content Analysis. Details are also provided about each of the variables used to interrogate the knowledge produced within the sociology of health and medicine.

The research questions

At the heart of this book is a question about whether there is *one* sociology of health and medicine, or many different sociologies spanning various countries, regions and institutions. The question might be posed this way:

> When disciplines are established in a new country, region or university, are these bodies of formal knowledge and sets of social practices merely transported across time and place, or do they undergo some radical metamorphosis, perhaps only retaining a name or other superficial resemblance to their past institutional form?

In the new global context, where education has become an exportable commodity and universities recognised as central mechanisms of economic development, questions about the operation of disciplines have become progressively more important. This makes it imperative to understand the processes of intellectual change. For this reason, a cluster of research questions have driven this comparative study of the sociology of health and medicine. Some of these have been addressed through the historical analysis of the first few chapters:

What is a discipline? What is a speciality? How do disciplines and specialities change over time? How is it possible for the knowledge base of a discipline to vary cross-culturally? What social factors shape the working lives of sociologists in the contemporary context?

In this second, empirical component of the study (discussed in this chapter and also the next), questions are asked about the speciality field of the sociology of health and medicine in three countries. The first of these questions are about sociological practices. These might be framed in this form:

What is a sociologist of health and medicine? How do they identify themselves? Where do they work? What proportion work in medical departments? Does their work context differ from country to country, context to context? Does this effect the intellectual work they do?

A second set of questions refers to the knowledge base of the sociology of health and medicine:

What is the sociology of health and medicine? What are its characteristics? Which theories and methodologies are the most common? Is it a universal disciplinary field or does it vary from one country to the next? Where are the boundaries of the discipline? Do these vary according to their institutional or national settings?

The study design

These various sets of empirical questions – about the *sociology* of health and medicine and the *sociologists* of health and medicine – require a two-pronged research design. The first research strategy, which focuses on the sociology of health and medicine, is aimed at obtaining a data set of the intellectual products of sociologists – their research publications – and analysing these using the methods of Content Analysis. The second strategy, which seeks to focus on *the sociologists* themselves, combines the data set of publications with a collection of (publicly available) demographic and institutional data pertaining to the authors of the publications. Statistical comparative analysis across the two kinds of information allows for insights into the different forms of sociology produced in each geographic, temporal and institutional setting. Thus the study will enable questions to be addressed about the nature of the sub-discipline and the characteristics of the sociologists within this speciality group.

The countries

As stated above, there is a small, relatively new, comparative litera-ture on the evaluation and assessment of the sociology of health and medicine. Its focus to date has primarily been the United Kingdom and the United States (Cockerham 1983, 2005b; Seale 2008). It is essential to study these two countries if the aim is to investigate the sociology of health and medicine, given the oft-repeated claim about the United States as the country of origin of the sub-field (Bloom 2002), and the sheer quantity of publications coming from the United Kingdom. Ini-tially it may not seem to make a lot of sense to include Australia as a third country in a comparative study. After all, Australia can neither claim to be the 'home' of the sub-field, nor to be as prolific in its pro-duction of sociological publications as the other two. Proportionally, Australia is a much smaller player. Nevertheless, in a world-wide study of citation counts in the major sociological journals, Australia takes fifth place, after the United States, the United Kingdom, Canada and Germany (Phelan 2000:354). In this sense, Australia 'punches well above its weight' on a *per capita* basis, even if it is not an equal third partner in the production of sociological research.

More importantly however, a three-way comparison (with Australia included) is a potentially fertile research design. Its inclusion offers not only a three-country study about national differences and simi-larities, but the chance to explore the processes of knowledge transfer and transformation. Australian sociology developed primarily through its connections with Britain and the United States. Many of the first Australian academics were from Britain or Europe, the earliest schol-ars undertook their advanced studies in either Britain or the United States, and for the most part, the research and teaching materials came initially from these countries. As such, the study presents an opportu-nity to investigate what happens to sociology when it is taken from the 'mother-country' and (re)produced in a smaller economy in a post-colonial locale. These forms of knowledge transfer are as distinctly under-studied in sociology as they are in the sociology of science.

There is an additional benefit from this comparative form of research design. The socio-historical linkages between the three countries are well established, and all share a common (formal) language, many elements of the same academic culture, and significant similarities in institutional settings. A research design offering a systematic comparison between Australian, American and British sociological publications is therefore likely to produce an homogenous data set comprised of some relatively stable, independent variables against which other important disparities can be measured.

The journals

The research design calls for the collection and analysis of a set of research publications by sociologists of health and medicine in three countries. The choice of academic journal articles rather than text books is based on the significant differences between these two forms of media. In the first place, books and journal articles are usually written with different audiences in mind. This ensures they differ in their style and approach to the subject matter. In the second place, books are not an optimum choice in a study seeking to identify disciplinary boundaries, because, compared with the authors of journal articles, the authors of books have the independence to direct their material towards other disciplines (or a broader readership), and while they must be accountable to publishers, are generally not open to the scrutiny of discipline-based associations, editors, and reviewers. This feature of 'surveillance' by disciplinary gate-keepers – which is found only in the case of journal articles – is essential if we are to capture data about disciplinary boundaries.

The identification of a small set of appropriate journals presented something of a challenge in this study. Given the aim to identify and describe the specialist field, the outcome may have been determined at the outset merely by the unreflexive selection of journals. In other words, there was a danger of presuming the nature of a health or medical sociologist, or, conversely, the nature of a health or medical sociology paper, and so defining the field before the study even began. This would have allowed the author to define the field and the discipline according to her beliefs and perspectives, rather than gathering empirical data to resolve – or at least address – the numerous (and heated) debates in the literature about the nature of sociology. Such debates litter the field, proposing different definitions of sociology, about what might constitute a sociological perspective or method (Abbott 2000; Holmwood 2007), and even whether sociology is a *product* of the world market or merely shaped by it (Freidson 1986a; Turner 1986a; Connell 2000). Narrowly defining the field in its initial stages would also have prevented a full empirical exploration of national disciplinary differences, because if the theoretical literature is correct, there are country variations in the discipline yet to be fully explored. Even among countries such as the United States, Britain and Australia, which share the English language, a research design must be sufficiently sensitive to differentiate between concepts which are transferable, and others which appear the same only on the surface, with their socio-cultural differences obscured through the commonality of formal language. Indeed it is possible that 'country variation' is too mild a term here: the research should not only indicate differences, but the design must offer the possibility for finding that sociology is not a universal, homogenous body of knowledge nor unified set of social practices.

With these considerations in mind, the study was designed to allow for definitions of the field to be outcomes of the research, rather than its origin points. The study thus began with the aim of collecting a set of research publications in which it could reasonably be expected to find materials produced by sociologists of health and medicine, but would also, importantly, include papers by others close to the boundaries of this field. This entailed envisaging the intellectual field as constituted by a central 'core' of sociological research papers – or several, perhaps overlapping 'cores' – and surrounded by an (almost infinite) field of intellectual work with increasingly less 'sociological' content. The outcome of this broadly targeted study would be a set of indications of where the 'core(s)' and the 'margins' of the discipline lay, and thus the location of the disciplinary boundaries for each country.

The task then, involved turning the researcher's gaze in the general direction of the sociology of health and medicine, and obtaining papers from sources where there was a high probability of finding appropriate material, rather than closely targeting a specific type of paper and potentially missing valuable material. This method of selecting materials relies to a significant extent on the disciplinary definitions held by journal editors and reviewers, and results in a mixed set of papers: some of which would be unquestionably accepted as belonging to the sociology of health and medicine if presented to a group of sociologists from any of the three countries. Other manuscripts, put to the consideration of the same group, would be subject to discussion and possible dissent over whether they might be not sociological but rather epidemiological, psychological or even mathematical. In other words, the object of the exercise was to assemble a collection with a 'core' of sociology of health and medicine papers, surrounded by others which would fit comfortably within the field of 'social science', but where there may not be consistent agreement about whether they conform to the sociology of health and medicine. The application of this research strategy would, theoretically at least, result in a collection of papers with room to locate the potentially varying definitions of sociology.

The same process of selection occurred with regard to the collection of 'health' and 'medical' papers. Rather than the researcher defining the field at the beginning of the study, the aim was to collect papers *assumed by others in the discipline* to be of a 'health' or 'medical' nature. This made it important to target journals where such papers would be found, but in a manner which would allow for the possibility of health being defined differently in various countries. (In other words, 'health' might be considered broadly in terms of physical, mental or social well-being in one location, but might elsewhere be more narrowly focused on biological functionality). If there are differences in the way health is regarded from one country to another, these various conceptualisations of health should be reflected in the papers themselves.

Designing the study in this way would also allow for the possibility of collecting a core group of authors who can be identified as 'sociologists of health and medicine', potentially surrounded by others who do not identify themselves, or are not identified in this way by others. In this way the resultant sample can allow for questions about whether 'sociologists of health and medicine' are a universal group, or culturally specific creatures, sharing few social characteristics or institutional features with other, similarly named groups in distant parts of the world.

With these issues resolved, the choice of journals was not difficult. The first journals to be selected were the health sociology journals of the professional associations in Britain, the United States and Australia. This meant the *Health Sociology Review* (HSR), a journal of *The Australian Sociological Association* (TASA); the *Sociology of Health and Illness* (SHI), a journal associated with the *British Sociological Association* (BSA); and the *Journal of Health and Social Behavior* (JHSB), associated with the *American Sociological Association* (ASA).

The reasoning behind the decision to select the journals connected with the national professional associations lay in the important role of these as 'boundary objects' for the professional associations. In a study seeking to ascertain the boundaries of the discipline, the best place to find a discipline's 'core' products should be in the journals under the jurisdiction of the associations. Admittedly, these journals are not fully controlled by the associations. Professional associations must maintain a balance between controlling a journal's content according to the strategic needs of the profession and the discipline, and allowing the journal to have editorial independence to ensure its credibility and legitimacy in the academic market-place. Nevertheless, these journals are potentially the richest source of 'core' disciplinary material.

This is particularly the case because of the important role of reviewers as 'boundary actors'. Each journal relies on a community of peer reviewers to ensure the papers conform to the unwritten rules of the discipline, and indirectly, the review process means that the journals of the professional association are also the most likely to reflect national distinctions in sociology. This is because their respective communities of reviewers are generally drawn from the membership of the national associations. Given that over the past two decades, the American *JHSB* has primarily published American papers and relied on American reviewers, the British *SHI* has primarily published British papers and relied on British reviewers, and the Australian *HSR* has primarily published Australian papers and drawn on Australian reviewers (though not to the same extent as the *JHSB* or *SHI*); the resulting data set should provide fertile material for the investigation of national differences.

This strategy of including the journals of the respective national associations was designed to ensure a 'core' of sociological papers on health and medicine. A second strategy was necessary though, to broaden the final yield by offering a richer assortment of papers over which there might be less disciplinary consensus (and therefore an arena in which the boundaries of the discipline might be found). For this purpose, a second set of journals was selected. This group comprised the *Journal of Sociology* (*JoS*), another journal of *TASA*; *Social Science and Medicine* (*SS&M*), an international journal with editorial offices in several countries; the *Australian and New Zealand Journal of Public Health* (*ANZJPH*); and refereed proceedings from the annual *TASA* conferences.

The inclusion of these additional journals significantly broadened the field of papers and produced a more heterogeneous group of papers for the final data set. This was particularly essential for the American authors, because it has been suggested that the *JHSB* is methodologically narrow in focus, skewed towards stress research, and hence does not accurately reflect American health sociology (Gold 1977:161; Clair *et al.* 2007:255). The second set of journals allows for American papers to be taken from four different journals, reducing the possibility of bias in the sample. A similar tactic was employed for obtaining the Australian sample. A reliance on the *JoS* or *HSR* is likely to have unnecessarily narrowed the inclusion of Australian sociologists of health and medicine, as it has been suggested these outlets are not fully representative of the Australian 'health sociology' group. For this reason, the search was extended to include a random selection of papers from the annual refereed conference proceedings (which are refereed by members of the Health Section). Overall, this broad selection of sources enhances the possibility of gathering manuscripts which reflect the disciplines of each country and allows for the location of disciplinary boundaries, but at the same time minimises the possibility of national differences being confounded by editorial differences specific to a given journal.

It is worth noting that many journals undergo changes in their titles over time. To avoid confusion, when the selected journals are discussed in this study, the current name of a journal is used, even if it had a different name over the period of the study (1990–2010). For instance, the *JoS* began its life as the *Australian and New Zealand Journal of Sociology* in 1965. It was given a new name in 1998 after the joint professional association was dissolved and the New Zealanders and Australians formed their own professional associations and journals. Similarly, *HSR* had its beginnings as the *Annual Review of Health Social Sciences* in 1991, and took on a new name in 2001. The *ANZJPH* has an even more complex history. Beginning publication as *Community Health Studies* in 1977, it became the *Australian Journal of Public Health* in 1991, and presented with its current title in 1995. The *JHSB* also has a pre-cursor, the journal of *Health and Human Behavior*, which operated from 1960 to 1966. Although the most recent names of these journals are used in tables and discussions throughout the text of this volume, when papers appear in the reference list at the rear of this monograph, they are assigned the journal title as it appeared at the time of publication.

The quantity of papers from each journal is shown in Table 4.1. The study contains a larger number of papers from Australia. This is the consequence of an explicit strategy to obtain papers from Australian sociologists of health despite their somewhat unusual publishing practices. Most Australian sociologists of health have a long-established practice of submitting papers to a broad array of publication outlets, though there are some who only publish in medical/nursing journals and the *TASA* proceedings. The inclusion of the *ANZJPH* and *TASACP* in the sample is an attempt to ensure a more representative group. Of course, any difference in the number of papers between the three countries is fully taken into account in all calculations throughout this study. The journal issues were selected randomly between the years 1990 and 2010, and the result is a study population of 811 papers, of which 361 are from Australia, 225 from the United Kingdom, and 225 from the United States.

Table 4.1 The journals, 1990–2010

	Australia		United Kingdom		United States		Totals	
Health Sociology Review (HSR)	202	56%	9	4%	8	4%	219	27%
Journal of Health and Social Behavior (JHSB)					89	40%	89	11%
Sociology of Health and Illness (SHI)	30	8%	213	95%	41	18%	284	35%
Social Science and Medicine (SSM)	16	4%			87	39%	103	13%
Journal of Sociology (JoS)	57	16%	3	1%			60	7%
Australian and New Zealand Journal of Public Health (ANZJPH)	8	2%					8	1%
TASA Refereed Conference Proceedings (TASACP)	48	13%					48	6%
Totals	361	100%	225	100%	225	100%	811	100%

Notes: (i) percentages may not total 100 due to rounding; (ii) the population of the table = 811; and (iii) the country of origin is derived from the affiliation provided by the first author of the paper, and indicates their place of employment at the time of publication.

The selection of papers

Papers were randomly selected from the list of academic journals referred to in Table 4.1. Refereed articles make up the majority of papers (96 per cent), with a few research notes, rejoinders and commentaries included where these offer a significant, analytical contribution, are fully referenced, and thus deserve treatment as an article. Editorials, book reviews and introductions are excluded.

The selection of papers from journals offering sociological *and* health-related materials was the least problematic (i.e. from *HSR* and *SHI*). In such cases it was assumed the papers were broadly sociological and health-related, and these were included without taking note of its author or title but with regard to the date of publication and the stated country affiliation of the first author (until the country quotas had been filled).

The selection of papers from some of the other journals was less straightforward. Some journals aim to draw papers from other disciplines or subjects other than health or medicine. Papers from these journals had to be more carefully selected. With regard to journals containing chiefly sociological papers, but where the subject matter is not restricted to health or medicine (e.g. *JoS*), an effort was made to gather papers according to very broad definitions of 'health' and 'medicine' during this selection process, so that the disciplinary or subject boundaries of *health* sociology were not presumed at the outset. A strategy of using the key words 'health' and 'medicine' was used to find suitable papers. (The set of 'key words' often found in journals next to the articles was ignored, as these are usually chosen by the authors and tend to be highly inconsistent and individualistic). The resulting papers are subsequently fairly diverse in their subject matter, examining topics such as the health system, the health industry, policy and regulation, the institution of medicine, the professions, medical and health knowledges, the allied health professions, complementary medicine, traditional healers or healing techniques, a broad variety of diseases and conditions as well as health research methodologies and health education/training issues. Although 'welfare' was not used in these key word searches, there appears to be a fairly permeable boundary between the welfare and health literatures, and some papers from the former were included where the authors also used the words 'health', 'medicine' or 'medical'.

Other journals in the selected group were obviously health-related, but multi-disciplinary (e.g. *SS&M*). In order to select *sociological* material from these journals (without being too prescriptive about the field), key word searches were also useful. The key words 'sociologist', 'sociology' and 'sociological' assisted to identify papers where the authors were located in sociology departments, as well as those where the author might use these terms to describe themselves, their approach, or the literature they might use.

As noted above, a primary criterion for the selection of papers was the country of origin. This was taken from the affiliation of the first author as stated in the manuscript. This might be considered the 'professional nationality' of an author, and may differ significantly from their personal nationality or citizenship. Although there are occasions when authors publish articles whilst holding the status of a visiting scholar or student in another country, in general, these country affiliations will reflect the country where the scholar holds an employment position. One of the consequences of classifying papers according to the author's 'professional nationality' is that where an individual's papers have been randomly selected on several occasions (as happens with some of the more prolific authors), they may, if they have worked in several countries (as some of them have), appear with a different country affiliation in each case. The significant majority of the authors on the data base however, are consistently found to have the same country affiliation for each of their papers. Moreover, the use of the *first author's country affiliation* as a fixed marker of nationality for the paper is valid for this research, given that the majority of papers originate in one country. Sociologists often publish by themselves (particularly in Australia), but even when they write with others, partners are usually from the same country. In this study population of 811 papers, 91 per cent of the Australian co-authored papers had both first and second authors from Australia. Among the UK papers, 93 per cent of co-authored papers had both first and second authors from the United Kingdom; and in the United States, the figure was a little higher at 95 per cent. This makes it quite valid to use the first author's country as a marker for the country of origin of each paper in the set.

The Content Analysis

Content Analysis has been described as 'the study of recorded human communications', and includes the use of a variety of materials including 'books, websites, paintings and laws' (Babbie 2010). The method of Content Analysis was selected for this research because it is an effective, unobtrusive method which doesn't put further pressure on already overloaded academics and practitioners to provide *other* sociologists with assistance in their research projects. It is also cost-effective (Berg 2007), and can combine both qualitative and quantitative methods. In this case, with its sociology of knowledge approach, the study requires a highly interpretive, qualitative methodology, but involves the analysis of both quantitative and qualitative forms of data. It is qualitative in approach, because it relies heavily on interpretive and inductive reasoning to identify the emergent themes and determine the categories in the research material. However, because the research process also draws on a set of theoretical frameworks (as outlined in the first chapter), the qualitative form of Content Analysis additionally involves deductive reasoning. In combination with the use of a *quantitative* form of Content Analysis, it becomes possible to draw causal, statistical conclusions from the data, allowing the researcher to effectively and systematically deal with a large volume of text. The *qualitative* components of Content Analysis, on the other hand, provide the capacity for tapping into the 'taken-for-granted' social worlds of a population that are not readily observable.

All researchers must consider issues such as reliability, validity and credibility in their research. Performing a valid Content Analysis necessitates a familiarity with the language and culture of the population under study, for without this, the data cannot be interpreted accurately (Hodder 1994). In this regard, the validity and reliability of the study rests, to some extent, on some personal qualities: namely that the researcher has travelled extensively, is a migrant who has lived in both Britain and Australia, has had many years of experience as an academic sociologist, and been the editor of *HSR* for six years. This said, the researcher has little in the way of formal languages other than English, and extending this study to Asian, European, or other countries which do not have English as their first language would require collaboration with sociologists with alternative language skills and a familiarity with the local academic culture. As this opportunity is not currently available, the study includes only three countries.

As discussed above, the Content Analysis for this study involved the retrieval of a population of scholarly articles from the selected journals. These papers were read closely, coded according to the framework set out in an extensive codebook, and recorded using the *Statistical Package for the Social Sciences*. Coding categories were established over a period of months, with the researcher continually revising the classifications and re-coding the papers. Each country was coded in turn, rather than as a mixed selection. This allowed for the development of a set of categories appropriate to each country. The need for a new set of categories became readily apparent as soon as work on another country began, and eventually entailed the re-coding of the first country's data to ensure a coherent and broad classification scheme which could cover the unique qualities, approaches and institutional contexts of sociologists from the three countries. Although this process was time-intensive, it was a major strength of the research strategy, because the extended, interactive process of working between the documents and the coding frame allowed the researcher to begin to understand and interpret the material from an early point in the research process. One of the products of this extended, reflexive, qualitative approach to the research was a coding frame highly sensitive to the subtle differences between the research papers of each country.

Moreover, this process of coding and re-coding over an extended period ultimately provides for a better overall result, giving the researcher time to reflect upon the material and follow new leads. It also assists with developing and sharpening any hypotheses for the study. For example, finding that the classification scheme constructed for the Australian papers was not suitable for either British or American authors forced an awareness of certain similarities and differences which had not previously been discussed in the literature. Although some national differences were expected, others were not. The greater interest in quantitative methodology among American sociologists is, for instance, well documented, but not differences in disciplinary affiliation, nor their intense interest in the problems of stigma and inequality. These issues are discussed at length in the next two chapters.

At the completion of the coding process, all articles were re-read and their codes checked to correct any mistakes with coding or data entry. A group of 150 papers was randomly selected to test the veracity of the coding scheme. In this second, independent, re-coding of the papers, four variables were found to have insufficient reliability, meaning they were not sufficiently stable or consistent (Neuman 2000:164). The four variables were adjusted and re-structured to improve their reliability, and thus validity, and all papers re-coded. A second, random sample of 100 papers was subsequently re-tested to ensure the adequacy of the new variables. These processes followed standard procedures for conducting and monitoring the quality of a Content Analysis. Ethical approval for the study was unnecessary, as it draws only on publicly available materials. Nevertheless, the study conforms to the ethical guidelines laid down by *The Australian Sociological Association*. The study was supported by small grants from the *Faculty of Arts* and the *School of Social and Political Sciences* at the University of Sydney.

Key variables

The demographic variables

The 'demographic' variables constructed for the purpose of the Content Analysis do not contain personal information (such as age or marital status), but professional information provided on the manuscripts and supplemented (where this was missing or inadequate), from institutional web pages, publicly available curriculum vitae's, press releases, biographies, library catalogues, and the publicity material from book and journal publishers.

1. *Gender*: The first variable is gender, and was inferred from the name of the author in most cases. Where this source was inconclusive, for instance with names such as 'Chris', a search on the Internet generally yielded photographs or other helpful descriptive material. In a few cases, where individuals changed gender over their lifetime, they were noted according to the gender they were using at the time of publication. Hence, if more than one of their papers is on the data base, their papers may appear under different genders.
2. *Number of authors*: A second variable was constructed to encapsulate the number of authors of each paper. It is common in some disciplines for authors to undertake research and write papers as members of large teams, and in others, for authors to work by themselves or with one colleague. This variable was designed to allow for such comparisons, and it was expected there would be some country differences, and also variations between the qualitative and quantitative research papers.
3. *Affiliation with a university*: A third variable pertains to whether the author is affiliated with a university or not. Various alternatives were noted, including a government department, professional organisation, community-based organisation, a corporate entity of some kind, an independent research unit, or private practice. (As it turns out, there are very few authors working outside the university system in this study population).
4. *Organisational context*: A fourth variable refers to the organisational context of the first author. Papers were coded according to the faculty, departmental or school affiliations provided on the manuscript, showing whether the authors were associated with discipline-based departments (such as sociology, anthropology, epidemiology etc.) or multidisciplinary units (the social sciences, health sciences, humanities, life sciences etc.). An extensive list of possible values was

constructed to ensure the variables would be sensitive to the diversity of organisational forms across the three countries.

During analysis, these affiliations would become a critical means for distinguishing between sociologists who work in sociology departments (or the arts or social sciences), and those employed within health or medical contexts. It was expected, given the extensive literature on the problems encountered by sociologists working in medical departments and hospitals, that different attitudes, perspectives and stances might be apparent in various institutional settings. For instance, it was suggested in the 1970s that sociologists working within medicine were less critical of medicine compared with others in the liberal arts or social sciences (Freeman *et al.* 1963; Freidson 1970b:42). This was the position of Robert Straus (1957), when he made a distinction between 'sociology *in* medicine' and the 'sociology *of* medicine'. Straus (1999:109) argued that a 'sociology *of* medicine', in which sociologists study the structures, organisation, values, relations and behaviours of medicine without adopting medical perspectives or values, is achieved more effectively by individuals 'operating from positions outside formal medical settings, such as those with primary appointments in departments of sociology'. Elliot Freidson offered a similar view. He argued, 'it would take an extraordinary person to be able to work full time in a medical setting and at the same time define his [or her] problems sociologically rather than medically' (Freidson 1978:128).

Forty-two years later Straus (1999:109–10) softened his position, suggesting it had become possible to work *with* medicine (and take its funding) without losing one's objectivity or capacity to criticise one's colleagues. This shift in Straus' position was a personal observation, not based on new data. Similarly Cockerham's (2005b:60) discussion of the recent decline in tension between sociologists employed inside and outside medical departments is not a view supported – or refuted – by empirical evidence. In the 1970s there were a number of calls for a 'sociology of medical sociology', where the influence of work contexts and funding arrangements for sociologists might be explored (Gold 1977; Greene 1978). The lack of knowledge about this problem was evident in Badgley's (1971:141) observation that there might be disadvantages to the sociologist working within medicine, but it is not clear why 'the objectivity of the sociologist is any more accurate or relevant when [s]he is an uninvolved bystander than when [s]he is an active participant observer'. Despite 50 years of expressions of concern over this matter, the question of whether work context continues to be an important determinant of the sociology of health and medicine has not previously been empirically addressed. Given that the relationship between social context and knowledge is a key focus of this volume, this fourth variable will be an important means to address the issue.

Citation patterns

Citations provide access to the communication system used by sociologists in different locations and circumstances. The list of citations accompanying a manuscript is an explicit statement which reveals the influence of others. These:

> ... citation inventories are used by authors to spread tentacles into other domains, reinforcing an argument, and sustaining the continuity of a disciplinary tradition as knowledge is shown to 'grow' through building on the work of others
>
> (Armstrong 2003:58).

Although citation patterns are often applied as indicators of performance in the current 'audit culture' (Najman and Hewitt 2003; Cheek *et al.* 2006), they also reveal important information about disciplines. Citation analysis tells us *which* subjects, authors and ideas are attracting notice in the discipline, and gives some indication of the *extent* of this notice. And it does this by paying attention to the individuals conducting the research, making note of the authors *they* cite, without having to rely on the original authors' observations or explanations.

There are a number of ways to examine citation patterns. For instance, worldwide electronic indexing systems (such as *Thompsons' Institute for Scientific Information or ISI*) indicate citation patterns and calculate impact factors. These have been used to provide data for studies of the sociology of health and medicine in a few cases (Chard *et al.* 1997; Armstrong 2003). Unfortunately, these have several drawbacks. One problem is the way they take note only of a narrow range of journals, and ignore books and policy documents. Another is that although they can give some indication of which groups are citing the reference works, they have their own, problematic means of defining disciplinary groups. In this study, where the very definition of the discipline is in question, existing citation mechanisms are inadequate. In its place is a procedure which captures the full range of reference materials cited by a group of authors: including books, conference materials, articles from both mainstream and marginal journals, and even unpublished papers. When tested against the demographic variables in this study, analysis will reveal any tendency for citation patterns to vary from one group of authors to another, from one country to the next, or one form of institution to another.

Even more importantly, citation patterns can be studied for what they tell us about the shape and nature of disciplines. Disciplines have many unique and identifiable practices, and members of a discipline might be identified on the basis that they, for instance, publish monographs rather than textbooks; write with multiple authors rather than individually; produce short papers in a 'report format' rather than long, discursive, highly descriptive pieces; or employ a specific theory or methodology. The disciplinary affiliation of a given individual may also be suggested according to whether they cite a particular key theorist or school of thought and disparage, ignore or criticise others. This is because citations are not simply references to the contributions of an individual scholar, but provide information about the network in which they are embedded (Najman and Hewitt 2003:76). As such, citations offer vital clues to understanding the sets of peer networks that constitute a discipline, for they can reveal particular ideas, concepts or 'lines of thought' which might be followed by one group but not another.

Relative to many of the sciences, sociology is often thought not to demonstrate a high level of 'consensus' concerning its methods and theoretical approaches. However, if we look beyond the often fierce disputes over method, and debates about the hierarchy of the sciences (Cole 1983; Fuchs and Ward 1994), and instead examine the trends and patterns of citation; it becomes apparent these are the consequences of social and structural factors which may have little to do with disciplinary 'consensus', agency or individual choice. The factors that determine citation patterns are complex, but they can be discerned. In an age of electronic communication, when it should be as easy to access the publications of a sociologist on the other side of the world as readily as those from the sociologist in the office next door, citation patterns are not random but highly patterned and an outcome of social and institutional context. Thus we can see academics selecting reference material largely on the basis of what they were exposed to as a student (a conservative approach that ensures inter-generational continuity of 'schools of thought' and the preservation of academic traditions); but also the significance of personal contact, because scholars prefer to draw on materials from *known* others, regardless of whether they met these individuals in formal conference settings, departmental hallways, or through social or familial networks. This more sociological understanding of the citation system makes it important to spurn the use of the pre-defined disciplinary codes of existing electronic indexing systems, and construct an analysis to address the association between citation patterns, and factors such as institutional context, gender, and nationality.

In this study, in an effort to reveal disciplinary boundaries, ascertain country differences in the reference materials used by sociologists, and also identify possible 'leaders' in the disciplinary field, papers were coded according to whether or not they cited the sociologists from a designated list. Multiple citations of the same author within a given paper were ignored, so that overall counts represent the number of papers in which an author was cited, not the number of times they were cited overall. This is an important distinction, because journal papers often function as quasi-curriculum vitae's, where it is standard practice for authors to include their own (relevant) papers or books. Counting multiple citations within papers would unnecessarily bias the statistics, as some reference lists are comprised almost wholly of the author's own publications.

The citation variable itself was constructed without the benefit of an automated process, but through the more time-consuming technique of identifying the authors who were frequently cited within the population of papers and continually adding to the list – and revising the coding on all previous manuscripts – until all commonly found authors had been included. This method enabled the collection of far more accurate data, as the researcher was able to identify the many cases where there were missed references, incorrect references, and the misspelling of author names. For instance, Graham Scambler's name is regularly spelled as Scrambler, and many authors seem unable to correctly spell Pierre Bourdieu. Sociologists also sometimes change their names (e.g. Australian sociologist Dorothy Broom has some publications under the name of Darroch, from a previous marriage, and others with Darroch-Broom; while Elizabeth Grosz has some publications under the name of Gross). Familiarity with the medical sociology literature made the task of sorting out these problems considerably easier, as did ready access to the Web. The latter provided publicly available lists of most authors' publications, enabling rapid checks to be made in those cases where authors have similar or very common names (e.g. G. Williams and P. Brown). Personal knowledge was also found to be important. For example, distinguishing between the works of Evan Willis and Eileen Willis, both Australian sociologists of health who also share a common middle initial, do not write together (and are not related to one another), is made easier given a long-standing familiarity with their work.

The coding frame for the citation analysis was completed over a period of 12 months. At the end of this process, a total of 409 names had been included. Most of these are sociologists (e.g. Bryan Turner, Evan Willis, Deborah Lupton, Pierre Bourdieu, Robert Merton, Donald Light), but quite a few come from other discipline areas and have become part of the sociological 'reservoir' of resources. For example, both Sigmund Freud (1938) and R. D. Laing make appearances, as do health economists John Deeble (2004) and Richard Scotton (the architects of Australian Medicare), and from the American context, a popular choice for papers focusing on matters of sexuality is Alfred Kinsey (particularly with regard to his classic text *Sexual Behaviour in the Human Male*, see Kinsey *et al.* 1948).

Sociological theories

Papers were coded to indicate the author's use of a specific theoretical framework. Up to two theories were coded for each manuscript. This variable was not a judgement about the quality of a paper, nor was coding based on a decision of the researcher, but taken from the author's statements about their theoretical framework or orientation. Many papers *were* theoretically framed, but did not contain explicit statements about their use of theory, and hence the researcher refrained from making inferences about the type of theory in use, even where this might easily be inferred. (These were coded as having no stated or readily apparent framework). Papers which did not use a specific *sociological* framework, but instead applied theoretical frameworks from other disciplines such as economics or psychology, were also coded as having no stated or readily apparent framework.

Examples of papers containing explicit statements about their theoretical perspective can readily be provided here. Madeleine Murtagh and Julie Hepworth (2003:190), who analyse general practitioners' meanings of the menopause, state:

> Our analytical framework employs post-structural concepts, including discourse and its constitution of objects/subjects, and technologies of power, based on Michel Foucault (Foucault 1972; Martin *et al.* 1988) and feminist post-structuralism
>
> (Weedon 1997).

As a consequence of this statement, and others of a similar nature, the paper has been coded as post-structuralist and feminist. Another paper, this time by Justin Waring (2007:164), is coded as Foucauldian, based on the author's statement that: 'I elaborate this argument, with

Foucault's (1991) concept of governmentality....'. A third paper, in this case coded as 'interpretist', comes from Lucy Biddle and colleagues at the University of Bristol. Examining non-help-seeking behaviour among young adults, Biddle *et al.* (2007:986) state, 'the research was conducted within the interpretive tradition'. A final example is provided from Derrol Palmer from the United Kingdom. This paper is coded as having a social constructionist perspective. In his introductory paragraph, Palmer (2000:663) explains:

> Although there are clearly ways in which sociological ideas have made an impact on psychiatry... this paper focuses on a seemingly powerful form of criticism which fails to do so; that is, the radical critique which has been articulated within the social constructionist perspective... I ... examine a key way that constructionist sociology has criticised psychiatric work...

From this last example it can be seen that an author may employ a theoretical framework in order to demonstrate its applicability, or

Table 4.2   The theoretical frameworks

Actor Network Theory	Marxism or political economy
Bourdieu'n (from Pierre Bourdieu)	Modernity, modernisation, modernism
Constructionist or social constructionist	Network analysis
Critical theory	Parsonian
Development or developmentalism	Professionalisation, de-professionalisation, etc.
Durkheimian	Post-modernist
Embodiment or the sociology of the body	Post-structuralist
Feminist	Queer theory
Fordism	Sociology of risk
Foucauldian	Social capital
Functionalist	Sociology of knowledge
Globalisation	Structural-functionalism
Habermasian	Structuralism
Industrial society or industrialisation	Structuration
Interactionist or symbolic interactionist	Taylorism, scientific management
Interpretist	Weberian
Other frameworks, often theories of the 'middle range' (e.g. ethnomethodology, phenomenology, masculinist studies, realism, reflexive-consumerism, ethnomethodology, social movements) or from unlisted theorists (e.g. Norbert Elias)	No framework stated or readily apparent

alternatively, show its shortcomings. Either way, it is coded for its use of this theoretical perspective. Table 4.2 provides the range of possible values for this variable.

The use of theory

Papers were also examined to ascertain the extent to which an author uses sociological theory or sociological concepts. As in the previous variable, this is not an assessment about how *well* authors employed these theories or concepts, but *whether* they contain sociological theories or concepts. Unlike the previous variable, this variable rests on the judgement of the researcher. Although the main focus is on theoretical frameworks, concepts are included, as a clear distinction between these is rarely found in sociological practice (e.g. some authors consider governmentality a concept, and others a theory). Four categories are employed:

1. *High use of sociological theory*: Papers in this category use a significant amount of sociological theory or concepts throughout the manuscript. In many cases, the paper is primarily theoretical, though some also contain empirical material.
2. *Some use of sociological theory*: Papers in this category employ a small amount of sociological theory or sociological concepts throughout the text, and may seek to test or illustrate these empirically. Theoretical development is generally not the primary aim of the paper, but is part of the discussion, at least at the beginning and end of the manuscript.
3. *Minimal usage of sociological theory*: Papers in this category merely mention a sociological concept or theory, but these are tangential to the main message or intent of the paper, and not integrated into the discussion or analysis.
4. *No use of sociological theory, or not applicable*: Papers in this category contain no sociological theory or concepts, and are instead about something else entirely, perhaps a methodological or statistical matter, or an opinion piece. Alternatively, papers may be highly conceptual or theoretical, but use theory and concepts from another discipline.

Examples can be offered to show how this variable is operationalised. Justin Waring's (2007) paper provides an illustration of the first category, where a 'high' level of sociological theory is employed throughout the paper. Waring utilises a Foucauldian framework to investigate the extent of regulatory change occurring in a British hospital. Although the manuscript contains empirical material (it is not simply a conceptual paper), the focus is continually returned to sociological concepts (governmentality, managerialism, ideology), as well as theories of regulation, control and surveillance, and thoroughly involves and integrates the sociological literature (Gramsci 1971; Foucault 1973; Freidson 1975; Larson 1977).

A second example of the 'high' use of sociological theory is provided by John Germov's (1995) article on medical fraud within the health care system. Germov, an Australian sociologist of health, bases his arguments around sociological concepts of managerialism and medical dominance, and embeds a small amount of empirical material within an extended discussion of the theories of de-professionalisation and proletarianisation. The reference list also contains a significant amount of material of a sociological, theoretical nature (e.g. Freidson 1970a, 1986b; Haug 1973; Braverman 1974; Braithwaite 1984; Bryson 1987; Hindess 1987).

A third example of a 'high' level of theory use can be found in Dufur *et al.* (2008), which is an empirical study, but offers a full discussion of the concept of social capital, uses data to explore and test the concept, and draws on a broad range of sociological material from the major sociology journals. Additional examples of papers in this category come from Kristin Barker (2008) from the United States, on medicalisation; and Simon Williams (2001) from Britain, on sociological imperialism.

The next category, 'some use of theory', is reserved for papers where theory is part of the discussion, but not a primary facet of the text. An example of a paper coded into this category is by Fabian Cataldo (2008) from the University of London, which employs the concept of citizenship from T. H. Marshall. Although this is a sociological concept, the emphasis is on the data (specifically, the HIV/AIDS programmes in Brazil) and much of the discussion concerns the issue of ethics. The approach also tends to be anthropological rather than sociological. Many of the reference materials are government and medical reports, and either multi-disciplinary or anthropological.

Examples can also be provided to illustrate the third category, 'minimal usage of theory'. These papers usually mention a sociological concept or theory, but do not explore or provide an extended discussion of these. Papers may be highly theoretical or conceptual, or may offer a sophisticated and innovative methodological approach, but neither sociological theory nor concepts are the objects of consideration. The paper by Hannah Knudsen and colleagues (2005) is a good case in point. Examining the possible effects of the violence of September 11, 2001 on mental health and alcohol consumption, this paper primarily employs psychological concepts (such as stress, distress, trauma, and 'negative psychological states'), and takes into account the psychological literature to discuss symptoms and possible impacts. The work of Èmile Durkheim is alluded to once (Knudsen *et al.* 2005:269) in referring to 'social integration', but the concept is not further explored or utilised. Reference materials are extensive, but do not include any of the major social theorists (except Durkheim 1951), and are taken primarily from medical or psychology journals.

A second example, this time from Australia, is the paper by Allan Borowski (2009). Here the issue is the uncertainty of retirement saving systems in an era of globalisation. Although Borowski uses the concept of globalisation to provide a focus for the paper, and indeed to integrate its various themes (e.g. changes in financial markets, changes in employment practices), it is raised in a rather superficial fashion, and explicated using multi-disciplinary rather than sociological literature. The reference list is primarily composed of newspaper reports, stock market announcements and financial articles/reports. A very small number of multi-disciplinary articles on policy are included, mostly the author's own. It is important to re-emphasise, at this point, that this is not a judgement on the quality of the article (or the importance of the topic). It is, on the contrary, a judgement about the *sociological* content of the article.

A third example of the minimal use of sociological theory or concepts comes from Rodrick Wallace (1993) of New York, USA. In this case the paper concerns AIDS and its capacity to impact negatively on urban minority neighbourhoods. Here the author uses a number of sociological concepts (such as social disintegration, social networks, socialisation, deviancy, social control), but applies these uncritically and without sociological discussion of their meaning. The reference materials are primarily from the medical, epidemiological and psychological literature, although there is one from the *American Sociology Review*.

The final category refers to papers which employ no sociological theory or concepts. There are quite a few, somewhat surprisingly, of these papers in the selected journals. Many may have been included in the sociological journals because of the information or insights they provide on subjects about which the editors or reviewers consider their readership should be aware. Journals also change over time as new editors are appointed, and some editors are more comfortable with inter-disciplinarity or multi-disciplinarity. The paper by Darrel Doessel (1992) is a case in point. In the early 1990s, the journal (*HSR*), published a broader range of papers than it did in later years, gradually becoming more focused on sociology and less multi-disciplinary. Doessel is an Australian-based economist, but his paper concerns a subject of some considerable public concern in the early 1990s. It discusses the number of trainee doctors required for the medical workforce and the best means of determining the appropriate training quota (quotas are regulated by government in Australia, because the state provides the finance for medical education). The paper, though obviously competent within the discipline of economics, and offering a sophisticated, methodological approach to the issue, nevertheless contains no sociological theory or concepts. As an indication of this, the reference list is composed entirely of economic papers and government reports.

A second example of a paper coded for the final category is from Shane Thomas *et al.* (1992). This paper argues the case for focus groups to be utilised in health research. It focuses on the benefits of the method, and is essentially multi-disciplinary in its approach. No specific references are made to sociology as a discipline, and the references could be used in any social science research. A third example is from R. Jay Turner and Donald Lloyd (1999). This article examines the stress process and the social distribution of depression in Toronto. Although it is a fully theorised paper, it offers no *sociological* theory. Admittedly, the authors use the concept of socio-economic status, but this is common to many disciplines. The paper does not follow a recognisably sociological approach to illness, but is representative of a significant number of papers which focus on the disease status of the individual, despite allowing for the social patterning of illness. For instance, the authors argue that individuals of 'lower socio-economic status have social relationships of lesser quality' (Turner and Lloyd 1999:377), and point to the finding that some individuals are exposed to 'fewer harmful experiences' and consequently tend to have fewer episodes of depression (Turner and Lloyd 1999:391). The reference materials drawn on for this study are primarily from the psychological, psychiatric and epidemiological literatures, though a few citations are from the *JHSB* and the *American Sociological Review* (*ASR*).

This last paper aptly illustrates the potentially contentious nature of this variable. How can it be that authors who discuss their subject matter as belonging within the genre of 'sociological stress research' (Turner and Lloyd 1999:375), can have their paper coded as 'not containing sociological theory'?

In a study of disciplines, their boundaries and the possibility of national differences in the placement of disciplinary boundaries; it is important to consider the extent to which authors might make use of sociological theories and concepts, so that different groups of papers (national or otherwise) might be distinguished. This is only one of several variables which sets out to achieve this. At this point it must be emphasised that any judgements about what constitutes a sociological approach are necessarily made from a specific standpoint, and in this case, from the standpoint of an *Australian* sociologist who works solely within one set of disciplinary boundaries and makes no claim to multi-disciplinarity (Collyer 2011a:322). The importance of standpoint to this study, and the impact of standpoint on the definition of the discipline and its borders, is discussed in further depth in subsequent chapters.

Applicable words

Some studies (e.g. Seale 2008) rely on an electronic keyword identification system to discern patterns in the field. However not all journals or journal issues contain key words, as it is a rather modern practice, and moreover, authors use very different logics to assign key words to their manuscripts. Combined with the multi-faceted nature of words, where a single word may have a multiplicity of possible meanings, this problem makes automatic key word searches an inappropriate tool for a study of disciplines and discipline boundaries. An alternative is to manually code papers according to a concept of 'applicable words'. Applicable words are assigned by the researcher rather than the author to indicate whether the paper contains sustained discussion about, or relies upon, a specified range of topics or concepts (such as death, disability, capitalism, class, gender or HIV/AIDS). Unlike 'key words', 'applicable words' do not necessarily refer to the essential focus of a paper, but to one of its many elements. In all, variables for 42 applicable words were constructed for this study.

Health or medical topics of focus

Two variables were assembled to address the question of the main topics or subjects of each paper. Each paper could be coded for two topics. These did not distinguish between a 'primary' and 'secondary' focus, but were simply two major areas of focus. Unlike 'applicable words', the choice of topic was restricted to a smaller list and this is represented in Table 4.3.

Table 4.3   Health or medical topics

CAM or traditional medicine	Medical sociology
Comparative health systems	Professions or occupations or work
Disabilities or disability	Sexualities or gender
Education or training	Specific diseases or conditions
Health inequalities	Technologies or therapies
Health research or methodology	The health industry
Health or welfare policy	The health or medical research sector
History	The health-welfare system
Inequality	The illness experience
Meanings or language	The media
Medicalisation	The patient or consumer
Medical or health knowledges	Other

Sympathy towards medicine

A set of variables was constructed to indicate whether a paper displays a sympathetic, rather than critical approach towards biomedicine. The point of this variable stems from discussions in the sociological literature (and discussed above), about the 'sociology *of* medicine' versus the 'sociology *in* medicine'. In this debate, it is argued by some, such as Robert Straus (1957), that working within medical departments or taking medical sponsorship is likely to lead to the adoption of medical values, perspectives and the definition of problems. The debate has continued since the 1950s, yet little hard evidence has been offered in this intervening period. This set of variables is offered as a means to address the issue.

Papers were coded as either critical or sympathetic towards medicine. The best way to explain the rationale behind the values for this variable is to offer examples. The first code – critical of medicine – is illustrated with a paper by Nicky Britten (2001). Here we find a discussion of the proletarianisation and deprofessionalisation theses drawing upon research into the nature of clinical autonomy given changes of prescribing patterns in the British context. Britten (2001:491) argues that although there have been challenges to clinical autonomy from a number of state interventions, these have not radically altered the working conditions of doctors as described in the proletarianisation thesis. In making her case, the language used by Britten is taken as an example of being critical towards medicine, as she liberally employs phrases such as 'medical dominance'; tells us that doctors 'do not give patients the information about their medicines that they both want and need' (Britten 2001:478); says that doctors 'fail to explore patients' treatment preferences' (Britten 2001:488); and uses words such as 'dominant' when describing doctors and 'rhetoric' with regard to the medical literature (Britten 2001:487). Britten also shows her sympathy with patients, rather than doctors, in the statement:

> The conflict with the State is more overt than the conflict with patients, who are the weaker party. In fighting two adversaries, the medical profession uses patients ('clinical need') when this suits its case, and blames patients ('patient demand') when they obstruct its own objectives
>
> (Britten 2001:490–1).

A second critical paper is on the subject of mainstream medicine in Trinidad by David Reznik and colleagues (2007) from the United States. The lack of sympathy of these authors with the growing trend towards the market form of medicine in Trinidad is clearly expressed in the summary statement:

> Overall, then, the individualism and the market logic behind medical globalisation appear to push growing numbers of otherwise healthy people into becoming patients who purchase unneeded healthcare goods and services on the medical market
>
> (Reznik *et al.* 2007:548).

The coding of this paper as 'critical' indicates that the category can be used where there is criticism of medical *doctors* (as there is in the paper by Britten, discussed above), but also where there is criticism of 'medicine' as an *institution*, a set of organised *practices*, or even a *body of formal knowledge*.

A third paper illustrating this 'highly critical category' is Dingwall's (2001) piece on the performative use of legends, myths, and rumours. Whole paragraphs of this paper are critical of medicine. For instance:

> Doctors are the successors of priests, witches and shamans whose work seeks to manage those mysterious forces which threaten to destabilise everyday life. All of these people are licensed, formally or informally, to look over the edge of chaos, to appreciate that the apparent solidity of everyday life rests on a swirl of occult forces – or at least forces which are treated as occult for all the practical purposes of our mundane existence. But this delving is simultaneously a source of benefit and a source of threat. Those who create order may

also exploit it for their own gain. The rest of us constantly struggle to derive the benefits available to us while recognising that we have a limited capacity to prevent those who are privy to this mysterious knowledge from taking advantage of our ignorance

(Dingwall 2001:196).

Dingwall's (2001:196–7) paper is about the way rumour operates as an informal mechanism with the capacity to provide a 'check' on the 'ambitions' of doctors. It exists alongside the many formal mechanisms which have been devised to prevent doctors from 'abusing the power they derive from their mysterious knowledge'. Criticism is also shown in his descriptions of doctors. For instance, transplant surgeons are described as rather unsympathetic to patients, for they see patients as 'having a selfish and irrational attachment to their bodies, and those of their loved ones, even when they [their bodies] are no longer in working order' (Dingwall 2001:195).

Other papers are less critical of medicine but nevertheless belong within this 'critical' category. An example is provided by Nick Fox and Katie Ward (2008), who are critical of the medical profession assisting in the legitimation of a condition as a disease and thus enabling the widespread 'pharmaceuticalisation of daily life' and allowing companies to exploit consumers/patients. The paper is less critical than the papers above, because the medical profession is shown to be co-opted by the industry rather than a primary driver of pharmaceuticalisation. The pharmaceutical industry uses the Internet to inform consumers or sell directly to them, often circumventing the general practitioners, and consumers are increasingly willing to 'adopt technology as a "solution" to a problem in their lives' (Fox and Ward 2008:861, 865). Other 'active' agents in the new distribution process are 'academic opinion leaders, patient advocacy groups, public health bodies and ethicists' (Fox and Ward 2008:861). In other words, the medical profession and the institutions of medicine are complicit in the process, but no longer directly responsible for the widespread consumption of medical products.

Examples may also be provided of papers 'sympathetic' towards medicine. Parry's (2004) examination of the interaction between patients and physiotherapists in the clinical context demonstrates the way physiotherapists manage the bodily incompetence of patients through subtle gestures of the body as well as through conversation. Countering conventional, sociological criticisms of the clinical context, Parry argues that the apparent failure of physiotherapists to attend to the needs of patients are actually strategies to avoid causing distress to patients, and devised to keep the patients' "'deviant identity" off the interactional surface' (Parry 2004:1002). Throughout the article there is an attempt to present the clinical context as a *negotiated* order, rather than one of dominance or fraught with tension. Parry states:

> We observed patients responding in keen 'compliant' ways to thera-pists' instructions, deferring to therapists' judgements about abilities and treatments, and often not engaging in talk about their physi-cal difficulties. Analysis, however, demonstrated that through these patterns of conduct, therapists and patients protected one another and the therapeutic process as a whole from the problematic and threatening implications which might arise from episodes of physical incompetence
>
> (2004:1001).

The inclusion of Parry's study is therefore an example of a high level of sympathy with medicine. It is also an indication of the way, in this study, the para-professions or allied professions are considered part of the institution of medicine, particularly for the purposes of this variable.

A second example of a 'sympathetic' view of medicine is offered by Collyer (2007). In this paper, Collyer (2007:250) defines the health sys-tem as composed of both the clinical services sector and the health industry, 'wherein the provision of clinical services is not a defining feature but only one of many areas of social activity'. The qualitative study investigates the significant issues faced by medical and health sector workers from the perspective of the workers themselves. Find-ing that workforce shortages are a key concern of the participants, the study focuses on the workers' constructions of the threat posed by the neo-liberal policies of the Australian government and the chronic under-funding of universities and public hospitals. The paper is essentially a vehicle for the medical scientists and medical professionals to put forward their views about the policy context and the management of key institutions, and the negative effect on the disciplines and occupa-tions which make up the health care system. The coding of this final paper as 'sympathetic' indicates that a paper in this category might be highly critical of the nation state or other social institution, but sympathetic towards medicine, medical or health workers, processes of medicalisation, or medical knowledge.

A number of papers were considered neutral towards medicine or not relevant, and these were put aside for the period of the current analy-sis. Papers in this group include Yang's (2007) study, which investigates the possibility of a relationship between depression and ageing. The paper belongs in this category because it focuses on locating statistical associations between symptoms, risk factors (such as socio-economic and physical health status) and specific age cohorts. It does not attribute blame or responsibility for these conditions to any group, institution, aspect of the social system or social practice. Equally 'neutral' is the study by Wen and colleagues (2005), which measures the relationship between social network density and health status in the city of Chicago; and also Browning and Cagney's (2003) study of the association between health status and neighbourhood affluence. This latter paper focuses on the potential for middle-class residents to provide the essential organisational and economic resources to support community institutions and promote a healthy environment for all residents. It does not address the category of medicine, either with regard to medical workers, medical knowledges, or the institution of medicine.

Funding and sponsorship

This variable is designed to denote whether an author has received funding or sponsorship from an external body, and where this funding may have originated. Papers were coded according to the following schema:

1) Funded study, but no funding body stated.
2) Funded study, with a neutral funding body or sponsor stated.
3) Funded study, with a health or medical funding body or sponsor stated.
4) Not funded, or not applicable (funding unnecessary given the nature of the paper).

Examples of neutral funding bodies are those which are not directed by health or medical bodies and unlikely to be controlled by medical interests or members of the medical professions. They include the Australian Research Council (Australia), the European Social Fund, the National Census Data Collections Agency (USA), and in general, university grants that are not tied to specific health or medical bodies, such as a University Graduate School Doctoral Dissertation Fellowship (USA), Arts Faculty Grants (Australia), or Australian Post-Graduate Awards (Australia).

Examples of health or medical funding bodies include the Medical Research Council (UK), the National Health and Medical Research Council (Australia), the Innovative Technologies Programme of the Economic and Social Research Council (UK), the Nottingham Community Health

NHS Trust (UK), the National Institute of Mental Health (USA), the Centre For Disease Control (USA), World Health Organisation, Royal College of Surgeons (Australia), Pharmacy Guild (Australia), Commonwealth Department of Health (Australia), or the Nuffield Trust (UK).

Methods

A variable was devised to distinguish between papers on the basis of their methods. The variable indicates an author's approach (i.e. qualitative, quantitative, or both qualitative and quantitative), and is based on the kind of data presented in the paper. If it involves the statistical analysis of measurable data, it is treated as quantitative. If it involves textual analysis of a date set, it is coded as qualitative. Papers are coded as 'non-empirical' where they are primarily issue-based, conceptual or theoretical; do not contain a study to report upon; do not involve fieldwork; or do not treat their archival, statistical information or library material *as* data.

Who is a sociologist?

University textbooks and even many journal articles contain definitive statements about 'what sociology is'. These commonly refer to sociology in terms of its content. For instance, Collins (1985:38) suggests sociology to be 'the general science of social phenomena', and for Lopez (1982:8), it is 'a body of information about society and the interactions of individuals and groups within it'. Equally, in answer to the question of 'who is a sociologist?', a frequent response is one who studies 'the facts of society *in the spirit of a philosopher*' (Small 1903:469). In other words, sociologists are assumed to be *what they teach*, or *the perspectives or methods* they might adopt towards their subject matter. From a sociology of knowledge approach however, we must examine the social context of sociology, the context in which sociologists work, and explore the relationships between these and the ideas, methods and perspectives of its practitioners. This means taking note of the variation in sociology and its practice from one social location to another, regarding it as a discipline and a profession (Freidson 1986a), and exploring the influence of patronage networks, reward systems and market forces (Turner 1986a:273); but also the broader relations of power including gender, class and ethnicity (Bryson 1986). From this position, sociology as a body of knowledge and as a practice might vary substantially from one context to the next, as will perceptions of the discipline. For instance, in Stein's (1977) study of the discipline, it was proposed that in America, where sociologists are employed in community colleges as well as universities, perceptions of the discipline vary significantly. In the community colleges, where most staff are involved in teaching, but rarely publish, the discipline is less likely to be based upon a unique set of perspectives and have a distinct set of boundaries (Stein 1977:31).

Such studies suggest that adequate definitions of sociology and its practitioners must take into account the *symbolic* aspects of the discipline (including the way it is perceived, its content, theories and methodologies), as well as the *social structures* that shape the institutional context within which sociology is practised. In this study, a number of variables have been constructed to capture some of the latter (e.g. institutional location, gender, country, funding arrangements), but an additional variable is needed to attend to the symbolic realm.

The variable created for this purpose is reliant on the way authors in the study population publicly present themselves with regard to their discipline. It allows papers to be coded according to the disciplines, intellectual fields and occupations used by authors to describe themselves professionally within the institutional setting in their publications, curriculum vitae's, press releases and on institutional websites.

Institutional websites are the more important sources of information for this variable, though these have to be supplemented with other materials because institutions vary in the extent to which they give staff members the autonomy to arrange their own website material. Publicly available biographies have been an excellent source of information for this study, offering insights into the professional activities and affiliations of the authors. A significant number of authors also provide full curriculum vitae's attached to their web pages, giving further details of disciplinary contributions and associations.

Analysis of this variable provides information about the disciplinary affiliations of our authors. It tells us how many of the authors in our study population, and which ones, are presented publicly as sociologists (and which are not), and identifies the other disciplines and intellectual fields that cluster around, and help to form, the disciplinary boundaries of sociology. The variable also offers information on the question of whether the disciplinary boundaries differ from one country to the next, and helps us to gauge the relative status of the discipline in each location.

The list of possible values for this variable is provided in Table 4.4. Note that the terms vary between disciplinary affiliations (e.g. sociology), occupations (e.g. nurse), and intellectual field (e.g. feminist studies). In many cases, but not all, the descriptors align with the qualifications of the individual. Individuals are also often described

Table 4.4 The disciplinary descriptors

Sociology (or Medical Sociology)	– and Health Systems Analysis	'Research Scientist'
– and Anthropology (or Medical Anthropology)	– and Medicine	Social Policy
– and Biology	– and Psychiatry	Social Research
– and Biomedical Ethics (or Ethics)	– and Public Health	Social Science (or Applied or Qualitative Social Science)
– and CAM	Archaeology (or Ethno-Archaeology)	Social Work
– and Communications	Business or Management Studies	Statistics
– and Criminology	Communications	STS (or the History and Philosophy of Science)
– and Demography	Criminology	Other Arts or Social Science Disciplines
– And Disability Studies	Cultural Studies	Other Disciplines (but not stated)
– and Economics	Demography	Other Health/Medical Disciplines
– and Education	Dentistry	'Women's Rights Activist'
– and Epidemiology (or Social Epidemiology)	Dietetics (or Nutrition)	Economics and Business Studies (or Accounting)
– and Feminist Scholarship/Studies	Economics	Economics and Health Policy
– and Geography	Education	Ethics and Public Health
– and Gerontology (or Social Gerontology)	Epidemiology (or Social Epidemiology)	Health Services and Social Policy
– and Health Policy	Ethics (or Bioethics)	Law and Medicine
– and Health Research	Feminist Scholarship (or Feminist Studies)	Medicine and Epidemiology
– and Health Services Research	Fine Arts (or Visual or Performing Arts)	Medicine and Health Research
– and History	Geography (or Human or Social Geography)	Medicine and History of Medicine
– and Journalism	Gerontology	Medicine and Political Economy
– and Management	Health Communications	Medicine and Public Health
– and Medicine	Health Economics (or Health Finance)	Medicine and Cultural History
– and Micro-Biology	Health Policy	Nursing and Qualitative Research
– and Natural Science	Health Research	Nursing and Development Studies

Table 4.4 (Continued)

– and Nursing	Health Science	Nursing and Feminist Research
– and Pharmacy	Health Services (or Health Administration)	Nursing and Health Research
– and Philosophy	History	Nursing and Health Economics
– and Policy (or Social Policy)	History of Science and/or Medicine	Nursing and Public health
– and Political Science	International Relations	Nursing and Women's Health
– and Population Health	Law (or Legal Studies)	Nursing and Social Science
– and Psychiatry	Linguistics	Nursing and Philosophy of Science
– and Psychology (or Social Psychology)	Medical Statistics	Pharmacy and Health Policy
– and Public Health	Medicine	Philosophy and Feminist Scholarship
– and Public Sector Management	Organisational Theory	Policy and Population Health
– and Public Services Management	Nursing (or Midwifery)	Political Science and Feminist Scholarship
– and Research Science	Occupational Therapy	Psychiatry and Public Health
– and Science and Technology Studies (or History and Philosophy of Science)	Pharmacy	Psychology and Feminism/Queer Studies
– and Social Policy	Psychiatry	Psychology and Public Health
– and Social Work	Psychology (or Social Psychology)	Psychology and Women's Health
– and Socio-Legal	Psychotherapy	STS and Feminist Scholarship/Studies
– and Statistics	Policy Studies (or Policy)	Social Science and Women's Health
– and University Teaching	Political Science	Social Work and Public Health
Anthropology (or Medical, Social, or Cultural Anthropology)	Population Health	
– and Education	Public Administration	
– and Feminist Scholarship/Studies/Sexualities	Public Health	
– and Gerontology	Qualitative Research	

Note: 'Medical' sociology in this variable includes other, similar descriptions such as 'sociologist of health' or 'health sociologist'. The label 'medicine' refers to a medical practitioner. Note also that terms such as pharmacy are inclusive of similar words such as pharmacist.

in various ways, differing somewhat between institutional websites, publishers' advertising materials, personal biographies and various professional media statements. In such cases, the more prevalent descriptors were used as a basis for the codes.

Up to two descriptors were coded for each author, for the use of a single disciplinary term appears to be insufficient in some contexts, and many authors explicitly position themselves across, or between, two established fields. For example, Kathryn Ehrich of King's College London, states on her website that she is 'a medical sociologist and anthropologist'. Similarly, Fran McInerney of the Australian Catholic University says she is 'a registered nurse and a sociologist', and Alexandra McCarthy of Griffith University, Australia, places herself as 'a registered nurse and sociologist'. It is expected that the question of whether one adopts the identity of a sociologist will be determined by a range of factors, including the professional standing of the discipline in a given country, the location of the individual within an institution, and the field one works within (or between). The adoption of a descriptor, whether this is a sociologist, health services researcher or something else, is often a critical factor in the success or otherwise of an application for a grant, promotion or an employment position.

Note also that neither this variable nor the one above is time sensitive. Authors may have changed their professional/disciplinary identity between the date of publication of their paper in the data set, and the time of this research study. The difficulties associated with ascertaining an author's identity *at the time of the publication* led to the decision to disregard potential changes in identity over time for the purposes of these variables. In this way, a paper published in 1991 and selected for the data set may show the author as identified as a sociologist for this variable, even though the author may not have fully adopted the identity of a sociologist until 2005 after the completion of their PhD, gaining employment in a sociology department, publishing in mainstream sociology journals and a sociology textbook, and joining the sociological association.

5
National Trends in the Sociology of Health and Medicine since 1990

The results of the Content Analysis of the publications of sociologists from three countries are presented in this chapter. Here the reader will find descriptions of the kind of sociology produced in the various national contexts, and an analysis of their many similarities and differences. Some of the findings confirm the views and impressions offered by leading practitioners within the sociological community, but others challenge conventional notions and provide new information about the practice of sociology in Australia, the United Kingdom, and the United States.

Institutional context

One of the key questions for this study has been about where sociologists of health and medicine work. An examination of the institutional affiliations provided with each of the published papers in our study population reveals that among health and medical sociologists working in Australia, the United Kingdom and the United States, the significant majority work within the university sector. Examining the location of first authors, we find 97 per cent of Australian-based authors, 96 per cent of individuals from Britain, and 92 per cent from the United States, working within a university or similar higher education institution. A small number in each country have other affiliations, indicating some country variations. For instance, six per cent (or 14/225) of the authors based in the United States are affiliated with research institutes. This is a phenomenon not commonly found within the sociology of health and medicine in Australia, and appears not to be common in Britain either, as only one of our authors from this latter country works in a research institute. Other country variations include the number of authors working in a community-operated or professional organisation (such as a pharmaceutical or consumer rights society). Among the Australian-based authors, 5/361 (or one per cent) work in this form of organisation, and we find no authors from the two other countries in this kind of unit. A few authors from each of the three countries work in government departments. The figures for this are one per cent (or 5/361 individuals) for Australia, three per cent (or 7/225) for Britain, and one per cent (or 3/225) for the United States.

Within the university sector, our sociologists are widely dispersed across many departments and schools. A small number of authors are located within devoted health or medical sociology units. The figures for this are one per cent (or 4/361 individuals) in Australia, three per cent (or 7/225) in Britain, and none in the American context. In all cases, these units are embedded within departments or schools of sociology and hence appear in the first row of Table 5.1. The table shows the departmental or school location of all authors in our study population. The largest group of authors, 29 per cent, are found within *named* sociology departments (e.g. Departments of Sociology or mixed units such as a Department of Sociology and Social Policy). The prevalence of named sociology departments is greater in America than elsewhere. At the same time, proportionally more of the authors from Australia and Britain are situated within departments carrying the names of various humanities and social science disciplines, as well as from multi-disciplinary units (often called schools of social sciences, social enquiry or similar).

The naming of the affiliated departments or schools of the first authors reveals a number of cultural and institutional variations. For instance, among authors working in this field of the sociology of health and medicine, disciplines (or intellectual fields) such as political science, gender studies, and cultural studies appear only in the Australian context, while demography is found only among authors from the United States. Likewise, authors giving their work designation as 'epidemiology' occur more often among the authors from Australia and Britain. The prevalence or dearth of these affiliations tells us two things. First, it says something about the availability of 'more appropriate' journals for authors working in intellectual fields such as gender studies. Second, it suggests the presence of disciplinary boundaries between the various fields, and the way these boundaries vary from country to country. For instance, epidemiology is a distinctly separate discipline in Australia. It has its own journals and departments, and its methods and perspectives are often criticised by sociologists as having a thoroughly biomedical approach to health and illness. In contrast, the

Table 5.1 Departments and schools

	Australia		United Kingdom		United States		Totals	
The humanities and social sciences								
Sociology	75	*21%*	47	*21%*	116	*52%*	238	*29%*
Anthropology	6	*2%*	3	*1%*	7	*3%*	16	*2%*
Demography					3	*1%*	3	*1%*
Political Science	7	*2%*					7	*1%*
Cultural Studies	1	*1%*					1	
Gender Studies	4	*1%*					4	*1%*
Science and Technology Studies (or similar)	3	*1%*	2	*1%*	3	*1%*	8	*1%*
Criminology or Law	3	*1%*					3	
Policy Studies	2	*1%*	5	*2%*	1		8	*1%*
Other allied disciplines (e.g. Human Geography)	11	*3%*	10	*4%*	3	*1%*	24	*3%*
Psychology	1		3	*1%*	1		5	*1%*
Business, Management or Economics	9	*3%*	2	*1%*			11	*1%*
General social sciences	78	*22%*	24	*11%*	10	*4%*	112	*14%*
Humanities (e.g. History)	4	*1%*			2		6	*1%*
Other departments								
Non-aligned disciplines (e.g. Forestry)	2	*1%*	1		1		3	
Not classifiable	2	*1%*					3	
The health and medical departments								
Socio-Health units	32	*9%*	20	*9%*	11	*5%*	63	*8%*

Sexual Health or Public Health	27	7%	7	3%	18	8%	52	6%
Epidemiology	12	3%	5	2%	1		18	2%
Health Financing, Planning, Admin or Services	2	1%	16	7%	9	4%	27	3%
General health sciences	29	8%	23	10%	7	3%	59	7%
Nursing or Midwifery	24	7%	16	7%	3	1%	43	5%
Pharmacy or Dentistry	2	1%	4	2%	3	1%	9	1%
Medicine (including Psychiatry)	13	3%	29	13%	19	8%	61	8%
Other health or medical	12	3%	8	3%	7	3%	27	3%
Totals	361	100%	225	100%	225	100%	n = 811	100%

Notes: (i) percentages may not total 100 due to rounding; (ii) population of the table = 811, i.e. all authors in the study; (iii) the country of origin is derived from the affiliation provided by the first author of the paper, and indicates their place of employment at the time of publication; and (iv) work designations are drawn from the affiliations provided by the authors on their manuscripts. Given the lack of common terminology for the units in which academics are located, either within or between the three countries, the labels that best described the author's discipline were selected and coded for each author. This was regardless of whether the work unit was called a school, department, centre or faculty. Hence an author with a designation of 'Department of Sociology, School of the Social and Political Sciences' was coded as 'Sociology'; as was an author with an affiliation of 'Research Centre of Work and Family, School of Sociology'.

boundaries between sociology and epidemiology are more permeable in the United States, where it can be studied as a speciality area within sociology departments. The likelihood of an epidemiologist working within a sociology department in Australia is very low, but much higher in the United States. This issue is discussed more fully below.

The departmental or school affiliations of the authors can be grouped for greater ease of analysis. Table 5.2 indicates the new categories. The table shows that approximately half the authors come from sociology and allied disciplines within the humanities and social sciences, though the proportion is smallest in the United Kingdom and largest in the United States. It also reveals the major differences between the countries. Fewer British-based authors come from the arts and social sciences, relatively greater numbers are drawn from medicine, and a healthy segment come from the allied health areas, health financing and planning. In Australia, only small numbers are drawn from outside the arts and social sciences. In America, sociology and the allied disciplines are the dominant source of papers for this field, with the other three areas fairly equally represented.

Gender

The composition of the discipline of sociology in each country varies considerably with regard to gender. Focusing on the first authors in our study population, 69 per cent of these are women in the Australian context, 51 per cent in the British context, and 50 per cent among the authors from the United States. These proportional differences remain the same even where we focus only on the authors who present themselves as sociologists on their Websites and in other public media. Here 69 per cent of the Australian sociologists are women, 49 per cent of the British sociologists, and 49 per cent of the Americans.

This examination of the study population suggests the discipline is a feminine one in Australia, but more equally structured by gender in the other two countries. We might ask whether this has changed over time, and examine the shift between the first decade of our study and the second. Interestingly, women first authors have increased from 62 to 75 per cent in Australia, and from 48 to 52 per cent in the United States between the 1990s and the 2000s, but remained at 51 per cent for the British authors. The larger shift in the Australian context is likely to be only partly explained by the continuing attraction of the field for women. More pertinent is the higher retirement rate among male sociologists during the recent decade. These men were the first cohort of

Table 5.2 Departments and schools – Aggregated

	Australia		United Kingdom		United States		Totals	
Sociology and allied disciplines (e.g. Anthropology, Geography, Gender Studies, Social Work, Policy Studies, History and Law)	194	54%	91	41%	145	64%	430	53%
Non-allied disciplines and Allied Health (e.g. Psychology, Business, the general health sciences)	100	28%	68	30%	26	12%	194	24%
Public Health, Epidemiology, Sexual Health, Mental Health, Health Financing, Health Services Planning	41	11%	29	13%	29	13%	99	12%
Medicine and medical services	24	7%	36	16%	25	11%	85	11%
Totals	359	100%	224	100%	225	100%	808	100%

Notes: (i) percentages may not total 100 due to rounding; (ii) population of the table = 808, i.e. all authors in the study with the exception of three for whom details of institutional affiliation were unclear or unknown; (iii) departments/schools by country, statistically significant (Pearson's chi-square = .000); (iv) the country of origin is derived from the affiliation provided by the first author of the paper, and indicates their place of employment at the time of publication; and (v) the departments and schools are drawn from the labels of the work units provided by the authors on their manuscripts.

academic sociologists in the country, often gaining their higher degrees in Britain (and sometimes America), but returning to take up tenured positions in sociology. Similar trends are not in evidence in the United States with its longer history of institutionally based sociology.

Disciplines and identity

In addition to the Content Analysis of the manuscripts, an examination of various Websites and other publicly available materials was undertaken to ascertain the disciplines with which the authors are associated. This data is displayed in Table 5.3. Comparing the three countries, 69 per cent of the Australian-based authors, 67 per cent of the British, and 77 per cent of the Americans are presented in these materials as sociologists. Many of the sociologists are identified, or identify themselves, as 'sociologists of health', 'specialists in the sociology of health or medicine', or 'medical sociologists'. This data is presented in the upper section of the table. British-based authors appear more comfortable with the label of 'medical sociologist', with the majority of the sociologists using this descriptor. The rate at which authors adopt an identification of sociologist appears to have shifted over time. Measuring this between the first decade (1990–9) and the second (2000–10), more American-based authors have come to adopt this descriptor, with the trend rising from 70 per cent in the first period to 83 per cent in the second (and yielding an average of 77 per cent over the two decades, as shown in the table). In the United Kingdom and Australia, the shift is in the opposite direction. In the earlier decade, 75 per cent of the Australians and 74 per cent of the British authors use this descriptor, but this falls to 64 per cent for these two groups by 2010.

If we examine the study population as a whole, we find some of our authors are portrayed as sociologists, others as sociologists combined with other disciplines or fields, and a few from a range of other disciplines or intellectual fields. In Table 5.4, these disciplinary affiliations are shown, with those holding a single, sociological identity separated from the others (there are 305 individuals with only a sociological identity). The rest of the table represents the range of other disciplines in our study population. Thus, if an individual has two identities, such as sociology and anthropology, or a single discipline that is not sociology, such as anthropology, these will be counted in the figures for anthropology. Looking at the table, we find that among the other disciplines, anthropology has a significant presence, as does psychology, nursing, feminist studies, public health and epidemiology. We find several important

Table 5.3 Discipline/field identities

	Australia		United Kingdom		United States		Totals	
Sociologist	105	35%	58	27%	99	45%	262	35%
Medical Sociologist	103	34%	87	40%	72	32%	262	35%
Other	95	31%	72	33%	51	23%	218	29%
Total	303	100%	217	100%	222	100%	742	100%
Sociologist or Medical Sociologist	208	69%	145	67%	171	77%	524	71%
Other	95	31%	72	33%	51	23%	218	29%
Total	303	100%	217	100%	222	100%	742	100%

Notes: (i) percentages may not total 100 due to rounding; (ii) population of the table = 742, i.e. all authors in the study with the exception of a few for whom details of discipline identity were unclear or unknown; (iii) disciplinary identity by country, statistically significant (Pearson's chi-square = .002); (iv) the country of origin is derived from the affiliation provided by the first author of the paper, and indicates their place of employment at the time of publication; (v) the disciplinary affiliations are drawn from publicly available materials such as institutional Websites; and (vi) the term 'medical sociologist' includes similar descriptors such as 'sociologist of health'.

Table 5.4 Discipline/field identities – In detail

	Australia		United Kingdom		United States		Totals	
Sociology or Medical Sociology (only)	135	51%	92	47%	78	39%	305	46%
The other disciplines/fields								
Anthropology	18	7%	18	9%	24	12%	60	9%
Psychology	8	3%	14	7%	24	12%	46	7%
Nursing	26	10%	17	9%	1	1%	44	7%
Feminist Studies	21	8%	9	5%	4	2%	34	5%
Public Health	16	6%	6	3%	14	7%	36	5%
Epidemiology	10	4%	3	2%	17	8%	30	5%
Medicine	6	2%	10	5%	11	5%	27	4%
Policy	8	3%	12	6%	5	3%	25	4%
Demography	1		1	1%	14	7%	16	2%
Economics, Finance or Business Studies	9	3%	4	2%	2	1%	15	2%
Health Services Research	3	1%	6	3%			9	1%
Gerontology	1		1	1%	6	3%	8	1%
Allied Health (e.g. Dentistry, Pharmacy)	2	1%	3	2%			5	1%
Population Health			1	1%	1	1%	2	1%
Total	264		197		201		662	

Notes: (i) due to the existence of dual descriptors (e.g. Anthropology and Nursing), totals may be greater than the number of authors for each country, will not total 100, and cannot readily be compared with the results of Table 5.3; (ii) population of the table = 662, i.e. all authors in the study except where disciplinary identity was unclear or unknown; (iii) the country of origin is derived from the affiliation of the first author, and indicates their place of employment at the time of publication; and (iv) the disciplinary affiliations are drawn from publicly available materials such as institutional Websites.

country variations, particularly with regard to anthropology, psychology, epidemiology and demography: all of which are more common among the American-based authors. Nursing and feminist studies are found more frequently among the Australian authors, and policy among those working in Britain.

Many authors (35 per cent or 263/742) use two disciplines or intellectual fields to describe themselves, such as a sociologist and health services researcher (a new category which seems to have emerged in the 1990s), or sociologist and epidemiologist. It is more common to use these dual descriptors in America (46 per cent) than in Britain (32 per cent) or Australia (30 per cent) (statistically significant, Pearson's chi-square = .000).

We start to find an explanation for this phenomenon when we compare the authors who present themselves as sociologists with those who affiliate more closely with other disciplines (e.g. with geography or medicine). This other group of authors, despite being interested in some of the same issues as the sociologists and submitting at least some of their manuscripts to the same set of journals, are more likely to use a single discipline affiliation than are the sociologists (i.e. 80 per cent of non-sociologists use a single-identity descriptor compared with 58 per cent of the sociologists). What this hints at is the possibility of 'sociologist' being a less valuable or useful label in the academic or policy market place, requiring a supplementary label of some kind. Hence one-third or more of our sociologists use a dual descriptor such as sociologist and health policy researcher. The phenomenon varies across the three countries, with the greatest disparity occurring in the United States, where 46 per cent of sociologists use a single descriptor compared with 80 per cent of the non-sociologists; but it also appears among the British authors (63 compared with 78 per cent) and Australians (65–81 per cent). This suggests a 'sociological identity' is quite insufficient in the American context relative to the other two countries.

It is also useful to take note of the kinds of disciplines the sociologists are combining with their own. Although 33 other disciplines were found to be joined with sociology across the whole study population, many were used by only one or a very small number of authors (such as sociology and cultural history, or sociology plus neuro-science). The more common of the dual descriptors, where they were combined with sociology, are displayed in Table 5.5.

If we examine the disciplines commonly combined with sociology (or medical sociology) in the study population as a whole (and

Table 5.5 Common, dual discipline/field descriptors

	Australia		United Kingdom		United States		Totals	
Sociology (or Medical Sociology) and:								
– Psychology (and Social Psychology)	2	4%	7	18%	22	28%	31	18%
– Nursing	17	30%	9	24%	2	3%	28	16%
– Epidemiology (and Social Epidemiology)	4	7%			14	18%	18	11%
– Health Policy or Health (Services) Research	9	16%	5	13%	4	5%	18	11%
– Anthropology (and Social, Cultural or Medical)	4	7%	6	16%	6	8%	16	9%
– Feminist Studies	12	21%	3	8%	1	1%	16	9%
– Demography			1	3%	13	17%	14	8%
– Public Health	5	9%	3	8%	6	8%	14	8%
– Medicine	2	4%	3	8%	4	5%	9	5%
– Gerontology (and Social Gerontology)			1	3%	5	6%	6	4%
– Population Health	1	2%			1	1%	2	1%
Total	56	100%	38	100%	78	100%	172	100%

Notes: (i) percentages may not total 100 due to rounding; (ii) population of the table = 172, i.e. all authors in the study with the identity of a sociologist plus at least one other discipline (with the exception of a few for whom details of institutional affiliation or discipline identity were unclear or unknown); (iii) the country of origin is derived from the affiliation provided by the first author of the paper, and indicates their place of employment at the time of publication; and (iv) the disciplinary affiliations are drawn from publicly available materials such as institutional Websites.

represented in Table 5.5), the more prevalent ones are psychology, nursing, epidemiology, policy, anthropology and feminist studies. Variations across the three countries are most stark with regard to psychology, nursing, epidemiology, health policy, feminist studies, demography and public health. The examination of the disciplines or intellectual fields that our authors have combined with sociology, and those which they have not, provides insights into the borders of the discipline, and reveals how these borders vary from country to country.

In Australia, the most common disciplines or intellectual fields to combine with sociology (or medical sociology) are nursing (30 per cent), followed by feminist studies (21 per cent) and health policy research (16 per cent). Fields poorly represented are psychology (four per cent), epidemiology (seven per cent) and population health (two per cent). This provides an initial indication that psychology, epidemiology and population health might be oppositional fields in the Australian context, while nursing, feminist studies, and policy are more compatible with the kind of sociology found in this country.

In the United States a very different picture emerges. In that country it is much more common to combine sociology (or medical sociology) with psychology (28 per cent), epidemiology (18 per cent) or demography (17 per cent). All three of these disciplines utilise statistical techniques, and these are skills the Americans take considerable care to cultivate. It is less common for these authors to merge sociology with nursing (three per cent), feminist studies (one per cent), or policy studies (five per cent). These patterns suggest a compatibility between *American* sociology and the fields of psychology, epidemiology and demography, but the possibility of an adversarial relationship between sociology and nursing, feminist studies, and policy studies.

The situation in Britain is different again. Here we find an affinity with psychology that is not as strong as found in the United States, but closer than in Australia. Likewise, there are more sociologists combining their discipline with nursing, policy, or feminist studies than in the United States, but not as many as we see in Australia. In each of these, Britain stands as an intermediary between the other two countries. However the pattern is broken when we look to anthropology, where there is a higher level of alliance than elsewhere; epidemiology, which does not appear as a partner discipline; and medicine, which is relatively well represented in the country.

Identities, work units and disciplinary boundaries

Stronger indications of the compatibility or otherwise of the disciplines, of the existence of disciplinary boundaries and the extent to which such boundaries are permeable, can be found by examining the departmental contexts in which our authors work.

Some of our authors work in sociology departments, but others in organisational units, only some of which are discipline-based. If we investigate the relationship between the disciplinary identities of the authors and their work contexts, we find the prevalence of 'sociological identities' is higher within sociology departments than elsewhere. This means 95 per cent of authors located within sociology departments or schools present themselves as sociologists compared with 61 per cent of those working elsewhere (statistically significant, Pearson's chi-square = .000).

There are some country variations in this matter, though the trend is similar. All the authors based in Australian sociology departments present themselves as sociologists, all but three authors in British sociology departments, and all but seven in the American sociology departments (statistically significant, Pearson's chi-square = .000). As revealed in Table 5.6, in America, the exceptions refer to one demographer, five medical anthropologists, and one ethicist/public health expert. In Britain, one of the non-sociologists is an archaeologist, and two are consistently referred to as 'research scientists'. The high level of sociologists employed within sociology departments suggests that (at least within the speciality area of health and medical sociology) the departmental system is functioning in all three countries as a means to ensure the survival of the discipline and enforce its borders by generally excluding non-sociologists.

Continuing with our focus on the sociology departments, we can also examine the dual disciplinary affiliations of the workers, and consider which fields are being combined with sociology. The figures in this same table add more evidence of the phenomenon already tentatively suggested with regard to country variations in the incompatibility of some disciplines. What is immediately noticeable is the way, in the Australian and British context, demography, psychology, gerontology, epidemiology and public health are barely represented when compared to the disciplinary affiliations of the authors from the United States. This reveals the possibility of some discordance between sociology and these disciplines in the former two countries, but not the latter.

Table 5.6 Discipline identities and the sociology departments

	Australia		United Kingdom		United States		Totals	
Sociology (or Medical Sociology)	51	88%	24	54%	58	51%	133	62%
Sociology (or Medical Sociology) and:								
– Anthropology (or Medical Anthropology)	1	2%	2	5%	1	1%	4	2%
– Demography					8	7%	8	4%
– Psychology	1	2%	1	2%	18	16%	20	9%
– Nursing	1	2%	1	2%			2	1%
– Policy (or Health Policy)	2	3%	1	2%			3	1%
– Epidemiology (or Social Epidemiology)	2	3%			6	5%	8	4%
– Criminology			1	2%			1	1%
– Feminist Sudies			2	5%	1	1%	3	1%
– Pharmacy			1	2%			1	1%
– Medicine			1	2%	1	1%	2	1%
– Science and Technology Studies			4	9%	1	1%	5	2%
– Public Services Management			1	2%			1	1%
– Socio-Legal Studies			1	2%			1	1%
– Gerontology (or Social Gerontology)			1	2%	4	4%	5	2%
– Public Health					3	3%	3	1%
– Social Work					1	1%	1	1%

Table 5.6 (Continued)

	Australia		United Kingdom		United States		Totals	
– Ethicist (or Biomedical Ethicist)					2	2%	2	1%
– Biology					1	1%	1	1%
– Disability Studies					2	2%	2	1%
Archaeology			1	2%			1	1%
'Research Scientist'			2	5%			2	1%
Demography					1	1%	1	1%
Anthropology (or Medical Anthropology)					5	4%	5	2%
Ethics and Public Health					1	1%	1	1%
Totals	58	100%	44	100%	114	100%	216	100%

Notes: (i) percentages may not total 100 due to rounding; (ii) the population of the table = 216, representing the number of individuals working in sociology departments/schools or faculties for whom disciplinary-identity affiliations could be found or readily ascertained. This represents 216/238 individuals known to be employed within the departments of sociology and captured within our broader study population; (iii) the country of origin is derived from the affiliation provided by the first author of the paper, and indicates their place of employment at the time of publication; (iv) the departments or work units are provided by the authors on their manuscripts; and (v) disciplinary identities are taken from publicly available materials such as institutional Websites.

The sociologists: Identity, method and theory

Different disciplinary identities have an effect on the way authors employ sociological theory and the methods they use in their studies. Taking the issue of methodology first of all, Table 5.7 offers a comparison of the methods employed by all authors in our study (the upper section of the table), with those identified as sociologists (the middle section), and the non-sociologists (the lower section). Irrespective of whether we focus on all authors or simply the sociologists or non-sociologists, it is evident that quantitative approaches are significantly more common among our American authors, and that both Australia and Britain are predominantly qualitative. These results are consistent with other studies of American sociology, which suggest a national propensity towards the quantitative approach to research (Cockerham 1983:1520; Clair *et al.* 2007:249).

Focusing on the middle section (the sociologists), we find that the Australian work differs a little from the British, as it offers more quantitative studies (nine compared with seven per cent), and also produces a higher number of mixed method studies (18 compared with seven per cent). The methodology of the American papers is highly polarised, and there is a relatively low level of qualitative papers.

Comparing the lower two sections of the table, we find the same general trends, but different country patterns. Sociologists working in Australia are less quantitative than the non-sociologists, engage in more qualitative work, and more inclined to combine both methods. In the United Kingdom, sociologists are less likely to favour the use of both methods, and more likely to be qualitative in their approach. In the United States a very different set of practices can be seen. In that country, sociologists are much more likely to favour the use of quantitative methods, less likely to combine methods, and significantly less likely to be qualitative in their approach to research.

A second issue we can examine is the use of sociological theory among sociologists and other authors. The prevalence of theory in sociological work has often been considered a key attribute of the discipline and one of the discipline's defining features. In this study, a comparison of the extent to which theory is used by all authors, sociologists, and non-sociologists is shown in Table 5.8. The uppermost section of the table indicates the use of theory by all authors in our study population. It is apparent that in general, the majority (51 per cent) of authors display a high use of sociological theory in their papers, and only 13 per cent use no sociological theory at all.

Table 5.7 Sociological identities and method

	Australia		United Kingdom		United States		Totals	
All authors								
Qualitative	151	70%	149	85%	54	34%	354	64%
Both Qualitative and Quantitative	33	15%	15	9%	10	6%	58	11%
Quantitative	32	15%	12	7%	96	60%	140	25%
Total	216	100%	176	100%	160	100%	552	100%
Sociologists only								
Qualitative	88	73%	90	87%	39	31%	217	62%
Both Qualitative and Quantitative	21	18%	7	7%	6	5%	34	10%
Quantitative	11	9%	7	7%	81	64%	99	28%
Total	120	100%	104	100%	126	100%	350	100%
Non-sociologists only								
Qualitative	41	65%	55	82%	15	48%	111	69%
Both Qualitative and Quantitative	8	13%	8	12%	4	13%	20	12%
Quantitative	14	22%	4	6%	12	39%	30	19%
Total	63	100%	67	100%	31	100%	161	100%

Notes: (i) percentages may not total 100 due to rounding; (ii) papers which do not involve the use of empirical research are excluded from all sections of the table. The upper section refers to the population of all authors engaged in empirical studies (552). The centre section refers to the population of authors identified as sociologists and engaged in empirical work (350). The lower section includes all authors in the study population not identifying as sociologists but engaged in empirical work (161); (iii) all sections of the table are statistically significant. Upper and centre sections (Pearson's chi-square = .000), lower section (Pearson's chi-square = .002); (iv) the country of origin is derived from the affiliation provided by the first author of the paper, and indicates their place of employment at the time of publication; and (v) disciplinary identities are taken from publicly available materials such as institutional Websites.

Table 5.8 Sociological identities and the use of theory

	Australia		United Kingdom		United States		Totals	
All authors								
High use of sociological theory	195	54%	132	59%	86	38%	413	51%
Some use of sociological theory	73	20%	57	25%	46	20%	176	22%
Minimal use of sociological theory	46	13%	30	13%	45	20%	121	15%
No use of sociological theory	47	13%	6	3%	48	21%	101	13%
Total	361	100%	225	100%	225	100%	811	100%
Sociologists only								
High use of sociological theory	135	65%	99	68%	66	39%	300	57%
Some use of sociological theory	40	19%	31	21%	30	18%	101	19%
Minimal use of sociological theory	18	9%	13	9%	38	22%	69	13%
No use of sociological theory	15	7%	2	1%	37	22%	54	10%
Total	208	100%	145	100%	171	100%	524	100%

Table 5.8 (Continued)

Non-sociologists only	Australia		United Kingdom		United States		Totals	
High use of sociological theory	22	23%	32	44%	19	37%	73	34%
Some use of sociological theory	22	23%	22	31%	14	28%	58	27%
Minimal use of sociological theory	22	23%	14	19%	7	14%	43	20%
No use of sociological theory	29	31%	4	6%	11	22%	44	20%
Total	95	100%	72	100%	51	100%	218	100%

Notes: (i) percentages may not total 100 due to rounding; (ii) the upper section of the table refers to the total study population (811). The centre section refers to the population of authors identified as sociologists (524). The lower section includes all authors in the study population not identifying as sociologists (218); (iii) all sections of the table are statistically significant. Upper and middle sections (Pearson's chi-square = .000), lower section (Pearson's chi-square = .002); (iv) the country of origin is derived from the affiliation provided by the first author of the paper, and indicates their place of employment at the time of publication; and (v) disciplinary identities are taken from publicly available materials such as institutional Websites.

When sociologists (in the centre section of the table) are compared with non-sociologists (the lower section of the table), a generally lower use of sociological theory is found among the non-sociologists (34 per cent of the non-sociologists compared with 57 per cent of the sociologists display a high use of theory). This higher prevalence of sociological theory in papers belonging to sociologists relative to authors identifying with other disciplines is a statistically significant association (Pearson's chi-square = .000).

In addition, there are notable country differences in the use of sociological theory. Focusing for a moment on the centre section of Table 5.8, sociologists from Australia and the United Kingdom display a much greater use of sociological theory than their colleagues in the United States (65 and 68 per cent of high users of sociological theory compared with only 39 per cent of the sociologists from the United States). Equally, only seven per cent of the Australian sociologists and one per cent of the British sociologists show no use of sociological theory, contrasted with 22 per cent of those from the United States.

A comparison may also be made between the sociologists and non-sociologists of each country. Focusing on the centre and lower sections of Table 5.8, we find very marked differences between the sociologists and non-sociologists in Australia, and also Britain, but remarkably similar trends for the United States. In other words, sociological theory appears to be a distinguishing feature of the discipline in Australia and Britain, but less so in the United States. This suggests much stronger disciplinary boundaries in the first two countries, and more permeable boundaries in the third.

Differences in methodology and the use of sociological theory among sociologists in the three countries need further investigation and explanation. While the adoption of a sociological identity in Australia and the United Kingdom is associated with the use of sociological theory, this does not appear to be the case for authors from the United States. The lower use of sociological theory and the similarity of usage between the sociologists and the non-sociologists from the United States are associated with a number of other factors. For one, in both Australia and the United Kingdom, the higher rate of theory use among sociologists is also found among those who engage in a greater number of sociological practices (such as attending sociological conferences). This doesn't occur in the United States, where regardless of sociological commitment, theory use remains at the same, relatively low level.

These unique results for authors from the United States make more sense when we conceptualise American sociology as significantly heterogeneous, or even polarised. Unlike the other two countries, which display considerable homogeneity across their academic, sociological communities, American sociology has long been a diverse and somewhat fractured discipline. This diversity is not apparent with regard to sociological practices, but is associated with variations in the use of theoretical frameworks and methods. If we conceptualise the American discipline as comprised of at least two, diverse forms of sociology, rather than one homogenous body of knowledge and practice, the differences between the three countries become more explicable.

The heterogeneity of American sociology makes it important to alter the way we compare the three countries. In Britain and Australia, the significant comparisons are between sociologists with non-sociologists. These two groups provide a set of diverse – and oppositional – sets of characteristics and practices. However among American authors, differences between sociologists with non-sociologists appear on some measures, but there is greater variation between some groups of sociologists and others. When the two groups of sociologists in America are identified, we find one of these producing a type of sociology not entirely dissimilar to that found in Britain and Australia. This group, like the British and the Australians, scores highly on the use of sociological theory, and also conducts qualitative, not just quantitative research.

There are a number of characteristics which define this first group. First, they are identifiable as sociologists. Second, they use single, rather than dual discipline descriptors. With the use of these two variables to distinguish the two groups, sociologists of health and medicine in the United States might be divided into two camps, with the first identified as USA (1), where its members use a single discipline descriptor, and the second identified as USA (2), where authors employ dual discipline descriptors. Some of the characteristics which differentiate the two groups are set out in Table 5.9. Re-examining the use of theory and the methodological approach of the countries, and this time also showing the different groups *within* the United States, we find that more sociologists from USA (1) use qualitative methods (44 per cent) compared with sociologists from USA (2) (20 per cent). Likewise, there is a much higher rate of the use of sociological theory from USA (1) (54 per cent) compared with USA (2) (26 per cent). With regard to both theory and method, the first group within the United States shows a much greater resemblance to the sociologists of Australia and Britain, than it does to the other American sociologists of USA (2).

Table 5.9 Divergent sociologies: Method and theory

Sociologists only	Australia		United Kingdom		United States		USA (1)		USA (2)	
Qualitative	88	73%	90	87%	39	31%	25	44%	14	20%
Both Qualitative and Quantitative	21	18%	7	7%	6	5%	3	5%	3	4%
Quantitative	11	9%	7	7%	81	64%	29	51%	52	75%
Totals	120	100%	104	100%	126	100%	57	100%	69	100%
High use of sociological theory	135	65%	99	68%	66	39%	42	54%	24	26%
Some use of sociological theory	40	19%	31	21%	30	18%	14	18%	16	17%
Minimal use of sociological theory	18	9%	13	9%	38	22%	15	19%	23	25%
No use of sociological theory	15	7%	2	1%	37	22%	7	9%	30	32%
Totals	208	100%	145	100%	171	100%	78	100%	93	100%

Notes: (i) percentages may not total 100 due to rounding; (ii) papers which do not involve the use of empirical research are excluded from the upper section of the table. The upper section (country comparison) is the population of all authors engaged in empirical studies, and who are identified as sociologists (350). The lower section refers to the population of authors identified as sociologists for whom disciplinary identity is known (524). For USA (1 and 2), the population in the upper section refers to sociologists who undertake empirical work (126). In the lower section, the population is composed of sociologists for whom disciplinary identity is known (171); (iii) 'method' is statistically significant for Australian, British and American authors (Pearson's chi-square = .000); 'theory' is statistically significant for Australian, British, and American authors (Pearson's chi-square = .002); for USA (1 and 2), 'method' by 'dual or single' field descriptor: statistically significant (Pearson's chi-square = .014); for USA (1 and 2), 'theory' by 'dual or single' field descriptor: statistically significant (Pearson's chi-square = .000); (iv) the country of origin is derived from the affiliation provided by the first author of the paper, and indicates their place of employment at the time of publication; and (v) disciplinary identities are taken from publicly available materials such as institutional Websites.

This study is not the first to acknowledge the diversity within American sociology. Although some (e.g. Lipset 1994) regard this as an outcome of political differences and ideological struggle, others, such as Leonard Pearlin (1992), see divergences in substantive interests, theoretical perspectives and methodology. Given the propensity of medical sociology to mirror the trends and developments of the larger discipline, Pearlin's (1992:2) reflections on the sub-field suggest the major division is between those 'who seek to reveal structure in social life' and those 'who seek to reveal the meaning in social life'. Although Pearlin (1992:2) argues that the 'structure seekers' and 'meaning seekers' do not refer to 'concrete groups with clearly delineated boundaries', this is contradicted by the evidence of this chapter. It may be the case that sociologists don't identity *themselves* as seekers of 'structure' rather than 'meaning', but there *are* different groups of sociologists working in the United States, and they use startlingly different sets of theories and methodologies. We might broadly differentiate between the groups on the basis of methodology, as Pearlin has done, but a more accurate division is achieved using the variable based on the 'dual versus single' discipline descriptors of the sociologists. There is of course a significant association between the discipline descriptors and methodology, for as we have seen in Table 5.9, the first group of American sociologists are higher users of qualitative methods and the second group of sociologists higher users of quantitative methods. Nevertheless, there are a number of other differences between the two groups of sociologists which can be demonstrated using the 'dual versus single' discipline descriptors, and these will be revealed throughout the rest of the chapter.

Authorship teams

The extent to which publications are sole authored, rather than produced by a team of collaborating authors, varies from country to country. Sole authorship is highest in Australia, and lowest in the United States. There is also a difference between papers authored by sociologists and non-sociologists, as sociologists are more likely to be sole authors, or collaborate with fewer individuals than non-sociologists. This information is displayed in Table 5.10, where 70 per cent of sociologists in Australia have published by themselves compared with 62 per cent of their non-sociological colleagues. Likewise, 55 per cent of the sociologists in the United Kingdom have published by themselves, compared with 38 per cent of the non-sociologists. The difference is smallest in the United States, where 40 per cent of sociologists and 39 per cent of the

Table 5.10 Authorship teams

	Australia		United Kingdom		United States		USA (1)		USA (2)	
Sociologists										
Number of authors										
One author only	146	70%	80	55%	68	40%	37	47%	31	33%
Two authors	38	18%	32	22%	53	31%	22	28%	31	33%
Three authors	16	8%	18	12%	29	17%	11	14%	18	19%
Four or more authors	8	4%	15	10%	21	12%	8	10%	13	14%
Total	208	100%	145	100%	171	100%	78	100%	93	100%
Non-sociologists										
Number of authors										
One author only	59	62%	27	38%	20	39%	16	39%	4	40%
Two authors	23	24%	18	25%	15	29%	10	24%	5	50%
Three authors	6	6%	12	17%	6	12%	6	15%		
Four or more authors	7	7%	15	21%	10	20%	9	22%	1	10%
Total	95	100%	72	100%	51	100%	41	100%	10	100%

Notes: (i) percentages may not total 100 due to rounding; (ii) the population of the table consists of all authors for whom disciplinary identity is known (sociologists = 524, non-sociologists = 218); (iii) number of authors by country, statistically significant (Pearson's chi-square = .000). Number of authors by sociological identity, statistically significant (Pearson's chi-square = .046). Number of authors by sociologists only, statistically significant (Pearson's chi-square = .000). Number of authors by non-sociologists, statistically significant (Pearson's chi-square = .010); (iv) the country of origin is derived from the affiliation provided by the first author of the paper, and indicates their place of employment at the time of publication. Statistical tests were unavailable for USA (1) and (2) due to the small number of papers in these categories; and (v) disciplinary identities are taken from publicly available materials such as institutional Websites.

non-sociologists publish by themselves. In other words, sole-authorship is a distinguishing feature of sociologists in Australia and Britain, but not the United States.

The differences within the United States are also shown in Table 5.10. A comparison between sociologists and non-sociologists from the United States is not particularly valid, given the small number of authors in the latter group. Nevertheless there is some indication of a tendency for non-sociologists (whether holding dual or single identity) from the United States to share similar characteristics in this matter to non-sociologists from the United Kingdom. The more informative aspect of the table is where sociologists in the first American group, USA (1), show greater similarity to the sociologists of Australia and the United Kingdom than they do with the sociologists of USA (2). In other words, we can locate one group of sociologists in the United States with a high rate of sole authorship and another group with a higher rate of collaborative authorship.

The proportion of sole authorship versus collaborative publishing among sociologists has changed a little over time, with a general rise in collaborative work of about ten per cent between the 1990s and the next decade across the three countries. As displayed in Table 5.11, there are differences between the two decades in each of the countries. In Australia we see a fall in the number of sociologists publishing by themselves (from 73 to 68 per cent), and although there is no growth in the number of papers published by three or more authors, there is a small shift (of 16–20 per cent) towards collaboration with one other person. In the United Kingdom, the rate of single authorship does not change over time, but there is a growth in the size of the teams undertaking collaborative work. In this country, the number of papers written by large teams of four or more authors increases quite dramatically from two per cent in the first decade to 15 per cent in the second. In the United States, the second decade sees a significant fall from 49 to 34 per cent in sole authorship, and a growth in large teams of writers from 6 to 16 per cent. These shifts in the United States occurred in both USA (1) and (2).

Citation patterns

In this study, the more common citations found in each paper were noted, and can be analysed to make a number of broad observations about the 'reservoir of ideas' among sociologists of health and medicine across the three countries. Table 5.12 displays the rates at which authors are cited in our study population for the three countries (with the

Table 5.11 Authorship teams over time

Sociologists only	Australia		United Kingdom		United States		USA (1)		USA (2)	
1990–9										
One author only	68	73%	29	56%	32	49%	14	58%	18	43%
Two authors	15	16%	16	31%	19	29%	8	33%	11	26%
Three authors	7	8%	6	12%	11	17%	1	4%	10	24%
Four or more authors	3	3%	1	2%	4	6%	1	4%	3	7%
Total	93	100%	52	100%	66	100%	24	100%	42	100%
2000–10										
One author only	78	68%	51	55%	36	34%	23	43%	13	26%
Two authors	23	20%	16	17%	34	32%	14	26%	20	39%
Three authors	9	8%	12	13%	18	17%	10	19%	8	16%
Four or more authors	5	4%	14	15%	17	16%	7	13%	10	20%
Total	115	100%	93	100%	105	100%	54	100%	51	100%

Notes: (i) percentages may not total 100 due to rounding; (ii) the population of the table consists of all authors identified as sociologists in the study population (524); (iii) authorship teams by country is statistically significant for 2000–10 (Pearson's chi-square = .000); and for 1990–9 (Pearson's chi-square = .051). Statistical tests for the two USA groups are unavailable given the small numbers of papers; and (iv) the country of origin is derived from the affiliation provided by the first author of the paper, and indicates their place of employment at the time of publication.

Table 5.12 Citations by country

	Australia	United Kingdom	United States	Total	USA (1)	USA (2)
Annandale, Ellen	5	16	2	23		1
Arber, Sara	3	14	5	22	1	1
Armstrong, David	13	28	6	47	3	2
Bauman, Zygmund	10	12	4	26	1	3
Becker, Howard	2	11	17	30	5	8
Beck, Ulrich	20	12	7	39	3	3
Bendelow, Gillian	2	11	2	15	1	
Berger, Peter	7	9	3	19	2	1
Berkman, Lisa	4	1	26	31	8	15
Blaxter, Mildred	8	24	5	37	2	1
Bloor, Michael	2	15	2	19	1	1
Bourdieu, Pierre	14	22	13	49	6	2
Broom, Dorothy	18	7	2	27		2
Brown, Phil	2	13	16	31	9	2
Bury, Mike	11	44	15	70	11	1
Busfield, Joan	3	12		15		
Calnan, Michael	11	25	2	38		
Chapman, Simon	11	1	2	14		1
Charmaz, Kathy	9	25	12	46	8	3
Clarke, Adele	1	6	8	15	4	3
Collyer, Fran	16		2	18		2
Connell, Raewyn (R.W.)	23	8	2	32	2	
Conrad, Peter	9	17	31	57	15	10
Corbin, Juliet	10	22	13	45	7	4
Denzin, Norman	7	10	5	22	4	1
Dingwall, Robert	2	25	2	29	1	1
Dohrenwend, Bruce			22	22	9	11
Douglas, Mary	12	15	4	31	1	1
Doyal, Leslie	7	12	5	24	2	
Durkheim, Emile	7	4	15	26	3	8
Elias, Norbert	5	12		17		
Engel, G.L.	4	5	5	14	2	3
Field, David	5	21	3	29	3	
Foucault, Michel	36	38	15	89	6	4
Fox, Nicholas	8	14	3	25	2	
Fox, Renee	4	5	14	23	6	5
Freidson, Elliot	14	24	31	69	17	9
Freund, Peter	3	8	5	16	2	2
Gabe, Jonathon	5	24	2	29	1	
Garfinkel, Harold	3	7	4	14	4	

Table 5.12 (Continued)

	Australia	United Kingdom	United States	Total	USA (1)	USA (2)
Radley, Alan	2	13	2	17	1	1
Riessman, Catherine	4	10	7	21		7
Rose, Nikolas	15	26	3	**44**	1	2
Ross, Catherine	2	2	34	38	15	16
Scambler, Graham	5	13	6	24	3	3
Seale, Clive	5	14	2	21	2	
Scheff, Thomas J.	3	4	8	15	5	3
Schutz, Alfred	2	11	3	16	3	
Sheper-Hughes, N.	1	9	8	18	2	1
Shilling, Chris	11	16	1	28		
Short, Stephanie	14			14		
Silverman, David	5	17	6	28	2	2
Sontag, Susan	6	6	4	16	2	1
Stacey, Margaret	2	17		19		
Starr, Paul	2	2	14	18	5	4
Stoeckle, John D.	2	1	11	14	4	4
Strauss, Anselm	23	55	29	**107**	17	9
Strong, Phil	2	19	3	24	1	2
Syme, S. Leonard	2	1	17	20	3	10
Szasz, Thomas S.	5	4	8	17	1	7
Thoits, Peggy	1	2	25	28	4	19
Townsend, Peter	1	12	2	15		
Treichler, Paula	3	4	11	18	5	3
Turner, Bryan	37	32	10	**79**	5	3
Turner, R. Jay		1	15	16	3	11
Verbrugge, Lois	1	4	25	30	7	17
Waitzkin, Howard	2	3	21	26	13	6
Weber, Max	11	7	11	29	5	5
White, Kevin	14	1		15		
Williams, Simon	13	32	8	**53**	5	
Williams, Gareth	10	42	11	**63**	8	2
Willis, Evan	38	1	2	**41**		2
Zola, Irving	8	11	18	37	5	8

Notes: (i) raw figures for Australia have been adjusted to ensure they are proportional to those of the United Kingdom and United States (i.e. 225 papers from each country). The number of papers coded for USA (1) was 78, and for USA (2) it was 92; (ii) figures for USA (1) and (2) refer to sociologists only, and are therefore not directly compatible with those from Australia, United Kingdom and United States, which are for all authors; and (iii) only the most highly cited authors are represented in this list.

less commonly cited authors removed and raw figures adjusted for Australia to ensure comparability). The most frequently cited authors are Anselm Strauss (107), Michel Foucault (89), Deborah Lupton (82), Bryan Turner (79), Anthony Giddens (78), Erving Goffman (71), Mike Bury (70), Elliot Freidson (69), Gareth Williams (63), Peter Conrad (57), Simon Williams (53), Talcott Parsons (51), Arthur Kleinman (51), David Mechanic (50), Pierre Bourdieu (49), David Armstrong (47), Kathy Charmaz (46), Juliet Corbin (45), Nikolas Rose (44), John B. McKinlay (42), and Evan Willis (41).

There are several features of these citation rates which are notable. First, two European theorists have made a strong impact in each of the three countries: Pierre Bourdieu and Michel Foucault. Second, authors in each country generally pay particular attention to a small number of authors who are based (or primarily based) in that country, and ignore the majority of authors from elsewhere. In other words, we are all rather inward-looking with regard to the sources of sociological knowledge. That said, the extent to which each country is 'closed' to the knowledge available elsewhere is variable. In the United Kingdom the highly cited *local* authors are Bryan Turner, Giddens, Bury, Gareth Williams, Simon Williams, Armstrong, Rose, Calnan, Blaxter, Field, Gabe, Kelly, and Dingwall. Some attention is paid to authors from other countries where these publish in *British* journals (e.g. Lupton, Connell), but also to individuals who regularly participate in local conferences, take up local appointments or otherwise collaborate with the locals. The proportion of highly cited local authors to 'foreign' authors is strongly in favour of the locals (a ratio of 11:6).

In the United States, the most highly cited local authors are Strauss, Goffman, Freidson, Parsons, Kleinman, Mechanic, Conrad, Charmaz, Corbin, McKinlay, Light, Ross, Pearlin, Berkman, Verbrugge, Link, Mirowsky, Thoits, House, Kreiger, Waitzkin and Dohrenwend. Little attention is given to authors from other countries, and few 'foreign' sociologists are published in American-based journals. The proportion of highly cited local authors to 'foreign' authors is very strongly in favour of the locals (a ratio of 50:6). The country is not entirely immune to outside influence however, as it is a country of migrants and when these come to work in the United States they may be given some attention, introducing variation in the otherwise very homogenous national programme of research (e.g. McKinlay was born in New Zealand, while Goffman was from Canada).

In Australia the most highly cited local authors are Lupton, Bryan Turner, Willis, Connell, Petersen, Broom, Collyer, Kellehear, Kippax,

White, Chapman, Short, and Lawler. Although local scholars are highly cited, significant attention is paid in this country to scholars from the United States and the United Kingdom. The proportion of highly cited, local authors to 'foreign' authors is very even (a ratio of 6:6). This is clearly the most open of the three countries, with most of the professional interaction flowing from Australia towards the other two countries. Very few Australian-based authors are cited in the United Kingdom and/or the USA journals. International impact, where it occurs, results from the strategic and sustained effort on the part of individual sociologists (sometimes assisted by university management). Important strategies include the submission of Australian work to international journals, international conference participation, the taking up of employment opportunities overseas (i.e. Bryan Turner, Connell, Petersen, Kellehear), and an engagement in research collaboration (e.g. Lupton, Broom, Willis). In the previous section, 'Authorship teams', we discussed the general trend towards increasing collaboration and a decrease in sole authorship over the recent decade. That trend, noticeable also in Australia, appears to have had some (though limited) impact in the extent to which Australian work is being cited in the other two countries.

A third point of note regards the 'two sociologies' of the United States. With the exception of Mike Bury, few authors from outside the United States are cited frequently by either group, and although they share Erving Goffman, Catherine Ross, and David Mechanic, the two USA groups are remarkably different. The highly cited authors in the USA (1) group are Strauss, Freidson, Conrad, Mechanic, Ross, Waitzkin, Light and Bury. In contrast, authors cited frequently by the USA (2) group include Pearlin, Thoits, Verbrugge, Ross, House, Link, Berkman, Mirowsky, Dohrenwend, Ray Turner, Phelan and Syme. The two groups clearly have different literatures to which they respond and contribute.

Moreover, where the citations of USA (2) are proportionally higher than those of USA (1), in most cases the author in question also has a low citation count among the authors from Australia and the United Kingdom. For instance, Lisa Berkman has a high citation count within the USA (2) group, a much lower one within USA (1), and a relatively low count from the authors of Australia and the United Kingdom. This also occurs with the sociologists House, Link, Mirowsky, Pearlin, Phelan, Thoits and Verbrugge. The opposite is not the case, for where the USA (1) group cite an author frequently, there is a similarly high rate from the authors of Australia and/or the United Kingdom (e.g. Bury, Conrad, Freidson, Strauss, Waitzkin and Gareth Williams). These figures confirm earlier indications of two very different sociologies within the

United States, because the kind of reference materials constructed by and applied within a discipline are a defining feature of that discipline. In addition, the markedly different kind of sociology conducted by USA (2) on the one hand, and the similarity between the reference materials of USA (1), Australia and the United Kingdom on the other, lends some support to the idea that the latter three groups share substantial features of their discipline.

Subjects, interests and concerns

There has been considerable debate about the extent to which there might be national differences in the kind of issues, problems, or subjects that sociologists study and write about. In this piece of research all papers were coded using the variable 'applicable words' in order to address this question. 'Applicable words' doesn't provide information about the *essential focus* of the papers: that matter is given attention in the next section of this chapter 'Medical sociology: Major areas of focus'. Instead, 'applicable words' gives us a sense of how often each subject is included within the population of papers. The use of this variable indicates that very few sociologists in the study population are interested in subjects such as religion (about four per cent of sociologists), social movements (about six per cent), social capital (about two per cent), globalisation (about two per cent), food or nutrition (about five per cent), children (about nine per cent), ageing (about five per cent), refugees (about one per cent), and youth (about two per cent). The more prevalent topics are presented in Table 5.13.

In this table, the issues are grouped into several categories for ease of analysis and presentation. The various areas of *shared* concern, where little difference appears from country to country, are those of 'death, euthanasia or hospice care', and the 'risks' of drugs, alcohol, HIV/AIDS and risk in general (about 11 per cent of the papers). Significant differences appear with the other categories however. In the uppermost section of the table is 'The work context'. Here we can see a proportionally greater level of interest among sociologists from Australia (average of 25 per cent), and also from sociologists in the first group of American sociologists relative to the second.

In the second section of Table 5.13, a similar trend appears, with significantly higher numbers of Australian sociologists writing about the subjects of 'masculinity, sexuality, gender and reproduction'. Note also the greater level of interest from USA (2), though this is with regard to 'gender' and 'reproduction' rather than 'masculinity' or 'sexuality'.

Table 5.13   Subjects and interests by country

(Sociologists only)	Australia		United Kingdom		United States		USA (1)		USA (2)	
The work context										
Doctors, the clinic, doctor–patient relationships	67	32%	48	33%	53	31%	30	39%	23	25%
Work	67	32%	40	28%	43	25%	22	28%	21	23%
Division of labour	38	18%	29	20%	19	11%	12	15%	6	8%
Medical dominance/power	63	30%	24	17%	25	15%	9	12%	16	17%
Nurses	22	11%	10	7%	2	1%	2	3%		
Average percent		25%		21%		17%		19%		15%
Sexuality										
Masculinity	14	7%	10	7%	5	3%	2	3%	3	3%
Sexuality	33	16%	13	9%	35	21%	12	15%	23	25%
Gender	86	41%	38	26%	18	11%	3	4%	15	16%
Reproduction (birth, contraception, abortion, etc.)	47	23%	22	15%						
Average percent		22%		14%		9%		6%		11%
Race and class										
Race, ethnicity or indigenous	24	12%	9	6%	28	17%	11	14%	17	18%
Class or socio-economic status	25	12%	14	10%	47	28%	23	30%	24	26%
Average percent		12%		8%		23%		22%		22%
Dying and death										
Death, euthanasia, hospice care	21	10%	18	12%	13	8%	6	8%	7	8%
Average percent		10%		12%		8%		8%		8%

Risks										
Drugs or alcohol	20	*10%*	21	*15%*	27	*16%*	17	*22%*	10	*11%*
HIV/AIDS	15	*7%*	7	*5%*	11	*6%*	6	*8%*	5	*5%*
Risk	31	*15%*	18	*12%*	17	*10%*	3	*4%*	14	*15%*
Average percent		*11%*		*11%*		*11%*		*11%*		*10%*
Knowledge, measurement										
Sociology (reflections on the discipline)	48	*23%*	25	*17%*	26	*15%*	11	*14%*	15	*16%*
Science and/or technology	59	*28%*	30	*21%*	36	*21%*	17	*22%*	19	*20%*
History	67	*32%*	25	*17%*	16	*9%*	8	*10%*	8	*9%*
Method or methodology	20	*10%*	6	*4%*	27	*16%*	9	*12%*	18	*19%*
Knowledge (truth, certainty, positivism, classificationism, etc.)	102	*49%*	64	*44%*	59	*35%*	24	*31%*	35	*38%*
Average percent		*28%*		*21%*		*19%*		*18%*		*20%*
The market										
Consumers, consumption	56	*27%*	31	*21%*	33	*19%*	24	*31%*	9	*10%*
Capitalism, the market, profit	30	*14%*	12	*8%*	15	*9%*	10	*13%*	5	*5%*
Average percent		*21%*		*15%*		*14%*		*22%*		*7%*

Notes: (i) percentages will not total 100 as this is a composite table with concepts calculated and coded separately. Papers were coded as either positive or negative for the relevance of each word. Percentages refer to the number of papers in that country which were coded positively for the word compared with the number of papers where it was not applicable (e.g. 22 papers from Australian first authors were coded positively for the word 'nurses', which was 22/208 papers = 11 per cent); (ii) all papers represented in this table are from first authors identified as sociologists ($n = 524$, i.e. 208 Australia, 145 UK, 171 USA (1) and 93 USA (2)); (iii) statistically significant differences were found for Australia, the United Kingdom, and the United States versus 'sexuality' (Pearson's chi-square = .000), 'reproduction' (Pearson's chi-square = .000), 'race' (Pearson's chi-square = .007), 'nurses' (Pearson's chi-square = .001), 'method' (Pearson's chi-square = .003), 'medical dominance' (Pearson's chi-square = .000), 'masculinity' (Pearson's chi-square = .002), 'knowledge' (Pearson's chi-square = .016), 'history' (Pearson's chi-square = .000), 'gender' (Pearson's chi-square = .000), and 'class' (Pearson's chi-square = .000); (iv) in general, statistical tests were unavailable for USA (1) and (2) due to the small number of papers in these categories. However statistically significant differences were found for USA (1) and (2) versus 'risk' (Pearson's chi-square = .015), 'reproduction' (Pearson's chi-square = .009), 'drugs' (Pearson's chi-square = .049), 'doctors' (Pearson's chi-square = .053), and 'consumers' (Pearson's chi-square = .000); and (v) the country of origin is derived from the affiliation provided by the first author of the paper, and indicates their place of employment at the time of publication.

The third section of the table concerns 'race and class'. These matters are of specific interest for the sociologists from the United States (23 compared with 12 from Australia and only eight per cent from the United Kingdom), and it is a subject matter equally shared across both American groups (average of 22 per cent).

The sixth section, on 'knowledge' and 'measurement', is of particular concern for the sociologists from Australia, though 'method', the fourth item in the list, is quite popular among those from the United States.

The final and seventh section on 'the market' is also dominated by the Australians and significantly favoured by the sociologists in the first group from the United States.

The presentation of the subjects of interest in this manner provides information about some of the similarities and differences between the sociologies of the three countries. It tells us first about our similarities: how we share concerns associated with the abuse of alcohol and other substances, and infectious diseases such as HIV/AIDS; the way we are preoccupied with 'the clinic' and the 'doctor–patient relationship' but generally neglect certain social groups including young people and refugees. But it tells us also about the differences, particularly the Australian interest in sexuality, knowledge, science, and truth, as well as in capitalism, the market, and consumption; and the American concern with race and class, and with method.

Medical sociology: Major areas of focus

The papers in our study population were examined and coded for their two main areas of focus, and the major categories are displayed in Table 5.14. Subjects which did not rate highly included health and the media (only two per cent of the papers), health education (about two per cent), complementary or alternative medicines (about three per cent), disabilities (about four per cent), and technologies or therapies (about five per cent).

Among the more prevalent topics of interest for the medical sociologists in our study population, we find some favoured by sociologists from Australia, others by sociologists from the United Kingdom, and others still by sociologists working in the United States. A few are common to all countries. In the uppermost section of Table 5.14 can be seen several topics of shared concern (and no significant differences from one country to the next). Note however, the greater interest displayed by sociologists within the first group from the United States (USA 1) with regard to both medicalisation and the health industry. (The health

Table 5.14 Medical sociology focus by country

	Australia		United Kingdom		United States		USA (1)		USA (2)	
Medical Sociology	28	*14%*	15	*10%*	20	*12%*	9	*12%*	11	*12%*
Medicalisation	9	*4%*	13	*9%*	15	*9%*	10	***13%***	5	*5%*
The health industry	12	*6%*	6	*4%*	12	*7%*	9	*12%*	3	*3%*
Gender or sexuality	25	***12%***	12	*8%*	8	*5%*	2	*3%*	6	*7%*
Research sector, health research or method	34	***16%***	9	*6%*	19	*11%*	9	*12%*	10	*11%*
Health or welfare policy	23	***11%***	8	*6%*	9	*5%*	3	*4%*	6	*7%*
The illness experience	21	*10%*	42	***29%***	17	*10%*	9	***12%***	8	*9%*
The patient	37	*18%*	56	***39%***	29	*17%*	19	***24%***	10	*11%*
Meanings or language	44	*21%*	45	***31%***	20	*12%*	15	***19%***	5	*5%*
Professions, occupations or work	33	***16%***	24	*17%*	13	*8%*	7	***9%***	6	*7%*
The health or welfare system	42	***20%***	26	*18%*	23	*14%*	13	***17%***	10	*11%*
Inequality	26	*13%*	10	*7%*	62	***36%***	23	*30%*	39	***42%***
Specific diseases or conditions	41	*20%*	20	*14%*	45	***26%***	19	*24%*	26	***28%***
Medical or health knowledges	37	*18%*	36	*25%*	32	*19%*	11	*14%*	21	***23%***

Notes: (i) percentages will not total 100 as this is a composite table with concepts calculated and coded separately. Papers could be coded for two topics of interest. Percentages refer to the number of papers in that country which coded positively for the concept compared with the number of papers where the concept was not applicable (e.g. 44 papers from Australian first authors were coded positively for the topic 'meanings or language', which was 44/208 papers = 21 per cent); (ii) all papers represented in this table are from first authors identified as sociologists (*n* = 524, i.e. 208 Australia, 145 UK, 171 USA, 78 USA (1) and 93 USA (2)); (iii) statistically significant differences were found for Australia, the United Kingdom, and the United States versus 'meanings' (Pearson's chi-square = .000), 'the illness experience' (Pearson's chi-square = .000), 'the patient' (Pearson's chi-square = .000), 'inequality' (Pearson's chi-square = .000), 'gender' (Pearson's chi-square = .039), 'specific diseases' (Pearson's chi-square = .021), 'the professions' (Pearson's chi-square = .026), 'policy' (Pearson's chi-square = .057), and 'research or method' (Pearson's chi-square = .014); (iv) in general, statistical tests were unavailable for USA (1) and (2) due to the small number of papers in these categories. However statistically significant differences were found for USA (1) and (2) versus 'meanings' (Pearson's chi-square = .005), 'health industry' (Pearson's chi-square = .034), and 'the patient' (Pearson's chi-square = .018); and (v) the country of origin is derived from the affiliation provided by the first author of the paper, and indicates their place of employment at the time of publication.

care industry is the category where we would find the paper by Donald Light (2001) on managed competition, while a paper such as the one from Peter Conrad and Valerie Leiter (2008) on medicalisation and the advertising of health products would be found in both categories).

In the second section of the table are included several topics of interest particularly to sociologists working in Australia, specifically 'gender or sexuality', a focus on the 'health research sector or methods', and 'health or welfare policy'. Sociologists in the other two countries do not display as much interest in these topics, though there is some sharing of concern with regard to the 'research sector or method' among the Americans. In this case the interest of the sociologists in the American context tends to be with 'method' rather than the 'research sector'. The greater interest shown by the Australians in the research sector itself is perhaps not unexpected. The issue has been a matter of concern for some time in the Australian context, with sociologists often commenting on the chronic shortage of funding for all types of research and the dominance of biomedicine in the allotment of research resources. Papers classified in this section might include an examination of the health research funding environment by Jeanne Daly (1998); and given that the category includes papers on the research process and methodology, Glennys Howarth's (1998) study of the emotional pressures of research would also be coded here. With regard to the slightly greater interest in 'gender or sexuality' shown by sociologists in the second USA group (relative to the first), this is largely due to their concern with 'gender' as opposed to 'sexuality'. Within this broad category, a greater number of the American papers explored matters connected with women's health, while the Australian papers more frequently concern issues of sexuality. This last set of papers includes works by sociologists such as Jane Edwards and Brian Cheers (2007) on the health of lesbian women in the rural sector, as well as Margie Ripper's (2008) investigation of the connections between sexuality and sperm donation.

The third section of Table 5.14 shows two topics of specific interest to a number of sociologists working in the United Kingdom: the illness experience and the patient. The extent to which sociologists of Britain have focused on these issues does not appear to be of great concern to members of the discipline, or is of lesser concern than the lack of quantitative analysis (Bechhofer 1996:584; Holmwood and Scott 2010:14), organisational analysis (Davies 2003:173), or the study of illness rather than health (Lawton 2003:33–6). The exceptions are from Scambler (2005:7), who points to the neglect of capital and power in British sociology, and Seale's (2008:686) summation of the field as bereft of a societal level of analysis. Papers coded in this category include Simon Williams (2000) on 'biographical disruption' and chronic illness, and Ann Adams and colleagues (2008) writing about patients, doctors and the diagnosis of heart disease. Note that these topics are also of proportionally greater interest to sociologists in the first group of sociologists from the United States than the second (12 compared with 9 per cent, and 24 compared with 11 per cent), indicating a greater similarity between USA (1) and the United Kingdom.

The fourth section shows a group of topics which are shared by sociologists from Britain and Australia but not particularly favoured among those from the United States. Papers focusing on 'meanings and language' are widespread among sociologists of Britain (31 per cent), and fairly common in Australia (21 per cent) but not so frequent in the United States (12 per cent). Likewise, the 'professions, occupations or work' is a topic shared among the first two countries, but not so much the United States (16, 17 and 8 per cent), and 'the health system' shows the same pattern (20, 18 and 14 per cent). With regard to all three topics, there is a relatively greater interest in the topics shown amongst the sociologists of the first group from the United States, emphasising the degree of similarity between these individuals and their overseas counterparts.

The final set of topics, displayed in the lowest section of the table, indicates the specific interests of the second group from the United States. While sociologists in USA (1) write about much of the same subject matter as those from the United Kingdom (including the illness experience, the professions, and meanings), this second United States group shows a proportionally greater concern with 'inequality', 'specific diseases or conditions', and, to a lesser extent, 'medical and health knowledges'.

Taken as a whole, Table 5.14 describes quite clearly the areas of common concern as well as the very different matters taken up by sociologists in the three countries, and vividly illustrates the diversity within the sociology of the United States. Although this diversity has often been discussed in terms of methodological differences, we can see that methods are only one of several areas of variation.

Sociological theories

Sociologists in the study population employ a wide range of theoretical frameworks. For ease of analysis and presentation, these were grouped into four categories: Conflict theories, Interactionist theories, Consensus theories, and Contemporary (and other) theories. The four categories bear only a passing resemblance to Randall Collins' (1985) model of the three sociological traditions, for the early model didn't include the theoretical developments of the contemporary era (specifically Post-Structuralism and Post-Modernism), and there are some problems with this model, particularly its assumption of a direct intellectual lineage between the 'classical period' of sociology and the contemporary era (cf. Collins 1985:4).

In the category of *Consensus theories* readers will find functionalism, Durkheimian theory (organicist, evolutionary, functionalist, and structuralist), Parsonian and Mertonian theories, developmentalism, Habermasian theory and theories of (cultural) globalisation.

The category of *Conflict theories* brings together macro-historical analysis of capitalism, of social stratification and political conflict, and stems essentially from the ideas of Karl Marx, Friedrich Engels and Max Weber. This group also includes Critical Theory, Feminism, Fordism, theories of the professions and the theory of Bourdieu.

Interactionist theories include those developed by George Herbert Mead, Charles Cooley, William Issacs Thomas, Herbert Blumer, Alfred Schutz, Harold Garfinkel and Erving Goffman. In this group readers will find Actor Network Theory, Social Constructionism, Interactionism, Symbolic Interactionism, Interpretism and Network Analysis.

The fourth category, *Contemporary and 'other' theories*, has been added to house the many recent additions to sociological knowledge. It is also used for 'other' theories: most of which are 'theories of the middle range' (Merton 1968:46), including Mike Bury's illness as a 'biographical disruption', as well as theories about social movements, technological change and innovation. This category includes Post-Structuralism, Post-Modernism, Embodiment, Foucauldian analysis, the Sociology of Knowledge, Queer Theory, theories of Risk and Modernity, Social Capital, and Structuration.

The classification of the theoretical frameworks into the four categories is to some extent, a subjective judgement, but it is also based on assessments discussed in the sociological literature. For example, Social Constructionism has been placed within the Interactionist Tradition because its tendency to focus on micro-interaction between groups and individuals in the scientific community and avoid the relations and structures of power has been a long-standing criticism of the framework (Martin and Richards 1995). A similar criticism has been made of Actor Network Theory (Collyer 1997b, 2003).

The outcome of these deliberations is revealed in Table 5.15. The consensus theories are the least favoured category, but more papers from

Table 5.15 Theoretical frameworks by country

(Sociologists only)	Australia		United Kingdom		United States		USA (1)		USA (2)	
Consensus theories	3	2%	3	3%	11	12%	3	6%	8	20%
Interactionist theories	18	13%	39	35%	27	28%	13	24%	14	35%
Conflict theories	56	39%	26	23%	29	31%	16	29%	13	33%
Contemporary and 'other'	65	46%	44	39%	28	30%	23	42%	5	13%
Total	142	100%	112	100%	95	100%	55	100%	40	100%

Notes: (i) totals may not add to 100 per cent due to rounding; (ii) all papers represented in this table are drawn from first authors identified as sociologists *and* using an explicit sociological theory. The numbers in the theory groups are smaller than in some other tables as many sociologists do not clearly state their intention to use a specific sociological theory; (iii) theoretical framework by country, statistically significant (Pearson's chi-square = .000). Theoretical framework by USA (1) and (2), statistically significant (Pearson's chi-square = .007); (iv) the country of origin is derived from the affiliation provided by the first author of the paper, and indicates their place of employment at the time of publication; and (v) disciplinary identities are taken from publicly available materials such as institutional Websites.

sociologists based in the United States use these theories (12 per cent) than those from Australia (two per cent) or the United Kingdom (three per cent). British sociologists tend to engage in greater numbers with interactionist (35 per cent) and contemporary theories (39 per cent); Australian sociologists to favour conflict (39 per cent) and contemporary theories (46 per cent), and sociologists from the United States are found in roughly equal numbers across interactionist, conflict and contemporary categories (28, 31, and 30 per cent). If we look closely at the final two columns, sociologists within the USA (2) group are the strongest supporters of the various consensus theories, while those in USA (1) show a high level of interest in the contemporary and 'other' theories, again indicating a set of shared perspectives between these sociologists and their Australian and British colleagues.

The funding of research

There are differences in the way research is funded across the three countries, and this has an impact on our authors. Although academics are given general institutional support for their research (access to library facilities, computer support, etc.), the extent of this form of support varies from one institution to the next and between countries. Moreover, additional, external funding is more commonly accessed in the United Kingdom and the United States than in Australia. These differences can be seen in the uppermost section of Table 5.16, where the rates at which our authors received funding was much lower in Australia (34 per cent) than in the United Kingdom (65 per cent) or the United States (62 per cent). In the Australian context, the general dearth of research funds encourages sociologists to undertake projects which can be done individually and on 'a shoe-string budget', and represents a significant barrier to large empirical projects.

If we compare the sociologists with the non-sociologists working within the sociology of health and medicine, we find that the first group are less likely to receive funding for their research in Australia and the United Kingdom. This situation differs in the United States, where sociologists are a little more likely to receive funding. These differences can be seen in the lower sections of Table 5.16.

When the *source* of funding is taken into account, we find that neutral sources are relatively more common in Australia and the United Kingdom, while *medical funding* is much more common in the United States. Indeed health or medical funding provides for 84 per cent of funded papers from the United States, compared with 64 per cent for the United

Table 5.16 External research funding

	Australia		United Kingdom		United States	
All authors						
Funded research	113	*34%*	121	*65%*	128	*62%*
Unfunded research	218	*66%*	66	*35%*	80	*39%*
Totals	331	*100%*	187	*100%*	208	*100%*
Sociologists						
Funded research	64	*34%*	74	*61%*	97	*62%*
Unfunded research	127	*67%*	47	*39%*	59	*38%*
Totals	191	*100%*	121	*100%*	156	*100%*
Non-sociologists						
Funded research	37	*43%*	44	*73%*	29	*58%*
Unfunded research	49	*57%*	16	*27%*	21	*42%*
Totals	86	*100%*	60	*100%*	50	*100%*

Notes: (i) percentages may not total 100 due to rounding; (ii) not all authors declared whether their research had been externally funded, or by whom. Hence the population of papers included in the calculations for the top section of the table is 726 rather than 811. Moreover, given the incomplete data for disciplinary identity, the lower sections of the table are based on even fewer papers: a total of 664; (iii) in the top section of the table, funding by country is statistically significant (Pearson's chi-square = .000). In centre and lower sections: for sociologists this is statistically significant (Pearson's chi-square = .000), for non-sociologists this is statistically significant (Pearson's chi-square = .001); (iv) the country of origin is derived from the affiliation provided by the first author of the paper, and indicates their place of employment at the time of publication; (v) information about the funding of research is taken from declarations made on the published manuscripts; and (vi) disciplinary identities are taken from publicly available materials such as institutional Websites.

Kingdom and only 55 per cent for Australia. These figures can be seen in Table 5.17.

Comparing sociologists with non-sociologists in our study population, we also find slightly more of the sociologists obtaining health or medical sponsorship than the non-sociologists in the United Kingdom and Australia, but not in the United States. This is further evidence of a quite different funding environment in the United States. This information is also found in Table 5.17.

Investigating this issue a little further, we find an association between the kind of funding received and the disciplinary identity of the author. Authors who identify themselves as sociologists or with one of the allied disciplines are less likely to receive medical funding than those who identify with one of the health or medical disciplines. We can examine

Table 5.17   External research funding and sponsorship

	Australia		United Kingdom		United States	
All authors						
Neutrally funded research	51	*45%*	44	*36%*	21	*16%*
Health or medical funding	62	*55%*	77	*64%*	107	*84%*
Totals	113	*100%*	121	*100%*	128	*100%*
Sociologists						
Neutrally funded research	27	*42%*	26	*35%*	17	*18%*
Health or medical funding	37	*58%*	48	*65%*	80	*83%*
Totals	64	*100%*	74	*100%*	97	*100%*
Non-sociologists						
Neutrally funded research	18	*49%*	17	*39%*	3	*10%*
Health or medical funding	19	*51%*	27	*61%*	26	*90%*
Totals	37	*100%*	44	*100%*	29	*100%*

Notes: (i) percentages may not total 100 due to rounding; (ii) not all authors declared whether their research had been externally funded, or by whom. Hence the population of papers included in the calculations for the upper section of the table is 362 rather than 811. In the lower sections, given the missing information about disciplinary identity, the population is further reduced, and totals are 235 and 110; (iii) for all authors, neutral/health funding by country, statistically significant (Pearson's chi-square = .000). For sociologists by funding, statistically significant (Pearson's chi-square = .002). For non-sociologists by funding, statistically significant (Pearson's chi-square = .004); (iv) the country of origin is derived from the affiliation provided by the first author of the paper, and indicates their place of employment at the time of publication; (v) information about the funding of a study is taken from the published manuscripts where available; and (vi) disciplinary identities are taken from publicly available materials such as institutional Websites.

this association by dividing papers along a continuum, with those published by authors who identify with sociology and its allied disciplines (anthropology, human geography, etc.) at one end, the semi-health disciplines (health sciences, health policy, etc.) in the middle, and the health and medical disciplines (including nursing, pharmacy, etc.) at the other. We find an increasing likelihood of health or medical funding and a lessening probability of neutral funding among authors who affiliate themselves with the health or medical disciplines. This information is displayed in Table 5.18.

This general tendency is noticeable for Australian papers and those from the United Kingdom. In the United States the same pattern emerges, but it is more difficult to verify statistically, as the numbers without funding are too small in our study population. These figures

Table 5.18   External research funding and sponsorship – By discipline

	Sociology and allied disciplines		Semi-health disciplines		Health and medical disciplines	
Australia						
Neutral funding	27	*56%*	16	*41%*	2	*15%*
Health or medical funding	21	*44%*	23	*59%*	11	*85%*
Totals	48	*100%*	39	*100%*	13	*100%*
United Kingdom						
Neutral funding	23	*50%*	18	*37%*	2	*9%*
Health or medical funding	23	*50%*	31	*63%*	20	*91%*
Totals	46	*100%*	49	*100%*	22	*100%*
United States						
Neutral funding	10	*15%*	10	*20%*	–	–
Health or medical funding	56	*85%*	40	*80%*	9	*100%*
Totals	66	*100%*	50	*100%*	9	*100%*

Notes: (i) percentages may not total 100 due to rounding; (ii) this table represents only authors who have funding for their research, and for whom the funding source is known. Not all authors declared whether their research had been externally funded, or by whom, nor is there full information about the disciplinary identity/affiliations of authors. Hence the population of papers is 100 for Australia, 117 for the United Kingdom, and 125 for the United States; (iii) funding by discipline for Australia is statistically significant (Pearson's chi-square = .026), for the United Kingdom statistically significant (Pearson's chi-square = .005). For the United States statistical calculations cannot be made as the numbers are too small in some cells; (iv) the country of origin is derived from the affiliation provided by the first author of the paper, and indicates their place of employment at the time of publication; (v) information about the funding of a study is taken from the published manuscripts where available; and (vi) disciplinary identities are taken from publicly available materials such as institutional Websites.

confirm long-standing ideas about the funding of the sociology of health and illness: that the funding for studies of health or medicine tends to be fiercely guarded by the medical disciplines, and it remains difficult for sociologists to garner essential support for research. Nevertheless, the extent to which this is true varies across the three countries. Among the Australian papers, in the group of disciplines that include sociology we find that 44 per cent have health or medical funding; in Britain, 50 per cent of this group have health or medical funding; and in the United States 85 per cent have health or medical funding. This suggests a relatively more permeable boundary between medicine and sociology in the United States than in the other two countries.

Objectivity, sympathy, and critical distance from medicine

All papers in the study population were coded according to the authors' perspective towards medicine. 'Medicine' in this case might be the medical profession, the institution of medicine, the discipline or intellectual field of medical knowledge, or practitioners of medicine. Papers were judged to be sympathetic towards the values or practices of medicine, or critical. Table 5.19 indicates the country differences in the papers. Note that the rate of criticism is proportionally highest among the Australian authors (93 per cent) and lowest among authors from the United Kingdom (76 per cent). British authors are the most sympathetic (24 per cent). There is, however, little difference between the rates from the United Kingdom and the United States.

Over the two decades of our study, authors in Australia and the United Kingdom have become generally less critical of the medical profession and more sympathetic (Pearson's chi-square = .000). In Australia, rates of criticism have shifted downwards from 95 per cent in the 1990s to 91 per cent in the 2000s; while in Britain, the rate fell from 83 to 73 per cent over the same period. Little change was observed in the United States, where 77 per cent of authors were critical in the first decade, and 78 per cent in the second.

The orientation towards medicine differs a little when we re-focus our analysis from the broader group of authors to those who identify as sociologists. Tests of association show that authors identifying as sociologists are more likely to be critical of medicine, while those who identify with other disciplines are more likely to be sympathetic. As described in Table 5.20, when the sociologists and non-sociologists are compared, we find a higher level of criticism and a lower level of sympathy among

Table 5.19   Orientation towards medicine

	Australia		United Kingdom		United States	
Sympathetic	17	*7%*	38	*24%*	31	*23%*
Critical	214	*93%*	118	*76%*	105	*77%*
Total	231	*100%*	156	*100%*	136	*100%*

Notes: (i) percentages may not total 100 due to rounding; (ii) population of the table = 523 (all authors for whom an orientation towards medicine was relevant to the paper and could be ascertained); (iii) orientation towards medicine by country, statistically significant (Pearson's chi-square = .000); and (iv) the country of origin is derived from the affiliation provided by the first author of the paper, and indicates their place of employment at the time of publication.

Table 5.20 Sociologists' orientations towards medicine

	Australia		United Kingdom		United States		USA (1)		USA (2)	
Sociologists										
Sympathetic	6	4%	21	21%	20	21%	7	15%	13	28%
Critical	131	96%	78	79%	74	79%	41	85%	33	72%
Totals	137	*100%*	99	*100%*	94	*100%*	48	*100%*	46	*100%*
Non-sociologists										
Sympathetic	7	13%	17	32%	11	27%				
Critical	47	87%	37	69%	30	73%				
Totals	54	*100%*	54	*100%*	41	*100%*				

Notes: (i) percentages may not total 100 due to rounding; (ii) population of the first set of columns = 479 (all authors for whom a disciplinary identity and orientation towards medicine could be ascertained for Australia, the United States, and the United States). Population for USA (1) and (2) = 171; (iii) there is a statistically significant association between the orientation towards medicine and an author's identity as a sociologist (Pearson's chi-square = .013), between orientation towards medicine and country (Pearson's chi-square = .000), and the orientation towards medicine for sociologists is statistically significant (Pearson's chi-square = .000). Statistical tests for USA (1) and (2) are not available due to the small numbers in these cells; (iv) the country of origin is derived from the affiliation provided by the first author of the paper, and indicates their place of employment at the time of publication; and (v) disciplinary identities are taken from publicly available materials such as institutional Websites.

sociologists in all three countries. When the population of authors from the United States is once again divided into two groups, we find more among the first group, USA (1), are critical of medicine (85 per cent) relative to the second group (72 per cent). Similarly, fewer from the first group are sympathetic towards medicine (15 per cent compared with 28 per cent). The first group, USA (1), displays an orientation towards medicine which has greater similarity to the sociologists of Britain and Australia. The second group, USA (2), is quite different with regard to the rates of sympathy and criticism.

The extent to which sociologists are critical rather than sympathetic towards medicine is very much dependent on a number of factors, one of which is whether or not their research has been directly funded by granting bodies or sponsors. Table 5.21 indicates the differences between funded and unfunded research for the three countries, focusing on the orientation of the sociologists. What is immediately obvious is the contrast between funded and unfunded research. Studies which have not required funding because they are theoretical rather than empirical; do not involve significant (and therefore costly) field work; or were not given external funding support are much more likely to be critical of medicine. The table indicates that 96 per cent of the authors without direct project funding are critical towards medicine compared with 77 per cent of those with funding. Likewise, only four per cent of the authors without funding are sympathetic towards the aims, perspectives or practices of medicine, compared with 23 per cent of those with sponsorship or funding. These figures are a clear indication of the potential dangers associated with funded research in matters of health or the health care sector.

Table 5.21   The funding of research and orientation towards medicine

(Sociologists only)	Unfunded research		Funded research		Totals	
Sympathetic	7	*4%*	29	*23%*	36	*13%*
Critical	157	*96%*	96	*77%*	253	*88%*
Totals	164	*100%*	125	*100%*	289	*100%*

Notes: (i) percentages may not total 100 due to rounding; (ii) population of table = 289 which is the number of sociologists in the study population for whom disciplinary identities are known, an orientation towards medicine can be ascertained, and for whom funding arrangements are relevant and known; (iii) funding by orientation towards medicine, statistically significant (Pearson's chi-square = .000); (iv) information about the funding of a study is taken from the published manuscripts. Not all papers provide this information; and (v) disciplinary identities are taken from publicly available materials such as institutional Websites.

Table 5.22 Orientation towards medicine by funding and country

(Sociologists only)	Unfunded research		Funded research	
Australia				
Sympathetic	2	*2%*	3	*9%*
Critical	87	*98%*	32	*91%*
Total	89	*100%*	35	*100%*
United Kingdom				
Sympathetic	3	*8%*	11	*23%*
Critical	33	*92%*	36	*77%*
Total	36	*100%*	47	*100%*
United States				
Sympathetic	2	*5%*	15	*35%*
Critical	37	*95%*	28	*65%*
Total	39	*100%*	43	*100%*
USA (1)				
Sympathetic			6	*26%*
Critical	17	*100%*	17	*74%*
Total	17	*100%*	23	*100%*
USA (2)				
Sympathetic	2	*9%*	9	*45%*
Critical	20	*91%*	11	*55%*
Total	22	*100%*	20	*100%*

Notes: (i) percentages may not total 100 due to rounding; (ii) population of the upper section of the table = 289 (i.e. all sociologists in the study population for whom details are available about funding and where an orientation towards medicine has been ascertained). For lower section, USA (1) and (2), population = 82; (iii) due to the small numbers in many of the cells, statistical tests are unavailable; (iv) the country of origin is derived from the affiliation provided by the first author of the paper, and indicates their place of employment at the time of publication; (v) information about the funding of a study is taken from the published manuscripts. Not all papers provide this information; and (vi) disciplinary identities are taken from publicly available materials such as institutional Websites.

The association between funding and orientation towards medicine can also be examined for the three countries. In Table 5.22 it can be seen that in Australia, where little research is funded relative to the other two countries, a higher level of criticism is nevertheless prevalent among sociologists of health and medicine (98 per cent) where research is unfunded, compared with funded research (91 per cent). A similar situation occurs in the United Kingdom, where 92 per cent of unfunded research is critical of medicine compared with 77 per cent of funded research. In the United States, unfunded research is similarly found to be much more critical than funded research (95 compared with 65 per cent), and less sympathetic towards medicine (five compared with 35 per cent).

Examining the two groups of American sociologists, we find the same pattern emerges, with unfunded research more critical than funded research. This occurs for both USA (1) and USA (2), but a trend can also be seen where the level of criticism is greater amongst the first group. This tells us that sociologists who identify solely as sociologists are more likely to be critical than those with a dual discipline affiliation when undertaking funded research.

A second factor which shapes the sociologists' orientation towards medicine is where they work within the university system. Sociologists working within sociology departments and other, allied discipline areas are more critical of medicine and less sympathetic, than those working in health-related areas. Table 5.23 illustrates these differences. Note also the way the table displays the disciplines categorised according to their distance from, or proximity to the workplace arena of medicine. This suggests the 'distance' from medicine in spatial and institutional terms provides for a decreasing acceptance of the biomedical model

Table 5.23   Sociologists, work units, and orientation towards medicine

(Sociologists only)	Sociology and allied disciplines		Non-allied disciplines, health and medicine	
Sympathetic towards medicine	20	*11%*	27	*19%*
Critical of medicine	164	*89%*	119	*82%*
Total	184	*100%*	146	*100%*

Notes: (i) percentages may not total 100 due to rounding; (ii) population of the table = 330 (i.e. all sociologists in the study population for whom details are known about their work unit and where their orientation to medicine is relevant and can be ascertained); (iii) orientation towards medicine by place of work, statistically significant for all authors (Pearson's chi-square = .000), for non-sociologists (Pearson's chi-square = .010), and for sociologists (Pearson's chi-square = .049); (iv) 'sociology and allied disciplines' includes disciplines such as anthropology, demography, political science, cultural studies, gender studies, policy studies, the humanities, and general social sciences; 'non-allied disciplines, health and medicine' includes psychology, business, socio-health units, nursing, the general health sciences, epidemiology, sexual health units, health services research and planning, the natural sciences such as biology plus various medical disciplines including psychiatry and community medicine; (v) information about the departments or work units is provided by the authors on their manuscripts; and (vi) disciplinary identities are taken from publicly available materials such as institutional Websites.

of health and illness, and the increasing likelihood of criticism of medicine. It implies that employment within the work units associated with health and medicine tends to encourage the adoption of medical values or perspectives, and conversely, employment within the critical disciplines (such as sociology and anthropology) promote less favourable orientations towards the medical establishment.

The association between the discipline in which an individual works, and their orientation towards medicine, remains strong whether they are working in Australia, the United Kingdom or the United States. There is a small amount of variation from country to country, and this is displayed in Table 5.24. In each case, individuals working in sociology,

Table 5.24 Orientation towards medicine by work context and country

	Sociology and allied disciplines		Non-allied disciplines, health and medicine	
Australia				
Sympathetic	4	*3%*	13	*12%*
Critical	116	*97%*	98	*88%*
Total	120	*100%*	111	*100%*
United Kingdom				
Sympathetic	6	*11%*	32	*31%*
Critical	47	*89%*	70	*69%*
Total	53	*100%*	102	*100%*
United States				
Sympathetic	13	*17%*	18	*31%*
Critical	65	*83%*	40	*69%*
Total	78	*100%*	58	*100%*

Notes: (i) percentages may not total 100 due to rounding; (ii) population of the table = 522 (i.e. all authors in the study population for whom full details are known about their work context and their orientation towards medicine); (iii) orientation towards medicine by work context, statistically significant (Australia, Pearson's chi-square = .015) (the United Kingdom, Pearson's chi-square = .006), (the United States, Pearson's chi-square = .048); (iv) 'sociology and allied disciplines' includes disciplines such as anthropology, demography, political science, cultural studies, gender studies, policy studies, the humanities and general social sciences; 'non-allied disciplines, health, and medicine' includes psychology, business, socio-health units, nursing, the general health sciences, epidemiology, sexual health units, health services research and planning, the natural sciences such as biology plus various medical disciplines including psychiatry and community medicine; (v) the country of origin is derived from the affiliation provided by the first author of the paper, and indicates their place of employment at the time of publication; and (vi) information about the departments or work units is provided by the authors on their manuscripts.

the social sciences or humanities are the most critical of medicine. Sociologists in the United Kingdom show the greatest disparity, with 89 per cent of sociologists employed in sociology and the allied disciplines expressing a critical view of medicine compared with 69 per cent of those from the health and medical disciplines. This represents a 20 per cent difference between the two groups. Focusing on sociologists in the United States, 83 per cent of those working in sociology, the social sciences or humanities are critical of medicine compared with 69 per cent of sociologists in the health and medical disciplines. This is a 14 per cent difference between the two groups. In Australia there is a nine per cent difference, with 97 per cent of sociologists working in the departments of sociology and allied discipline areas critical of medicine compared with 88 per cent of those in the health and medical departments.

The picture presented by this data could hardly be clearer. Although sociologists as a group generally offer a critical perspective on medicine, their place of work – the disciplines or departments – as well as the acceptance of funding for their research, shape their perspectives and orientation towards the medical profession, the institutions of medicine, and medical knowledges.

6
Old Roads and New Pathways: Reflections, Conclusions and a Way Forward

This book began with some key questions about the sociology of health and medicine. We asked for a definition of the speciality field, for information about the individuals and groups working within its boundaries, about possible national differences in sociological knowledge about health and medicine, and whether there might be variations in organisational or institutional practices from one country to the next. The quest for answers has taken us on a journey through the history of the discipline in three countries and included an empirical study of a set of research publications from its practitioners.

The whole endeavour has been situated within the principles set out in the programme of the sociology of knowledge. This has brought into focus the social and cultural processes behind scholarly knowledge, and led to an examination of the institutions and social structures within which that knowledge is produced, exchanged, legitimated and transmitted. This search for the connections and inter-connections between scholarly knowledge, social practices, institutions and social structures has revealed new knowledge about sociology and its speciality, the sociology of health and medicine.

Central to the study has been a re-conceptualisation of the nature of disciplines. The conventional approach has been to define a discipline as a cognitive domain or 'parcel' of formal knowledge which immanently 'emerges' or 'unfolds' over time and differs from others in subject matter, perspective or methodology. This is the approach taken in most introductory textbooks of sociology. As a consequence, sociology has been granted an identity based on its 'object' of study, usually described as the realm of 'the social' (Wilson and Kolb 1949:59; Naegele 1965b:148). Such approaches continue to have value in orienting students towards the discipline and encouraging a common disciplinary identity among practicing sociologists, but are inadequate for the theorising of disciplines. Indeed, the lack of reflexivity about the discipline has been a point of contention, albeit mainly from individuals critical of the 'mainstream' (e.g. Gouldner 1970; Connell 1997).

In the post-Kuhnian era, when the social sciences can no longer be viewed as offering ever-progressive, cumulative steps towards the 'truth'; it is increasingly imperative for disciplines to be regarded as *social* forms produced through *social* processes. Yet only a handful of sociologists have raised questions about whether disciplines even *have* legitimate 'objects' of study and unique methodologies (Therborn 1976:424, 426), and whether there might be inherent difficulties in regarding the scholarly landscape in terms of cognitive divisions:

> The differentiation of disciplines...will rarely map onto any scheme of intellectual differentiation. Attempts to differentiate disciplines by their concern with particular and exclusive intellectual problems are doomed to failure. Real life is messier than our intellectual schemes
> (Scott 2005:137).

Putting aside the more conventional approaches of the past, disciplines have been theorised within this volume as multi-dimensional social forms. Primarily sites of social relations, created over time through the interaction of individuals and groups, disciplines have been shown to provide members with the opportunity for meaningful activity, forms of identity and 'ways of life'. Within these dynamic, constantly shifting domains, human actors construct and re-fashion the terrain upon which they operate, and act to defend and maintain the boundaries between themselves and other disciplinary sites. As institutional forms, disciplines have been shown to structure the behaviours, roles, rules and norms of human actors, and regularise and pattern these into an hierarchical ordering of individuals and groups. Moreover, as domains of social action and social structure, disciplines are themselves situated within a broader social field and thus subjected to the organising effects of other social structures. As such, they operate within the institutions of the capitalist social system, organising academic labour and the production of valuable resources for national and global markets.

Disciplines and specialities

This theoretical framework has provided for new definitions of the relationship between disciplines and specialities. In the past, disciplinary 'specialities' have been considered mere divisions of larger, formal bodies of knowledge with their own areas of study and specific sets of problems (e.g. Akers 1992:4). Set apart from the disciplinary 'core', specialities were said to address unique sets of concerns and problems, and have their own orientation towards sociological practice, being 'applied' rather than 'theoretical'. This was the view adopted during sociology's early professionalisation period and expounded in its programmatic statements (e.g. Merton 1959, 1968; Parsons 1959, 1965; Shils 1965). In more recent times, specialities have been regarded as a practical means for managing extensive spans of literature and producing more accessible networks for members.

In this volume, these assumptions about disciplines and their specialities have been challenged. Rather than consider the sociology of health and medicine as simply a part of the larger discipline and distinguished by an alternative orientation to the sociological knowledge base; this study investigated the internal boundaries between specialities and their parents and demonstrated their construction to be fundamentally *social*. Viewing specialities as sites of social action with a specific *social* relationship to the parent discipline, we focused instead on the hierarchical arrangements and relations of power within the disciplinary field. In sociology, perhaps more so than other disciplines, speciality areas are often found at the bottom of the hierarchical social order. As we have seen, this order is maintained largely through internal boundary-work, with privileged groups able to more effectively control the resources of the discipline, setting out the tasks, roles and relative status positions of its constituents. Although accepting the overall legitimacy of the knowledge base and the discipline's leadership, the specialities are often a source of friction within the discipline, seeking more equal representation in the general journals, adequate resources from the professional associations, and appropriate space within the conference programmes. Indeed, the constant competition for legitimacy and better representation within the field – by actors who accept its essential structure, rules and values – provides the discipline with an essential vitality in its struggles with other disciplines, but at the same time preserves its hierarchical order and the privileges of those at the top.

This more dynamic conception of disciplines and their specialities repudiates the notion of differences stemming solely from the speciality's knowledge base or any inherent incapacity to contribute to 'core' disciplinary knowledge. It speaks instead of the social relations of disciplines, of the nature of their boundary relations, and even tells us something about the competitive environment within which they are located. Of course, conflicts within the discipline of sociology which involve one or more of the specialities are a curious form of struggle, as specialities are not necessarily distinct 'groups' of sociologists. At any given moment, there may be more individuals who have contributed to the work of a specialty than there are individuals who work solely within the speciality arena. Moreover, most sociologists operate within several internal disciplinary spaces, and loyalties tend to be flexible, varying from one situation to the next. We have seen this in practice with regard to some of the disciplinary disputes discussed in previous chapters. Sociologists will fight for their speciality areas, as they did over the *Health Sociology Review (HSR)*, where specialists rallied to support the editors to achieve equal representation in the professional association. Yet these same sociologists will be united with their protagonists on other issues. Sociology is an arena with many fracture lines, and one of its unique features is the way members can simultaneously belong to several fractions. This is not to minimise the ferocity of disciplinary disputes, but just to suggest some of their complexity:

> The cautionary note...is as follows: scientific communities do divide and fight over paradigms. They also divide and fight over issues of professional power, status and material privilege. These two sources of confrontation may fuse into a single dynamic for conflict, but they are not necessarily fused
>
> (Lengermann 1979:195).

From this conception of the complex social relations of the field, we can see specialities sharing similar external boundary-relationships with their parent. For example, the relations with the state or private sector, the university, and with many of the disciplines (perhaps anthropology or physics) are similarly configured for both sociology and its specialities, and as a consequence, all members of the discipline tend to utilise similar discursive defences and draw on common professionalisation strategies when under challenge. Indeed the commonality of the border relations for sociologists and sociologists of health and medicine identifies all members as part of the same discipline, rather than as *separate* disciplines. These shared border relations encourage all members of a discipline (including members of its specialities) to adopt similar social practices (such as publishing in sociological journals, joining sociological associations, and attending sociological conferences), and to pay attention to a broad but nevertheless generally specifiable *sociological* literature.

Yet the *internal* relations of the disciplinary field are not homogenous across all its specialities. There are some specialities which fall entirely within the disciplinary field: perhaps the study of class or ethnicity offers appropriate examples. On the other hand, specialities situated between two disciplines (e.g. the sociology of medicine, social psychology, economic sociology, political psychology, or sociological epidemiology) tend to be associated with a rather different set of social relations and practices. Practitioners who are fully engaged in these boundary areas (i.e. specialists) are under a requirement to work two borders: an *internal* one with other sociologists, where they must display an interest and competence in the issues and theories declared 'central' to the discipline (and defend themselves against claims of being 'atheoretical' and 'applied'); and an *external* one directed towards the other discipline (perhaps medicine or psychology), where they must deploy the full flexibility of their discursive repertoire to establish their worth. As we have argued in earlier parts of this book, few practitioners are able to make regular and effective contributions to both fields and meet two sets of – often contradictory – professional and disciplinary obligations. Hence specialities often form in situations where significant numbers are working the same borders, facing similar problems and challenges. In this sense, specialities are a *defensive mechanism,* a vehicle established by members under threat within their own discipline – and yet not entirely welcomed into the other discipline – and a means to ensure the contributions of its members will be valued according to the rules of the speciality, rather than entirely by its parent.

The necessity to 'work on two fronts' is in evidence in the historical accounts provided in Chapters two and three, where sociologists employed in departments of medicine or engaged in joint research found it difficult to gain the respect of colleagues from their own discipline as well as medicine. These individuals encountered problems with obtaining tenure and promotion: difficulties exacerbated by a system of academic publishing which sets out discipline-specific criteria and rules for ascertaining and rewarding 'good' scholarship. In the results of our empirical study described in Chapter five, the publications of the sociologists of health and medicine reveal a more positive dimension to the efforts of those working in the border areas between medicine and sociology. Focusing on the citation patterns in these publications, we found sociologists have constructed a knowledge base which pays attention to the parent discipline yet also promotes the speciality. For instance, among the commonly cited authors we find sociologists such as Michel Foucault, Pierre Bourdieu, Anthony Giddens, Juliet Corbin,

Erving Goffman and Nikolas Rose; few of whom could be readily identified as specialists of medical sociology. Revisiting the same list of highly cited sociologists we find many others who have made their career mostly within the speciality: Mike Bury, Peter Conrad, Deborah Lupton, John McKinlay, Mildred Blaxter, David Mechanic, Evan Willis, Irving Zola, Catherine Ross, Sarah Nettleton and Alan Petersen. A similar pattern can be found when we examine the topics of interest among sociologists in the speciality. While there is some interest in subjects of exclusive concern to sociologists of health and medicine (e.g. medicalisation, specific diseases, and the illness experience), many other papers explore the connections between health/illness and issues of general interest within the discipline (e.g. work, language, professions, inequality and sexuality).

What does this tell us about the sociology of health and medicine? It suggests that despite the challenges of 'working on two fronts', many sociologists have been able to do so successfully. There has, in the past, been widespread concern about the specialist field as possibly 'out of touch' with the central questions of sociology, yet the results of this Content Analysis do not support this. The strong representation of both specialist and generalist figures in the citation lists, and the interest in specialist subjects as well as those from the mainstream (e.g. work, class, sexuality, consumption), instead indicate a healthy diversity of interests within the field.

The results of the historical and empirical studies in this book also offer new insights into the nature of specialities and disciplines. Though specialities are often regarded in negative terms – as fragmenting the discipline, making it difficult to differentiate 'good' sociology from 'bad', and weakening the capacity of the discipline to maintain its territory and uphold the uniqueness of the sociological perspective (e.g. Pearlin 1992; Pescosolido and Kronenfeld 1995:6; Bird *et al.* 2000:8) – specialities need also to be seen in a more positive light. Some leading commentators have paused to examine the more constructive possibilities of specialities, seeing their capacity for 'creative integration' (Levine 1995), a more 'playful' sociology that explores research which others may regard as 'useless' (de Vries 2003:35), and a chance to bring new voices into the discipline, new theories and epistemologies, new research questions, and the foundations for new theoretical frameworks (Fitzgerald *et al.* 1995). These positive aspects become evident when specialities are regarded as essentially social forms rather than cognitive divisions within disciplines. We *could*, of course, choose to retain a conventional conception of disciplines as fixed intellectual spaces, permanently fractured by cognitive disputes and differences, and internally divided by a number of specialities each occupied by sociologists isolated from one another and the disciplinary 'core'. Alternatively, understood as social forms, disciplines and specialities are dynamic sites and structures, peopled by sociologists with multiple loyalties and interests, operating across the internal boundaries of the discipline between 'core' and 'speciality', wearing different 'hats' and flexibly working the discourses and protecting and extending disciplinary boundaries. From this perspective, specialities throw up tensions and contradictions, demand resources and compete for attention; but they also build new alliances, pose new theoretical and policy problems, offer new solutions, and contribute to the overall vibrancy of the discipline by continually negotiating and extending its external boundaries.

Sociology's external borders

In the historical analysis of the three national sociologies, we have seen how the professionalising disciplines of medicine and sociology established separate spheres of operation during the first half of the twentieth century. In the process, sociology was complicit in the production of a new definition of health as the absence of physical malady, and in an individualised, mono-causal, bio-physical model of illness. It was not until the second half of the twentieth century that sociologists returned to the sociological critiques of this reductionist approach to ill-health – critiques which had been evident in the much earlier work of Frederich Engels, Florence Nightingale, Emile Durkheim and others – and began to establish a more sustainable presence within the institutions of medicine.

In each of the three countries, the borders between the disciplines of sociology and medicine, which had become largely impermeable from the 1930s, eventually began to be transformed in association with the strengthening of sociology itself. As the discipline of sociology professionalised, developed a unique identity and increased in status, its practitioners became more effective at establishing collegial rather than subordinate relations with medicine. In each country, sociology was given assistance in this task from other disciplines, the state, the private sector and the university system. In the United States, the capacity of sociology to engage with medicine in the research arena and influence its educational curriculum was boosted systematically from the 1950s with the availability of both private and public forms of funding, by legislative changes making research a more viable activity for medical schools, and the post-war expansion of the university system. Likewise, in the United Kingdom, the subordinate position of sociologists shifted in the 1970s (somewhat later than the United States) in conjunction with significant growth in the university sector, government directives to educate rather than merely train medical students, and dedicated research funding from the state. In the Australian context, sociology was boosted from the late 1960s with increases in government funding, the general expansion of the university system and the influx of mature students. Over the next two decades, the relations between sociology and medicine became more collaborative, with sociology appearing more regularly in the medical curriculum through its alliances with nursing, community medicine and public health.

Sociology has of course many other disciplines on its boundaries. In the 1930s, American sociology successfully differentiated its approach from that of medicine, but also acted to halt the threat of encroachment from economics. In this case (and as described in Chapter three), debates between institutional and neo-classical economics provided an opportunity for sociology to trespass into its territory. With neo-classical economics declaring its intention to focus on only some aspects of reality, it left an intellectual space for sociology to occupy (i.e. areas of social life not determined by the economy). Parsons' adoption of the methodological schema of neo-classical economics in 1937 was, according to Camic (1987), a strategic act of professionalisation. The middle decades of the twentieth century were, in all three countries, periods of relatively successful collaboration with economics and medicine; for both disciplines (perhaps begrudgingly) allowed space for sociology to ply its trade. The field altered dramatically from the 1980s however, as border relations with orthodox economics grew hostile. With health care services increasingly conceived as an expense rather than an investment on the part of governments, sociologists began to struggle for opportunities to enter the discursive territory of health and health policy. In the face of a concerted and widespread movement to spread pro-market policies in the health care sector, to encourage the privatisation of the *NHS* (Pollock and Price 2011) and Australian Medicare (Collyer and White 2001; Harley *et al.* 2011), and to strengthen and extend market control in the United States (Jasso-Aguilar and Waitzkin 2011); the broad response of sociologists in all three countries has been to 'turn inward', suppress their critique of capitalist medicine, and focus on less contentious arenas such as the illness experience, issues of measurement, and the unequal distribution of specific forms of illness. Once again sociology has retreated from overt confrontation. This time it has become complicit in the new conception of ill-health as a consequence of individual risk-taking and irresponsibility. And, as occurred on previous occasions, alterations in the political and economic environment have forced a response from disciplinary actors. Some have found opportunities to engage in 'dual production' (i.e. research produced for peers as well as political or economic actors) (Albert 2003:178), some have retreated into (politically safer) areas of research (e.g. the patient experience), while others have bravely entered developing areas such as health services research, where the field is dominated by either economics or medicine and sociological critique is muted.

Although the dynamics of the political and market context have always had an impact on disciplines and disciplinary actors, many have expressed concern over the future of the current disciplinary landscape. There are a few who see it as relatively secure. Andrew Abbott (2001:152), for example, sees little likelihood of a forthcoming challenge to the foundational ideas of Marx, Freud, Weber or Durkheim, and considers the current layout of disciplines safe from fundamental structural change. This is because, in acting as the primary hiring agents for their universities and recruiting from within their own discipline, these actors protect and promote the discipline (Abbott 2001:126). Yet this book suggests the autonomy of the university sector has been dramatically reduced within the past handful of decades. Where the professoriate once dominated the institutions in the United Kingdom and Australia (Butler *et al.* 2009), and university presidents the institutions of the United Sates (Collins 1985:41); the influence of the trans-national corporations and the impacts of fierce cross-national competition have radically altered the publishing market (Agger 2000), placing pressure on academics to produce 'relevant' knowledge which can be used by private capital (Kurasawa 2002:337). With foreign policy and business alliances now more critical to an institution's success than the merit of an individual's record of scholarship, it is thus questionable whether academics are still the primary 'hiring agents' in the universities. Even when functioning in this capacity, they are unlikely to do more than 'rubber-stamp' decisions made by others; for disciplinary needs are increasingly over-ridden by more pressing institutional objectives.

In our study, these pressures for change are most evident in the United States, where there is less state regulation of the university sector and significantly more private funding of research and research positions. In that country, sociology has fractured into two major groups. One of these has opted for 'dual production', as signified by their adoption of twin professional identities (e.g. sociologist-psychologist).

This increases their marketability, enabling them to build a career by producing knowledge for private capital as well as their peers. This knowledge is more quantitative than the sociology of others in the United States, contains less sociological theory, is less likely to engage with contemporary theories, more likely to incorporate consensus theories, more likely to be sympathetic towards medicine, and less likely to tackle issues of health consumption or the contentious topics connected with the health market.

National differences

Our empirical study of journal publications indicated both similarities and differences in the practice of sociology between the three countries. Almost all authors publishing in the key health and medical sociology journals work within universities. In the United States, the majority are employed in named departments of sociology, making it quite different to the other two countries. The rest of the sociologists in the United States are widely dispersed across departments of many other disciplines, with the only other notable areas being public health and medicine. In Australia the pattern is quite different. This country has the lowest number of sociologists within medicine, with the majority scattered across sociology, the social and health sciences, and various social or sexual health units including nursing. The pattern is similar in the United Kingdom, though there are more within medicine and health financing/planning.

The distinctive concentration of sociology as a work site for sociologists in the United States is matched by a higher proportion of American authors in our study population identifying as sociologists or medical sociologists. We also find quite different disciplinary alliances in the United States. When the disciplinary identities of the study population were examined, it became evident that sociologists in the United States were far more likely to regard themselves as a sociologist and either a psychologist, epidemiologist or demographer. In contrast, sociologists in the United Kingdom who used two identities were more likely to choose between psychology, nursing, health policy/research or anthropology; and Australians to select from nursing, health policy/research or feminist studies. The significantly closer association between sociology and the sciences – the disciplines of psychology, demography and epidemiology – in the United States, compared with either Britain or Australia, indicates very different boundary patterns internationally, with the United States as a unique case.

These variations in the external boundary-relationships of sociology are associated with national differences in the production of sociological knowledge, for a mutuality of interests across disciplinary boundaries suggests a compatibility between their knowledge bases, social practices, and perhaps their organisational arrangements. In our empirical study for instance, we find the relatively closer relationship between sociology and psychology in the United States to be linked with a greater sociological interest in concepts and topics such as stigma and deviance. Although these concepts/topics were of interest to sociologists in Australia and the United Kingdom some decades ago, in recent decades they are more commonly found in the discipline of psychology. The strength of American interest in these areas has been noted also by others, for it has been said that the discipline has a strong focus on mental health and psycho-social stressors, and well-integrated with social psychology (Levine 1995:3; Clair *et al.* 2007:255). We find a similar linking between knowledge and external boundary relations with regard to some of sociology's other boundaries. For example, the more distant boundary-relations between nursing and sociology in the United States are reflected in the proportionally lower level of interest in the work context of nurses in that country. Likewise, the much more permeable boundaries between epidemiology and sociology in the United States roughly mirror the proportional levels of interest in 'specific diseases' in each country.

Variations in the external border relationships are also allied with divergent sociological *practices* (e.g. working in research teams rather than independently), and with the dissimilar *organisational* and institutional placement of individuals. Thus, for example, the much stronger relationships between sociology and psychology, and sociology and epidemiology in the United States, have produced not merely collaboration between the disciplinary fields, but some merging of sociological territory with the neighbouring field and the adoption of some of its methods, concepts, subjects and social practices into sociology itself. While this incorporation process may initially be confined to the sociological speciality, over time, as we have seen with other forms of sociological knowledge (e.g. grounded theory, theories of the professions, statistical methods) and practice (e.g. the introduction of large research teams, measuring 'performance' according to an individual's success with obtaining grants rather than scholarship); these new knowledges and practices tend to become established in all aspects of the disciplinary field. Indeed, where there is extensive excursion into the territory of another field, the dominant discipline may dispense with its practitioners and adopt its skills and practices as its own. It is not difficult to find examples of this, for many sociology courses are taught by non-sociologists within medical faculties in all three countries. Less common in the United Kingdom and Australia (but pervasive in the United States) is the practice of teaching epidemiology and psychology within sociology departments. In the case of the United States, the sharing of territory by sociology and psychology has been evident for some considerable time, for social psychology was the first sociological speciality to be established within the *American Sociological Association* (*ASA*).

What do these differences in the external disciplinary boundaries mean for the production of sociological knowledge in each country? They show that where the borders between sociology and medicine are more permeable, as they are in the United States, their knowledges and practices are likely to show greater similarities, and sociology to be more accommodating of medical values and less controversial or critical in its approach. Where, on the other hand, the borders show a rigidity, there is less opportunity for interaction and collaboration, and, at the same time, sharper differentiation between their knowledges and practices. In the United Kingdom, and even more so in Australia, where disciplinary boundaries between sociology and the statistical and medical sciences (e.g. epidemiology, psychology, demography) are relatively impermeable, sociological knowledge has retained the distinct critical edge we first encountered with Marx, Durkheim, Weber and the other early sociologists.

These findings indicate the strong relationship between the institutional context of a discipline and its knowledge base. Previous studies have pointed to differences in the knowledge bases of the various disciplines (whether with regard to their objects of knowledge, methodologies, significant concepts or theoretical perspectives), and theorised these as the drivers of divergent disciplinary practices. This study, in contrast, has investigated the social practices and institutional setting as causal agents underpinning the variations in the cognitive products of sociologists. This possibility has been explored in two ways: (1) by investigating the disciplinary identities adopted by sociologists and (2) the disciplines they are employed within. This focus on the differences in social relations rather than knowledge content has provided a map of the more important disciplines at the boundaries of sociology, showing where they are rigid and where they are more permeable, and where they vary from one country to the next. Of course, the current data set provides information only about sociologists of health and medicine, and it is possible, and indeed likely, that sociology's external boundaries may vary a little when the different disciplinary specialities are taken into account. However even this brief study gives us an insight into the importance of the institutional context for understanding the inter- and intra-disciplinary disputes over knowledge, and it tells us something of how disciplinary fields are formed and maintained through their social relationships, their alliances and hostilities, their oppositions and compromises.

Identity, inclusion and exclusion

One of the aims of this study was to explore sociology in its current manifestation rather than define, *a priori*, its terrains and boundaries, tensions and debates, its people and forms of organisation. The study was designed so that without having to ask, our authors could nevertheless tell us what they called themselves, and show us what theories, topics and reference materials they saw as important to the discipline. Other studies have been done – often by the professional associations – to discover the factors encouraging individuals to become sociologists or stay within the discipline. Instead of gathering statements about the reasons and motivations driving the actions of sociologists, this study has sought answers through continually teasing out the connections between sociological knowledge, identity and institutional context. In the process, the study has discovered quite a bit about the way sociologists construct their disciplinary identity and practice their craft.

The discipline – as a site of social action and a social structure – is a significant aspect of the sociologists' social and institutional context. Disciplines encourage conformity to a set of often unspecified social rules. In this study, individuals working within departments of sociology (i.e. discipline-based departments) are shown as more likely to adopt the identity of a sociologist, attend sociological conferences, have qualifications in sociology, write for sociological journals, and use sociological theory in their papers. This suggests the critical importance of discipline-based departments (rather than multi-disciplinary units) for the ongoing sustainability of the sociological project.

Disciplines also function in conjunction with professional associations. Professionalisation practices have assisted sociologists to bargain in the academic marketplace, gain space within the university system, and hold onto a defined territory of formal knowledge. Disciplinarity, on the other hand, has involved a process of construction of the social and cognitive resources of sociology and put these into play in negotiations over territory and legitimacy. As such, it is disciplinarity that provides sociologists with their relative status positions within the sociological community, their roles and tasks within the university system, and defines the content and boundaries of their knowledge base. The two processes – disciplinarity and professionalisation – operate together to shape the working lives of sociologists. The reverse is also true. The norms and interests of the membership, often closely aligned with theoretical perspectives developed within the sociological knowledge base, influence the activities of sociologists and so have an impact on the discipline as a profession. This becomes evident when the professional association provides subsidies to minorities, runs childcare services, offers scholarships, or makes public statements about issues the members hold dear. In other words, sociologists configure their *professional* practices according to the values embedded in the discipline of sociology itself.

The entwining of professionalism and disciplinarity enables disciplines to function effectively as systems of social control. This becomes evident when individuals or groups fail to conform to 'sociological norms', or when debates arise over the discipline's successes and failures, trends and developments. There have been many examples of both of these over the decades. One of the more notable of the former arose in the 1980s in the United Kingdom, when sociology was under attack from the conservative Thatcher government. In the midst of this, two prominent sociologists made headlines in the media with their criticisms of the 'Left-Wing' bias of sociology: David Marsland and Julius Gould. Both were called to task for their actions by the *British Sociological Association (BSA)*, and Gould subsequently resigned (Platt 2002:190). The response from the discipline and the profession is evidence of institutional processes at work, where apparent 'deviations' from expected behaviour are addressed to re-establish the social order.

Many examples can also be found of the second type: decades of claims about the 'lack of coherence' or 'fragmentation' of the discipline; about its failure to grapple with the 'big questions' and the 'real' world of policy and public affairs (Mechanic 1993:96; Bird *et al.* 2000; Clair *et al.* 2007); its narrow concentration on the industrialised, first world (Hafferty and Light 1995:148); and the tendency for the specialities to be 'applied' or 'atheoretical' (Scambler 2005:7; Seale 2008). While such claims need to be taken seriously, in this volume, rather than signs of the inadequacies of individuals or groups, they are seen as the discipline and the profession in action. Taking note of the social and institutional conditions under which the works were produced, we traced, for instance, the tendency towards accepting the definitions and perspectives of medicine back to the phenomenon of contract research and the direct support of health agencies or medical institutions. And rather than condemn individuals for their lack of objectivity and for taking 'the King's shilling', these were seen as a response to the pressures on academics to increase their citation scores: a situation which Graham Scambler (2005:6) regards as a taming or 'colonisation of the academic imperative'. The response of the discipline, as a regulatory system, has not been uniform. Some disciplinary actors have sought to distance the 'applied' work of the speciality from the disciplinary 'core', preserving the ideal image of sociology as a critical and independent discipline. This reaction was perhaps most evident in Britain during the 1970s, though it continues to reappear in the contemporary context, particularly in Australia. In other parts of the discipline the new practices appear to have become 'normal practice' and regarded as evidence of successful adaptation. This latter response is more evident in the United States where sociology is often entwined with social psychology or epidemiology.

Disciplines are often the vehicles through which institutions such as universities or the state bestow legitimacy, deploy resources for sociologists, control their activity and possibilities for promotion, and organise their daily workloads. Departmental structures are important in this process. Offering an individual employment within a department can, in itself, be an acknowledgement of disciplinary identity and a mark of official acceptance. In an ongoing sense, a department is an institutional administrative apparatus that assists a discipline to ensure compliance with norms and standards of behaviour and output, and makes its credentialisation and training processes possible. By insisting on specific degree structures and the teaching of courses, institutions can make it difficult for groups to break away to form new disciplines (Butler *et al.* 2009). Together, the discipline and the department define what counts as merit and academic 'success', and offer (different kinds of) sanctions for 'failure' or lack of output.

This tells us that disciplines are *Janus-Faced*. They operate as vehicles of inclusion as well as exclusion. On the one hand, they are capable of providing members with an identity, meaningful goals, and a set of practices which unite individuals and groups across continents. On the other hand, they are a means of exclusion, determining who can call themselves a sociologist and what can be said and done in the name of the discipline. Of course, disciplines are not in themselves responsible for the entirety of these exclusions; after all, the structures of inequality, the opportunities for corruption, the tendencies towards poor decision-making, prejudice and irrational, unethical behaviour, cut through into this arena as they do in all aspects of social life. Nevertheless there are some characteristics peculiar to disciplinarity. These are the discourses and practices defining the intellectual arena and protecting its boundaries. They operate on individuals, encouraging compliance, conferring identity but also subjecting many – particularly those from the working class or minority groups – to an anxiety about one's suitability as a sociologist and member of this elite group. They also operate at a local or national or even international level, shaping the size and strength of the sociological community, producing specific kinds of politics and mechanisms of governance, and determining the placement of the disciplinary boundaries.

These discourses and practices mean the configuration of the discipline differs to some extent in each location. In the United States, for instance, medical sociology is viewed by many as a discipline in its own right, whereas in Australia, with its much smaller academic community, it is seen as a speciality field of the discipline. This reminds us that disciplines and disciplinary boundaries are *social artefacts*. The very notion of what a discipline is, and indeed what a speciality field is, varies from country to country as well as over time. In some locations the boundaries are relatively permeable and the territory extensive. This appears to be the case for sociology in the United States. In contrast, the boundaries for sociology in Australia are rigidly controlled and the territory remains small. This is *not just a facet of the smaller population*, but a consequence of the (local) 'rules' of the discipline. These do not allow for much multi- or inter-disciplinary scholarship, do not give value to works produced outside the university (e.g. for the policy community), and rarely bestow approval on works popularising sociology for the general market.

The more stringent rules of the discipline in the Australian context are, in part, the result of its unique historical conditions of settlement. Devoid of a culture of science as the pursuit of 'gentlemen' and amateurs (as it was in Britain during the eighteenth and nineteenth centuries), or a corporate imperative secured through a cult of individualism (as evident in the United States from the later nineteenth century); Australian scholarship has long displayed an intolerance for expertise without authorisation, whether this be from the colonial state, or, more recently, the imprimatur of the professions or the disciplines. Moreover, given that the brief and intense process of institutionalisation is an experience still in living memory of its senior practitioners, 'protectionism' of sociology's borders continues to be encouraged within the discipline. This rigidity of its boundaries has significant implications for the viability of the discipline, for many individuals who would, in another country, be included as a sociologist are not granted this identity in Australia. Individuals finding that the discipline won't publish their papers, won't give them grants, won't give them regular employment, and won't recognise their expertise are likely to find other disciplines, other social networks and reference groups, and other conferences and publishing venues where they are made welcome.

One sociology of health and medicine or three?

One of the questions threading through this volume has been whether there is only one sociology of health and medicine or perhaps several, each with unique characteristics and flourishing largely independently. We have already noted the many national variations in the practice and organisation of sociology, and the implications these have for the knowledge base of the discipline and its speciality. The question still remains about whether these national variations are sufficient to conclude the existence of three distinct sociologies.

We may be tempted to say yes to this question if disciplines and specialities are regarded as discrete domains of formal knowledge, each with characteristic 'traits' and logics that distinguish them from others. From such a perspective we could simply add together the commonalities, and subtract any dissimilarities to find an answer to our question. This was very much the mid-twentieth-century view of disciplines, and remains the more conventional approach, for it assumes sociology has a 'core' or 'essence' which provides it with coherence and an integrity that can be threatened by difference and divergence. It is a conception of sociology continually making an appearance in contemporary debates, particularly when the issue of the profusion of sub-fields arises, for it is asserted that these will lead to a disintegration of the 'controlling centre' of the discipline (cf. Pearlin 1992:1). As an approach, it focuses on the protection and preservation of the sociological heritage, and is generally associated with an internalist position on disciplinary or intellectual change, where radical, structural change can be prevented by maintaining the intellectual traditions (cf. Collins 1998; Abbott 2001:152). The major shortcoming of this older approach is its failure to acknowledge the inherently *political* nature of disciplinarity. Questions about the universalism (or otherwise) of the sociology of health and medicine are only partly 'technical' ones: for disciplines are, as we have argued in this volume, social forms. This means debates about variations in the knowledge base or practices of sociology are about whose voices *should* be heard, and which methods, practices and perspectives *should* be marginalised rather than tolerated, encouraged, and institutionalised across the domain. As such, they are revealing of the extent to which hegemony has been achieved across the discipline.

Though the older conception of sociology was successful as a professional strategy of unification in previous decades, it is no longer *politically acceptable* for one model of sociology to be explicitly imposed on all practitioners, and it is increasingly improbable that one would be tolerated – without resistance – in the current context. As suggested by Pescosolido and Kronenfeld (1995:16), the older form of industrial society has ended, and our social institutions are no longer meeting individual and societal needs. This calls for a re-alignment of 'the original agendas of sociology, medical sociology and policy':

> We stand at a transition between social forms. The society that created the opportunity for the rise of a dominant profession of medicine, for a new discipline of sociology, and for a spin-off of the subfield of medical sociology, is undergoing major change. As the larger social system unravels in the face of rapid social change, established problems, solutions, and understandings are challenged because they do not successfully confront current realities
>
> (Pescosolido and Kronenfeld 1995:9).

The alternative, argued throughout this book, is an emphasis on disciplines as sites of social practice and forms of social structure. We no longer need to see disciplines as being 'one single thing', but instead as heterogeneous social forms with regard to knowledge, practice and organisation. As collectivities and sites of social action, disciplines are held together through their social relations, common professional objects, and shared disciplinary identities. Their structures have developed over time, taken on an institutional form through decades of social and political action: some of it deliberate and strategic, much of it conducted without consideration of the implications for the discipline's future. From this perspective, sociology is understood reflexively as a socio-historical product, open to the possibilities of change:

> ... sociology is not an eternally valid 'form of knowledge'. Neither does it hold exclusive property rights in a pre-constituted field of

'the social'. Rather, sociology as we find it: an untidy and developing network composed of concepts, arguments, models, exemplary studies, associations, journals and practitioners – living and dead. The elements that make up this odd assemblage are not bound together by any 'logic', but neither are they randomly distributed and associated. Moving through time, the disciplinary network acquires the status of a tradition – or set of traditions – through citation and self-reference. On that basis, the question of our disciplinarity is the question of the extent to which we continue to link our activities in research and teaching to the elements of that network

(Crook 2005:425).

Conceiving disciplines in this way enables us to see the sociology of health and medicine in a new light. We see specialities and disciplines as products, not only of the social actions of their members, but of cross-disciplinary and even cross-national relations. In the early twentieth century in the United States, and the 1960s and 1970s in Australia and the United Kingdom, sociologists often spoke of the dearth of culturally appropriate materials for research and teaching and the difficulty of obtaining translations of key sociological works. Calls for greater diversity in the concepts and problems of sociology have also been a persistent, if small and irregular part of sociological debate. Alvin Gouldner's (1970) challenge to the restrictive and narrow orthodoxy of sociology lies alongside the feminist critiques of the same period. These debates have taken on a new intensity in the past decade, as claims for a more reflexive, and culturally appropriate sociology have begun to be heard from the sociologists of marginalised nations (Akiwowo 1999; Alatas 2001, 2006a, 2006b; Connell 2007; Keim 2011).

In this study, we have seen certain commonalities in the sociology of health and medicine across the three countries. Some of these commonalities are the lingering evidence of a past set of hegemonic ideas, practices and forms of organisation which were taken up in the local context through contact with more powerful, authoritative individuals, groups, and texts. Details about precisely *how* these hegemonic processes occurred are often sketchy, as few sociological writings analyse the actual processes of adoption. Nevertheless it is broadly accepted that the discipline was dominated by specific groups and nationalities in certain historical periods. For instance, between 1945 and 1965 American sociology was internationally dominant, imposing the theories of Merton and Parsons and the survey methods of Lazarsfeld on sociologists in other countries including Britain and Australia (Platt 2010:125). During the same period, the United States was also the centrifugal point for the sociology of health and medicine, at least for British and Australian sociologists. In recent decades there has been a growth in local products in both countries. For sociologists in the United Kingdom, French theory has been an important influence; while for those in Australia, developments in Britain have been more influential than those of the United States.

In the current context, world sociology has become more fragmented and diverse than it has been for the past 60 years. Even in the United States, where parochialism is rife (Scambler 2005:5; Clair *et al.* 2007:255), little interest is shown in other methods, theories, or specialities (Levine 1995:2; Pescosolido and Kronenfeld 1995:8) and little is known about forms of sociology beyond the national border; at least two forms of sociology appear to be flourishing (despite being seen as a 'problem' more often than an asset). Elsewhere the trend is also towards a healthier diversity of sociologies. Though few distinctive *national* schools can be identified, there are many groups drawing from their unique socio-geopolitical context to critique and engage with mainstream sociological ideas and methods.

Some of this diversity has been made evident through this study of the speciality field of the sociology of health and medicine. Despite the national differences pointed out in the sections above, it would be overstating the case to conclude that three distinct national sociologies are in evidence. Conceiving disciplines primarily as social forms rather than discrete parcels of formal knowledge means taking into consideration the social relations and social identities of the social actors within these sites. And this tells us that rather than three national sociologies, we see two main social forms for the speciality. One shares permeable, soft boundaries with psychology, epidemiology and public health; the other has closer ties to anthropology, the allied health sciences, and the policy and social sciences. Neither variation has entirely permeable boundaries with medicine or economics, indicating ongoing social action on all sides to protect the parent discipline – and its specialties – from incursion. Both forms flourish within the United States, but only the latter appears to have taken up significant territory in the other two countries.

What does this pattern of disciplinary relations and structures tell us about dominance and hegemony within the speciality? It suggests that sociology is no longer led by the visions and strategies of one small group within an identifiable geographic locale; yet the speciality and the discipline continue to be constrained and hierarchically organised. In the contemporary context, the capacity of small groups of social actors to shape the direction of the discipline and its specialities is less certain. New spaces and forms of resistance are possible in the new technological context, for self-publishing and electronic publishing opportunities have proliferated, as have other means to connect with one another internationally. With the advent of new global publishing conglomerates, and new market-based mechanisms (such as electronic indexing and citation systems), certain forms of sociology and sociological practices, and the status positions of sociologists from the leading universities in the dominant countries have been confirmed within the new system. Compared with the sociology of the mid-twentieth century, this one *is* more diverse, it *is* multi-paradigmatic, and it tends to be lead by a larger network or coalition of actors and groups rather than a small circle of individuals. It is, in effect, evidence of a shift in control from the individual and the group to the hegemony of key institutional actors within an increasingly dominant marketplace.

This shift in the relations of power brings radical change for the discipline, pressing sociologists to breach the historically constructed boundaries between it, economics and medicine. Given the salience of these boundaries for the knowledge base of the speciality, it is perhaps not surprising that the sociology of health and medicine is criticised for reflecting a narrow range of concerns, theories and methodologies. 'Health' continues to be largely defined by medical definitions of disease, and little sociological work explores the many notions of *good* health, nor challenges the dominant view of ill-health as a consequence of individual risk-taking and irresponsibility. Moreover, much of the work on health inequalities simply ignores class or race except as descriptive categories for the measurement of differences. And much more can be done to investigate the structural barriers that block access to health services and prevent radical improvements to health care systems. Why are there so many complaints about the narrowness of the speciality field? Why does it fail to tackle some of the more significant problems? Why is so little notice taken of the health of the third world? By examining the speciality as a social form, and taking more note of the structures which determine its content and direction, it becomes possible to see the constraints on our actions. Like all social actors, sociologists of health and medicine are hampered by a lack of opportunities, by our class and ethnicity, our gender, and the barriers of language. Other disciplines are still more powerful and lock us out of debates. These same factors – and many others – limit the possibility of more variants of the sociology of health and medicine emerging.

A way forward

No social group can plan for the future without a sense of who they are and what they do. This book has taken a small step in this direction by offering a description of the boundaries of one of sociology's specialities and an indication of its major features. Like those in other disciplines, sociologists face an uncertain future. The unrelenting pressures of the global marketplace are re-fashioning the universities and other institutions which have supported our research and teaching, and it is likely, indeed quite probable, that one day, the disciplinary landscape will be virtually unrecognisable to those most familiar with its twentieth-century form.

How might we ensure the survival of the sociology of health and medicine in the midst of these changes? This volume has provided an alternative way of understanding ourselves as sociologists as well as the speciality we work within. We can now see the field as inherently social, where our actions and thoughts are shaped by the same social forces we study daily. This greater reflexivity can assist us, as sociologists of health and medicine, to – in the words of Elliot Freidson – face our 'self-mystifications' and our own 'myths', be cautious about offering criticism which is essentially moral outrage and condemnation, put more effort into constructively indicating how things might be different to the way they are, and making an effort to be 'self-conscious and systematic no matter what the theoretical school' (Freidson 1983:212, 219). This advice seems very appropriate in an era when many new voices are beginning to be heard in the international arena. We can use such reflexivity to assist in finding opportunities to break down the barriers that constrain our actions, and build a better discipline while we work towards improving the health and well-being of the world's peoples.

This seems an appropriate opportunity to put the final words to this book. In earlier pages I spoke of the 'magic' of sociology – the wonder of which has not been dispelled by theorising the very sociological processes that create and sustain the discipline. I trust that my current and future colleagues, when faced with the difficulties of academe and the world of medicine, may find a little of their own sociological magic in their journeys through the discipline.

Notes

1 Theoretical Frameworks and Beginnings

1. In the United Kingdom, the majority of universities have been, and continue to be public or state institutions, and the private sector is insignificant. Only *Buckingham University* is privately owned, though it might be argued that *Oxford* and *Cambridge*, with their large endowments and reserves, are able to operate *as if they were* private institutions, as they are not as dependent on the state for funding (for more information, see Fulton and Holland 2001:302).
2. Australian universities are also primarily state institutions. Some belong to the Catholic Church, though student fees in these universities are publicly subsidised as they are in the state institutions. Only Bond University is fully private.
3. The term professor is reserved throughout this text for individuals within the university holding the highest academic rank. It is not used in the American sense for a teacher in the university system. In Australia and Britain, junior academic staff are known as lecturers. Staff with PhDs are given the title of Doctor, but this is largely dispensed with if they are promoted to, or appointed to, the rank of Professor or Associate Professor. Professors may be given a department to run, in which case they are usually said to 'hold a chair', or the title may simply denote their rank. In some cases they are given a 'personal chair', which indicates their rank without the responsibility of running a department. An academic who is given the title of professor in an honorary capacity when undertaking a particular role, for example as Vice-Chancellor, cannot legitimately retain this once the role has been relinquished.

2 Past and Present: Three National Sociologies of Health and Medicine

1. Information about the medical sociology research centres can be found on the *BSA* website: http://www.britsoc.co.uk/medsoc (accessed November 2010).
2. Information about the Foundation for the Sociology of Health and Illness and the *BSA* Medical Sociology Group can be found on the website: http://www.shifoundation.org.uk (accessed November 2010).
3. Indeed, the Medical Section continued as a significant dimension of the national association, even after the withdrawal of the New Zealand sociologists from the federal body and the separation of *SAANZ* into two independent units in 1988: *The Australian Sociological Association* (*TASA*) and the *Sociological Association of Aotearoa* (*New Zealand*).
4. Basil Hetzel, who graduated in medicine from *Adelaide University* in 1944, became the Foundation Professor of Social and Preventative Medicine at

Monash University in 1968. His 1974 book *Health and Australian Society* subsequently sold nearly 40,000 copies.

5. With the exception of six years between 2004 and 2009 when the author was the Editor-in-Chief of the *Health Sociology Review*.

3 Disciplines, Professions and Specialities

1. Both disciplines and their speciality areas contain many of the same social actors, often sharing similar relationships with institutions and other disciplines. Under certain conditions however, significant differences may emerge between the disciplines and specialities with regard to their relationships with other institutions or disciplines – particularly with medicine – and some of these will be explored in subsequent chapters.

2. For example, Dugald Baird, the Professor of Midwifery at the *University of Aberdeen*, was interested in social class differences in childbearing matters and began to recruit, from about 1948, researchers from various fields, including dieticians, sociologists, pathologists and statisticians for his department (Jefferys 1997:134). Likewise, nursing, which expanded during and after the Second World War, became receptive to sociology in the United States in the 1950s. It turned from its previous focus on educational psychology towards sociology, providing a 'critical locus' for the developing field (Olesen 1974:6). Both Robert Merton and Everett Hughes served as consultants to nursing organisations during these years. Departments of public health and community medicine have been instrumental since the 1970s in the United States in providing a disciplinary space for medical sociologists (Bloom 2000:26).

3. A recent development has been the creation of the Council of the Humanities and Social Sciences (CHASS). Unlike the office of the Chief Scientist and the Chief Medical Officer, CHASS has no official role and is poorly funded.

4. As this publication goes to press, announcements have been made by the Australian government that the journal ranking process is to be discontinued. I have allowed the text to remain however, as the damage to many journals has been quite irreparable.

References

Abbott, A. (1995) 'Things of Boundaries', *Social Research* 62(4): 857–82.

Abbott, A. (2000) 'Reflections on the Future of Sociology', *Contemporary Sociology* 29(2): 296–300.

Abbott, A. (2001) *Chaos of Disciplines*, The University of Chicago Press: Chicago.

Abend, G. (2006) 'Styles of Sociological Thought: Sociologies, Epistemologies, and the Mexican and U.S. Quests for Truth', *Sociological Theory* 24: 1–41.

Abernathy, W. and Utterback, J. (1978) 'Patterns of Industrial Innovation', *Technology Review* 80(7): 78–89.

ABS (2002) *Education and Training Indicators, Australia Catalogue No. 4230.0*, Australian Bureau of Statistics: Canberra.

Abrams, P. (1968) *The Origins of British Sociology 1834–1914*, Chicago University Press: Chicago.

Adams, A.; Buckingham, C.D.; Lindenmeyer, A.; McKinlay, J.B.; Link, C.; Marceau, L. and Arber, S. (2008) 'The Influence of Patient and Doctor Gender on Diagnosing Coronary Heart Disease', *Sociology of Health and Illness* 30(1): 1–18.

Agger, B. (2000) *Public Sociology: From Social Facts to Literary Acts*, Rowman Littlefield: Lanham.

Akers, R.L. (1992) 'Linking Sociology with Its Specialities: The Case of Criminology', *Social Forces* 71(1): 1–16.

Akiwowo, A. (1999) 'Indigenous Sociologies: Extending the Scope of the Argument', *International Sociology* 14(2): 115–38.

Alatas, S.F. (2001) 'The Study of the Social Sciences in Developing Societies: Towards an Adequate Conceptualisation of Relevance', *Current Sociology* 49(2): 1–26.

Alatas, S.F. (2006a) 'The Autonomous, the Universal and the Future of Sociology', *Current Sociology* 54(1): 7–23.

Alatas, S.F. (2006b) *Alternative Discourses in Asian Social Science*, Sage: London.

Albert, M. (2003) 'Universities and the Market Economy: The Differential Impact on Knowledge Production in Sociology and Economics', *Higher Education* 45(2): 147–82.

Albury, R. (1989) 'Inquiry into Ethics: The Australian Senate and Human Embryo Experimentation', *Australian Journal of Social Issues* 24(4): 269–84.

Alcorso, C. (1989) 'Migrants and the Workers' Compensation System: The Basis of an Ideology', *Australian and New Zealand Journal of Sociology* 25(1): 46–65.

Alexander, J.C. (1997) 'General Introduction', in Alexander, J.C.; Boudon, R. and Cherkaoui, M. (eds), *The Classical Tradition in Sociology: The American Tradition*, Volume 1, Sage: London, pp. i–xv.

Amsterdamska, O. (2005) 'Demarcating Epidemiology', *Science, Technology and Human Values* 30(1): 17–51.

Ancich, M.; Connell, R.W.; Fisher, J.A. and Kolff, M. (1969) 'A Descriptive Bibliography of Published Research and Writing on Social Stratification in Australia, 1946–1967', *Australian and New Zealand Journal of Sociology* 5(1): 48–76.

Anderson, D.S. and Western, J.S. (1967) *An Inventory to Measure Student's Attitudes*, University of Queensland Press: St Lucia.

Annandale, E. (1998) *The Sociology of Health and Medicine*, Polity Press: Cambridge.

ANZJS. (1965a) 'Notes and Announcements', *Australian and New Zealand Journal of Sociology* 1(1): 62–7.

ANZJS. (1965b) 'Notes and Announcements', *Australian and New Zealand Journal of Sociology* 1(2): 132–6.

ANZJS. (1967) 'Notes and Announcements', *Australian and New Zealand Journal of Sociology* 3(2): 151–6.

ANZJS. (1970) 'Notes and Announcements', *Australian and New Zealand Journal of Sociology* 6(1): 70–3.

ARC. (2010) *Ranked Outlets*, Australian Research Council, http://www.arc.gov.au/era_journal_list.htm [accessed 2010].

Armstrong, D. (1980) *An Outline of Sociology Applied to Medicine*, Butterworth-Heinemann: Bristol.

Armstrong, D. (1982) 'The Doctor–Patient Relationship: 1930–80', in Wright, P. and Treacher, A. (eds), *The Problem of Medical Knowledge: Examining the Social Construction of Medicine*, Edinburgh University Press: Edinburgh, pp. 109–22.

Armstrong, D. (1987) 'Bodies of Knowledge/Knowledge of Bodies', in Jones, C. and Porter, R. (eds), *Reassessing Foucault*, Routledge: London.

Armstrong, D. (2000) 'Social Theorising about Health and Illness', in Albrecht, G.; Fitzpatrick, R. and Scrimshaw, S. (eds), *The Handbook of Social Studies in Health and Medicine*, Sage: London, pp. 24–35.

Armstrong, D. (2003) 'The Impact of Papers in Sociology of Health and Illness', *Sociology of Health and Illness* 25: 58–74.

Aron, R. (1971) 'Modern Society and Sociology', in Tiryakian, E. (ed), *The Phenomenon of Sociology: A Reader in the Sociology of Sociology*, Meredith: New York, pp. 158–70.

Ashley, J. (1976) *Hospitals, Paternalism and the Role of the Nurse*, Teachers College Press: New York.

Atkinson, P. (1977) 'Becoming a Hypochondriac', in Davis, A. and Horobin, G. (eds), *Medical Encounters*, Croom Helm: London, pp. 17–31.

Atkinson, P. (1981) *The Clinical Experience: An Ethnography of Medical Education*, Gower: Westmead.

Atkinson, P. (1995) *Medical Talk and Medical Work: The Liturgy of the Clinic*, Sage: Thousand Oaks, CA.

Atkinson, R.J. (2010) 'Bibliometrics Out, Journalmetrics In!' *HERDSA News*, 32(1), http://www.roger-atkinson.id.au/pubs/herdsa-news/32-1.html. [accessed 2010].

Babbie, E. (2010) *The Practice of Social Research*, Wadsworth, Thomson Learning: Belmont.

Badgley, R. (1971) 'The Sociology of Health: Some Questions', *The Milbank Memorial Fund Quarterly* 49(2): 133–57.

Badgley, R.F. and Bloom, S.W. (1973) 'Behavioural Sciences and Medical Education: The Case of Sociology', *Social Science and Medicine* 7: 927–41.

Baer, H. (1981) 'The Organisational Rejuvenation of Osteopathy: A Reflection of the Decline of Professional Dominance in Medicine', *Social Science and Medicine* 15A: 701–12.

Bagley, C. (1976) 'Sociology and Social Ethics of Abortion', *Ethics in Science and Medicine* 3(1): 21–32.

Baker, C. (1983) 'The "Age of Consent" Controversy: Age and Gender as Social Practice', *Australian and New Zealand Journal of Sociology* 19(1): 96–112.

Baker, C.M.A. and Manwell, C. (1981) 'Honesty in Science: A Partial Test of a Sociobiological Model of the Social Structure of Science', *Search* 12: 151–60.

Baldock, C. (1994) 'Sociology in Australia and New Zealand', in Mohan, R. and Wilke, A. (eds), *International Handbook of Contemporary Developments in Sociology*, Greenwood Press: Westport, CT, pp. 587–622.

Baldock, C. and Lally, J. (1974) *Sociology in Australia and NZ*, Greenwood Press: Westport.

Barber, B. (1959) 'The Sociology of Science', in Merton, R.K.; Broom, L. and Cottrell, L. (eds), *Sociology Today: Problems and Prospects*, Basic Books: New York, pp. 215–28.

Barker, K. (2008) 'Electronic Support Groups, Patient-Consumers, and Medicalisation', *Journal of Health and Social Behavior* 49(1): 20–36.

Barnes, B. (1977) *Interests and the Growth of Knowledge*, Routledge and Kegan Paul: London.

Bates, E.M. (1977) *Models of Madness*, University of Queensland Press: St Lucia.

Bates, E.M. (1979) 'Decision Making in Critical Illness', *Australian and New Zealand Journal of Sociology* 15(3): 45–54.

Becher, T. (1989) *Academic Tribes and Territories: Intellectual Enquiry and the Cultures of Disciplines*, Open University Press and the Society for Research into Higher Education: Milton Keynes.

Bechhofer, F. (1996) 'Quantitative Research in British Sociology: Has It Changed Since 1981?' *Sociology* 30(3): 583–91.

Becker, H.S.; Geer, B.; Hughes, E.C. and Strauss, A. (eds) (1961) *Boys in White: Student Culture in Medical School*, University of Chicago Press: Chicago.

Bell, D. (1974) *The Coming of Post-Industrial Society: A Venture in Social Forecasting*, Heinemann Educational: London.

Bell, D. (1979) 'The New Class: A Muddled Concept', in Bruce-Briggs, B. (ed), *The New Class?* Transaction Books: New Brunswick, pp. 169–90.

Ben-David, J. (1965) 'The Scientific Role: The Conditions of Its Establishment', *Minerva* 4(1): 15–54.

Ben-David, J. and Collins, R. (1966) 'Social Factors in the Origins of New Science', *American Sociological Review* 31: 451–65.

Benton, T. (1978) 'How Many Sociologies?' *The Sociological Review* 26: 2.

Berg, B.L. (2007) *Qualitative Methods for the Social Sciences*, Pearson: Boston.

Berger, P. and Luckmann, T. (1984 [1966]) *The Social Construction of Reality: A Treatise in the Sociology of Knowledge*, Penguin: London.

Berger, P. and Pullberg, S. (1966) 'Reification and the Sociological Critique of Consciousness', *New Left Review* 35(1): 56–71.

Berkman, L.F. and Breslow, L. (1983) *Health and Ways of Living: The Alameda County Study*, Oxford University Press: New York.

Betts, K. (1976) 'The Ovulation Method of Contraception', *Australian Journal of Social Issues* 11(1): 1–14.

Betts, K. (1980) 'Wanted and Unwanted Fertility: Victoria 1971 to 1975', *Australian Journal of Social Issues* 15(3): 194–208.

Betts, K. (1981) 'Ex-Nuptially Conceived Births: A Note on Measurement', *Australian and New Zealand Journal of Sociology* 17(3): 53–6.

Biddle, L.; Donovan, J.; Sharp, D. and Gunnell, D. (2007) 'Explaining Non-Help-Seeking amongst Young Adults with Mental Distress', *Sociology of Health and Illness* 29(7): 983–1002.

Billings, J.S. (1888) 'The History of Medicine', *Boston Medical and Surgical Journal* 118: 29.

Bird, C.; Conrad, P. and Fremont, A. (2000) 'Medical Sociology at the Millennium', in Bird, C., Conrad, P. and Fremont, A. (eds), *Handbook of Medical Sociology*, 5th edition, Prentice Hall: New Jersey, pp. 1–10.

Blackwell, E. (1902) *Essays in Medical Sociology*, 2 volumes, Ernest Bell: London.

Blane, D. (1985) 'An Assessment of the Black Report's Explanations of Health Inequalities', *Sociology of Health and Illness* 7(3): 423–45.

Blane, D. (2003) 'The Use of Quantitative Medical Sociology', *Sociology of Health and Illness* 25: 115–30.

Blaxter, M. (1990) *Health and Lifestyles*, Tavistock: London.

Bloom, S.W. (1963) *The Doctor and His Patient*, Free Press: New York.

Bloom, S.W. (1986) 'Institutional Trends in Medical Sociology', *Journal of Health and Social Behavior* 27(3): 265–76.

Bloom, S.W. (1990) 'Episodes in the Institutionalisation of Medical Sociology', *Journal of Health and Social Behavior* 31(March): 1–10.

Bloom, S.W. (2000) 'The Institutionalisation of Medical Sociology in the United States, 1920–1980', in Bird, C.; Conrad, P. and Fremont, A. (eds), *Handbook of Medical Sociology*, Prentice Hall: New Jersey, pp. 11–31.

Bloom, S.W. (2002) *The Word as Scalpel*, Oxford University Press: New York.

Bloom, S.W. (2005) 'The Relevance of Medical Sociology to Psychiatry', *The Journal of Nervous and Mental Disease* 193(2): 77–84.

Bloor, M.; Samphier, M. and Prior, L. (1987) 'Artefact Explanations of Inequalities in Health', *Sociology of Health and Illness* 9(3): 231–64.

Booth, C. (1902) *Life and Labour of the People in London*, Palgrave Macmillan: London.

Boreham, P.; Pemberton, A. and Wilson, P. (1976) *The Professions in Australia*, University of Queensland Press: St Lucia.

Borowski, A. (2009) 'The Certainty of Uncertainty', *Health Sociology Review* 18(4): 364–78.

Boston Women's Health Book Collective (1973) *Our Bodies, Ourselves*, Simon and Schuster: New York.

Bottomley, W.J. (1974) 'The Climate of Opinion in Australasian Sociology', *Australian and New Zealand Journal of Sociology* 10(1): 64–9.

Boulton, M.; Tuckett, D.; Olson, C. and Williams, A. (1986) 'Social Class and the General Practice Consultation', *Sociology of Health and Illness* 8(4): 325–50.

Bourdieu, P. (1969) 'Intellectual Field and Creative Project', *Social Science Information* 8: 89–119.

Bourdieu, P. (1984) *Distinction* (Translated by Nice, R.), Harvard University Press: Harvard.

Bourdieu, P. (1993) *Sociology in Question* (Translated by Nice, R.), Sage: London.

Bourke, H. (1981) 'Sociology and the Social Sciences in Australia, 1912–1928', *Australian and New Zealand Journal of Sociology* 17(1): 26–35.

Bourke, H. (2005) 'Social Scientists as Intellectuals', in Germov, J. and McGee, T. (eds), *Histories of Australian Sociology*, Melbourne University Press: Carlton, 145–69.

Bower, H.M. (1960) 'The Hospitalisation of the "Criminal Insane" in Victoria', *Medical Journal of Australia* 47(2): 41–7.

Bower, H.M. (1964) 'Old Age in Western Society (Part One)', *Medical Journal of Australia* 2(August 22): 285–92.

Bower, H.M. (1972) 'Psychiatry and Political Thought', *Australian and New Zealand Journal of Psychiatry* 6(3): 191–6.

Bower, H.M. (1986) 'Diagnosis and Differential Diagnosis', in Walters, W. and Ross, M. (eds), *Transsexualism and Sex Reassignment*, Oxford University Press: Melbourne.

Braithwaite, J. (1984) *Corporate Crime in the Pharmaceutical Industry*, Routledge and Kegan Paul: London.

Bramson, L. (1971) 'The Rise of American Sociology', in Tiryakian, E. (ed), *The Phenomenon of Sociology*, Meredith: New York, pp. 65–80.

Braverman, H. (1974) *Labor and Monopoly Capital*, Monthly Review Press: New York.

Brint, S. (1985) 'The Political Attitudes of Professionals', *Annual Review of Sociology* 11: 389–414.

Britten, N. (1991) 'Hospital Consultants' Views of Their Patients', *Sociology of Health and Illness* 13(1): 83–97.

Britten, N. (2001) 'Prescribing and the Defence of Clinical Autonomy', *Sociology of Health and Illness* 23(4): 478–96.

Broad, W. and Wade, N. (1982) *Betrayers of the Truth*, Simon and Schuster: New York.

Broom, D.H. (1991) *Dammed If We Do*, Allen and Unwin: Sydney.

Broom, D.H. (1995) 'Masculine Medicine, Feminine Illness', in Lupton, G. and Najman, J. (eds), *Sociology of Health and Illness*, Palgrave Macmillan: South Melbourne, pp. 99–112.

Broom, L. (1964) Opening Address, *Sociological Association of Australia and New Zealand*, 22nd October, Australian National University: Canberra.

Brown, G. (1959) 'Social Factors Influencing Length of Hospital Stay of Schizophrenic Patients', *British Medical Journal* 2: 1300–4.

Brown, G. and Harris, T. (1978) *The Social Origins of Depression*, Tavistock: London.

Brown, G.; Bone, M.; Dalison, B. and Wing, J. (1968) *Schizophrenia and Social Care*, Oxford University Press: London.

Browning, C.R. and Cagney, K.A. (2003) 'Moving Beyond Poverty', *Journal of Health and Social Behavior* 44(4): 552–71.

Brownlea, A. (1977) 'New Surbia – A Disquieting Synergy', in Hicks, N. (ed), *Proceedings of the Annual Meeting of the Australian and New Zealand Society for Eidemiology and Research in Community Health*, May 1977, University of Adelaide. ANZSERCH: North Adelaide, pp. 328–43.

Bryson, L. (1986) 'How Academic Is an Academic Trade? A Response to Turner', *Journal of Sociology* 22(2): 283–4.

Bryson, L. (1987) 'Women and Management in the Public Sector', *Australian Journal of Public Administration* XLVI(3): 259–72.

Bryson, L. (2005) 'Some Reflections on Australian Sociology and Its Political Context', in Germov, J. and McGee, T. (eds), *Histories of Australian Sociology*, Melbourne University Press: Carlton, pp. 29–48.

Bullough, B. (1972) 'Poverty, Ethnic Identity and Preventive Health Care', *Journal of Health and Social Behavior* 13(4): 347–59.

Bulmer, M. (1985) 'The Development of Sociology and of Empirical Social Research in Britain', in Bulmer, M. (ed), *Essays on the History of British Sociological Research*, Cambridge University Press: Cambridge, pp. 3–35.

Bulmer, M. (1992) 'The Growth of Applied Sociology after 1945', in Halliday, T.C. and Janowitz, M. (eds), *Sociology and Its Publics*, University of Chicago Press: Chicago, pp. 317–45.

Burawoy, M. (2005a) '2004 ASA Presidential Address – for Public Sociology', *American Sociological Review* 70: 4–28.

Burawoy, M. (2005b) 'The Return of the Repressed', *Annals AAPSS* 600: 68–85.

Burton, C. (1977) 'Rejoinder to "Social Contracts amongst Surburban Housewives" ', *American Journal of Sociology* 12(4): 316–17.

Bury, M. (1982) 'Chronic Illness as Biographical Disruption', *Sociology of Health and Illness* 4(2): 167–82.

Bury, M. (1986) 'Social Constructionism and the Development of Medical Sociology', *Sociology of Health and Illness* 8(2): 137–69.

Bury, M. (1991) 'The Sociology of Chronic Illness', *Sociology of Health and Illness* 13(4): 451–68.

Butler, G.; Jones, E. and Stilwell, F. (2009) *Political Economy Now!*, Darlington Press: Sydney.

Buxton, W. and Turner, S.P. (1992) 'From Education to Expertise', in Halliday, T.C. and Janowitz, M. (eds), *Sociology and Its Publics*, University of Chicago Press: Chicago, pp. 373–407.

Caldwell, J.C. (1984) 'Fertility Trends and Prospects in Australia and Other Industrialised Countries', *Australian and New Zealand Journal of Sociology* 20(1): 3–22.

Calhoun, C. (1992) 'Sociology, Other Disciplines, and the Project of a General Understanding of Social Life', in Halliday, T.C. and Janowitz, M. (eds), *Sociology and Its Publics*, University of Chicago Press: Chicago, pp. 137–95.

Calhoun, C. and Van Antwerpen, J. (2007) 'Orthodoxy, Heterodoxy, and Hierarchy', in Calhoun, C. (ed), *Sociology in America*, University of Chicago Press: Chicago, pp. 367–410.

Callan, V. (1980) 'Family Size Attitudes and Use of Contraception in Sydney', *Australian and New Zealand Journal of Sociology* 16(3): 90–6.

Callon, M. (1995) 'Four Models for the Dynamics of Science', in Jasanoff, S.; Markle, G.E; Petersen, J.C. and Pinch, T. (eds), *Handbook of Science and Technology Studies*, Society for Social Studies of Science and Sage: London, pp. 29–63.

Calnan, M. and Johnson, B. (1985) 'Health, Health Risks and Inequalities', *Sociology of Health and Illness* 7(1): 55–75.

Calnan, M.; Silvester, S.; Manley, G. and Taylor-Gooby, P. (2001) 'Doing Business in the NHS', *Sociology of Health and Illness* 22(6): 742–64.

Camic, C. (1979) 'The Utilitarians Revisited', *American Journal of Sociology* 85(3): 516–50.

Camic, C. (1981) 'On the Methodology of the History of Sociology', *American Journal of Sociology* 86(5): 1139–44.

Camic, C. (1987) 'The Making of a Method', *American Sociological Review* 52(4): 421–39.

Camic, C. (1995) 'Three Departments in Search of a Discipline', *Social Research* 62(4): 1003–33.

Camic, C. (1997) 'Introduction', in Camic, C. (ed), *Reclaiming The Sociological Classics*, Blackwell: Oxford, pp. 1–10.

Camic, C. and Xie, Y. (1994) 'The Statistical Turn in American Social Science', *American Sociological Review* 59: 773–805.

Cant, S.L. and Calnan, M. (2008) 'Using Private Health Insurance', *Sociology of Health and Illness* 14(1): 39–56.

Carr-Saunders, A.M. and Wilson, P.A. (1964 [1933]) *The Professions*, Oxford University Press: London.

Cartwright, A. (1975) *How Many Children?* Routledge and Kegan Paul: London.

Cartwright, A. and Anderson, R. (1981) *General Practice Revisited*, Tavistock: London.

Cass, B. (1983) *Why So Few?* Sydney University Press: Sydney.

Casswell, S. and Smythe, M. (1983) 'Alcohol Consumption by Women', *Australian and New Zealand Journal of Sociology* 19(1): 146–52.

Cataldo, F. (2008) 'New Forms of Citizenship and Socio-Political Inclusion', *Sociology of Health and Illness* 30(6): 900–12.

Cawte, J. (1964) 'A Psychiatric Service in the North', *Australian Journal of Social Issues* 2(1): 20–32.

Chadwick, E. (1842) *Report on the Sanitary Condition of the Labouring Population of Great Britain* (edited, and with an introduction by Flinn, M.W.), University Press: Edinburgh.

Chard, J.A.; Lilford, R.J. and Court, B.V. (1997) 'Qualitative Medical Sociology', *Journal of the Royal Society of Medicine* 90: 604–9.

Charles, E. (1934) *The Twilight of Parenthood*, Watts and Co: London.

Charmaz, K. (1991) *Good Days, Bad Days*, Rutgers University Press: New Brunswick, NJ.

Cheek, J.; Garnham, B. and Quan, J. (2006) 'What's in a Number?' *Qualitative Health Research* 16(3): 423–35.

Cheek, J.; Shoebridge, J.; Willis, E. and Zadoroznyj, M. (1996) *Society and Health*, Longman: Melbourne.

Cherkaoui, M. (1997) 'General Introduction', in Boudon, R.; Cherkaoui, M. and Alexander, J. (eds), *The Classical Tradition in Sociology. The European Tradition*, Volume 1, Sage: London, pp. i–xvi.

Chernew, M.E.; Hirth, R.A.; Sonnad, S.; Ermann, R. and Fendrick, A.M. (1998) 'Managed Care, Medical Technology, and Health Care Cost Growth', *Medical Care Research and Review* 55(3): 259–88.

Chimisso, C. (2000) 'The Mind and the Faculties', *History of the Human Sciences* 13(3): 47–68.

Chomsky, N. (1972) *Problems of Knowledge and Freedom*, Barrie and Jenkins: London.

Clair, J.M.; Clark, C.; Hinote, B.P.; Robinson, C.O. and Wasserman, J.A. (2007) 'Developing, Integrating, and Perpetuating New Ways of Applying Sociology to Health, Medicine, Policy, and Everyday Life', *Social Science and Medicine* 64: 248–58.

Clark, A.W. and Yeomans, N. (1969) *Fraser House*, Springer: New York.

Claus, L. (1983) 'The Development of Medical Sociology in Europe', *Social Science and Medicine* 17(21): 1591–7.

Clausen, J. (1959) 'The Sociology of Mental Illness', in Merton, R.K.; Broom, L. and Cottrell, L.S. (eds), *Sociology Today, Problems and Prospects*, Basic Books: New York, pp. 485–508.

Cock, P.; Hay, C.; Gidlow, B. and Willmott, B. (1979) 'The Indigenisation of Sociology in Australia and New Zealand', *Australian and New Zealand Journal of Sociology* 15(3): 69–76.

Cockerham, W. (1983) 'The State of Medical Sociology in the United States, Great Britain, West Germany and Austria', *Social Science and Medicine* 17(20): 1513–27.

Cockerham, W. (2005a) 'Medical Sociology and Sociological Theory', in Cockerham, W. (ed), *The Blackwell Companion to Medical Sociology*, Blackwell: Victoria, pp. 3–22.

Cockerham, W. (2005b) 'Medical Sociology at the Millennium', in Scambler, G. (ed), *Medical Sociology* (Volume One, The Nature of Medical Sociology), Routledge: London, pp. 55–78.

Cockerham, W.C. (1978) *Medical Sociology*, Prentice-Hall: Englewood Cliffs.

Cole, S. (1983) 'The Hierarchy of the Sciences', *American Journal of Sociology* 89: 140–65.

Collins, R. (1985) *Three Sociological Traditions*, Oxford University Press: New York.

Collins, R. (1986) 'Is 1980s Sociology in the Doldrums?' *American Journal of Sociology* 91(6): 1335–55.

Collins, R. (1998) *The Sociology of Philosophies*, The Belknap Press of Harvard University Press: Cambridge.

Collyer, F.M. (1993) Interview with Herbert Bower, unpublished transcript.

Collyer, F.M. (1994) 'Sex-Change Surgery: An "Unacceptable" Innovation?' *Australian and New Zealand Journal of Sociology* 30(1): 3–19.

Collyer, F.M. (1996a) 'Understanding Ulcers: Medical Knowledge, Social Constructionism, and Helicobacter Pylori', *Annual Review of Health Social Science* 6: 1–39.

Collyer, F.M. (1996b) 'Frankenstein Meets the Invisible Man: Science, Medicine and a Theory of Invention', *Electronic Journal of Sociology* 2(2): 1–23.

Collyer, F.M. (1997a) 'The Port Macquarie Base Hospital: Privatisation and the Public Purse', *Just Policy* 10: 27–39.

Collyer, F.M. (1997b) 'Technological Invention: Postmodernism and Social Structure', *Technology in Society* 19(2): 195–205.

Collyer, F.M. (1998) 'Privatisation on the Agenda', *The Australian Journal of Hospital Pharmacy* 28(2): 108–11.

Collyer, F.M. (2003) 'Theorising Privatisation', *Electronic Journal of Sociology* 7(November): 25pp.

Collyer, F.M. (2007) 'A Sociological Approach to Workforce Shortages', *Health Sociology Review* 16(3–4): 248–62.

Collyer, F.M. (2008) 'Max Weber, Historiography, Medical Knowledge, and the Formation of Medicine', *Electronic Journal of Sociology*, http://www.sociology.org/contents.html.

Collyer, F.M. (2010) 'Origins and Canons: Medicine and the History of Sociology', *History of the Human Sciences* 23(2): 86–108.

Collyer, F.M. (2011a) 'Reflexivity and the Sociology of Science and Technology', *The Qualitative Report*, 16(2): 316–40.

Collyer, F.M. (2011b) 'The Sociology of Health and Medicine in Australia', *Politica Y Sociedad* 48(2): 101–18.

Collyer, F.M. and White, K.N. (1997) 'Enter the Market: Competition, Regulation and Hospital Funding in Australia', *Australian and New Zealand Journal of Sociology* 33(3): 344–63.

Collyer, F.M. and White, K.N. (2001) *Corporate Control of Healthcare in Australia*, Discussion Paper No. 42, Australia Institute, Australian National University: Canberra.

Comaroff, J. (1976) 'A Bitter Pill to Swallow', *Sociological Review* 24: 2.

Comaroff, J. (1977) 'Conflicting Paradigms of Pregnancy', in Davis, A. and Horobin, G. (eds), *Medical Encounters*, Croom Helm: London.

Comaroff, J. (1982) 'Medicine: Symbol and Ideology', in Wright, P. and Treacher, A. (eds), *The Problem of Medical Knowledge*, Edinburgh University Press: Edinburgh, pp. 49–68.

Congalton, A.A. (1963) *Nurses' Evaluation of Occupational Status and Other Studies*, New South Wales College of Nursing: Sydney.

Congalton, A.A. (1969) *Status and Prestige in Australia*, Cheshire: Melbourne.

Congalton, A.A. (1976) *The Individual in Society*, Wiley: North Ryde.

Congalton, A.A. and Najman, J.M. (1971) *Nurse and Patient: A Sociological View*, F.S. Symes: Sydney.

Connell, R. (1997) 'Why Is Classical Theory Classical?' *American Journal of Sociology* 102(6): 1511–57.

Connell, R. (2000) 'Charting Futures for Sociology', *Contemporary Sociology* 29(2): 291–6.

Connell, R. (2006) 'Core Activity', *Journal of Sociology* 42(1): 5–23.

Connell, R. (2007) *Southern Theory*, Allen and Unwin: Crows Nest.

Connell, R.W. and Dowsett, G.W. (eds) (1993) *Rethinking Sex*, Temple University Press: Philadelphia, PA.

Connell, R. and Wood, J. (2002) 'Globalisation and Scientific Labour', *Journal of Sociology* 38(2): 167–90.

Connell, R.; Wood, J. and Crawford, J. (2005) 'The Global Connections of Intellectual Workers', *International Sociology* 20(1): 5–26.

Conrad, P. (1988) 'Worksite Health Promotion', *Social Science and Medicine* 26(5): 485–9.

Conrad, P. (1992) 'Medicalisation and Social Control', *Annual Review of Sociology*, Annual Reviews: Palo Alto, CA.

Conrad, P. and Kern, R. (eds) (1981) *The Sociology of Health and Illness*, St. Martin's Press: New York.

Conrad, P. and Leiter, V. (2008) 'From Lydia Pinkham to Queen Levitra', *Sociology of Health and Illness* 30(6): 825–38.

Cook, J.A. and Wright, E.R. (1995) 'Medical Sociology and the Study of Severe Mental Illness', *Journal of Health and Social Behavior* 35(extra issue): 95–114.

Cooke, H. (1993) 'Boundary Work in the Nursing Curriculum', *Journal of Advanced Nursing* 18: 1990–8.

Cooper, D.G. (eds) (1967) *Psychiatry and Anti-Psychiatry*, Paladin: London.

Cooter, R. (1982) 'Anticontagionism and History's Medical Record', in Wright, P. and Treacher, A. (eds), *The Problem of Medical Knowledge*, Edinburgh University Press: Edinburgh, pp. 87–108.

Coser, L. (1965) *Men of Ideas*, Free Press: New York.

Cox, C. and Mead, A. (1975) *A Sociology of Medical Practice*, Collier-Macmillan: London.

Crane, D. and Small, H. (1992) 'American Sociology Since the Seventies', in Halliday, T.C. and Janowitz, M. (eds), *Sociology and Its Publics*, University of Chicago Press: Chicago, pp. 197–234.

Cravens, H. (1978) *The Triumph of Evolution*, University of Pennsylvania Press: Philadelphia, PA.

Crook, S. (2005) 'Change, Uncertainty and the Future of Sociology', in Germov, J. and McGee, T. (eds), *Histories of Australian Sociology*, Melbourne University Press: Carlton, pp. 419–28.

Crothers, C. (2005) 'History of Sociology in New Zealand', in Germov, J. and McGee, T. (eds), *Histories of Australian Sociology*, Melbourne University Press: Carlton, pp. 67–80.

Crozier, M. (2005) 'Society Economised', in Germov, J. and McGee, T. (eds), *Histories of Australian Sociology*, Melbourne University Press: Carlton, pp. 123–43.

Currie, J. and Vidovich, L. (1998) 'The Ascent toward Corporate Managerialism in American and Australian Universities', in Martin, R. (ed), *Chalk Lines*, Duke University Press: Durham, pp. 112–44.

Dahrendorf, R. (1980) 'On Representative Activities', in Gieryn, T.F. (ed), *Science and Social Structure*, Series 2, Volume 39, The New York Academy of Sciences: New York, pp. 15–28.

Daly, J. (eds) (1996) *Ethical Intersections*, Allen and Unwin: St. Leonards.

Daly, J. (1998) 'The Micropolitics of Qualitative Health Research Funding', *Annual Review of Health Social Science* 8: 19–25.

Daly, J.; Green, K. and Willis, E. (1987) *Technologies in Health Care*, Australian Government Printing Service: Canberra.

Daly, J.; McDonald, I. and Willis, E. (1992) *Researching Health Care*, Routledge: London.

Daniel, A. (1990) *Medicine and the State*, Allen and Unwin: Sydney.

Darby, D. (1977) 'Self Help and Self Medication in Health Care', *Australian Journal of Social Issues* 12(3): 208–23.

Davies, C. (2003) 'Some of Our Concepts Are Missing', *Sociology of Health and Illness*, 25th Silver Anniversary Issue: 172–90.

Davis, A. and Horobin, G. (eds) (1977) *Medical Encounters*, Croom Helm: London.

Davis, F. (eds) (1969) *The Nursing Profession*, Wiley: New York.

Davis, F. (1972) *Illness, Interaction, and the Self*, Wadsworth: Belmont, CA.

Davis, M.M. (1971 [1921]) *Immigrant Health and the Community*, Paterson Smith: Montclair.

Davison, G. (2003) 'The Social Survey and the Puzzle of Australian Sociology', *Australian Historical Studies* 34(121): 139–62.

Dawe, A. (1970) 'The Two Sociologies', *British Journal of Sociology* 21(2): 207–18.

Daykin, N. and Clarke, B. (2000) 'They Still Get the Bodily Care', *Sociology of Health and Illness* 22(3): 349–63.

Deeble, J. (2004) 'Twenty-Five Years of Australian Economics', *The Australian Economic Review* 37(1): 1–2.

de Lepervanche, M. (1989) 'Breeders for Australia', *Australian Journal of Social Issues* 24(3): 163–82.

Dempsey, D. (2008) 'ART Eligibility for Lesbians and Single Heterosexual Women in Victoria', *Health Sociology Review* 17(3): 267–79.

Den Hollander, A.N.J. (ed) (1971) *Diverging Parallels*, E.J. Brill: Leiden.

Dent, M. (1990) 'Organisational Change in Renal Work', *Sociology of Health and Illness* 12(4): 413–32.

Devereux, E. (1961) 'Parsons' Sociological Theory', in Black, M. (ed), *The Social Theories of Talcott Parsons*, Prentice Hall: New Jersey.

de Voe, J.E. and Short, S.D. (2003) 'A Shift in the Historical Trajectory of Medical Dominance', *Social Science and Medicine* 57: 343–53.

de Vries, R. (2003) 'Protecting Our Virtues', *Medical Sociology News* 29(3): 35–8.

Dewdney, J. (1989) 'The Australian Health Care System', in Lupton, G. and Najman, J. (eds), *Sociology of Health and Illness*, Palgrave Macmillan: South Melbourne, pp. 71–100.

Diesendorf, M. (ed) (1976) *The Magic Bullet: Social Implications and Limitations of Modern Medicine – An Environmental Approach*, Society for Social Responsibility in Science (ACT): Canberra.

DiMaggio, P. and Powell, W.W. (1983) 'The Iron Cage Revisited', *American Sociological Review* 48(2): 147–60.

Dingwall, R. (1976) *Aspects of Illness*, St. Martin's Press: New York.

Dingwall, R. (1977) *The Social Organisation of Health Visitor Training*, Croom Helm: London.

Dingwall, R. (2001) 'Contemporary Legends, Rumours and Collective Behaviour', *Sociology of Health and Illness* 23(2): 180–202.

Dingwall, R.; Heath, C.; Reid, M. and Stacey, M. (eds) (1977) *Health Care and Health Knowledge*, Croom Helm: London.

Doessel, D. (1992) 'Policy and Empirical Evidence', *Annual Review of Health Social Science* 2: 34–52.

Donahue, S. (1976) 'Research Into Community Health – An Accepted Dichotomy', in Hicks, N. (ed) *Proceedings of the Annual Meeting of the Australian and New Zealand Society for Eidemiology and Research in Community Health*, May 1976, University of Queensland. ANZSERCH: North Adelaide, pp. 222–5.

Donnison, J. (1977) *Midwives and Medical Men*, Heinemann: London.

Dowsett, G.W. (1996) *Practicing Desire*, Stanford University Press: Stanford.

Doyal, L. (1979) *The Political Economy of Health*, Pluto Press: London.

Duff, J. (1973) 'Politics and the Medical Profession', *Australian and New Zealand Journal of Sociology* 9(3): 50–4.

Dufur, M.J.; Parcel, T.L. and McKune, B.A. (2008) 'Capital and Context', *Journal of Health and Social Behavior* 49(2): 146–61.

Durkheim, É. (1951 [1897]) *Suicide*, Free Press: New York.

Durkheim, É. (1933) *The Division of Labor in Society*, Palgrave Macmillan: New York.

Durrington, L.; Lupton, G.; Najman, J.M.; Sheehan, M.; Payne, S. and Western, J.S. (1979) 'A Comparison of Spinal Manipulation by Medical Practitioners and Chiropractors', *Australian Journal of Social Issues* 14(2): 126–33.

Edwards, J. and Cheers, B. (2007) 'Is Social Capital Good for Everyone?' *Health Sociology Review* 16(3): 226–36.

Egger, G. (1978) 'Medical Nemesis and Economic Health, or Economic Nemesis and Medical Health', *Australian Journal of Social Issues* 13(4): 287–301.

Ehrenreich, B. and English, D. (1973) *Complaints and Disorders*, Feminist Press: Old Westbury, NY.

Ehrenreich, J. and Ehrenreich, B. (1971) *The American Health Empire*, Vintage: New York.

Elinson, J. (1985) 'The End of Medicine and the End of Medical Sociology?' *Journal of Health and Social Behavior* 26(4): 268–75.

Elling, R.H. (1989) 'The Political-Economy of Workers Health and Safety', *Social Science and Medicine* 28(11): 1171–82.

Elston, M.A. (1977) 'Women in the Medical Profession: Whose Problem?' in Stacey, M.; Reid, M.; Heath, C. and Dingwall, R. (eds), *Health and the Division of Labour*, Croom Helm: London.

Encel, S. (1970) 'Medicine and Society', *Social Science and Medicine* 4: 147–52.

Encel, S. (1984) 'Sociological Education', *Alumni Papers* 1(3): 4–9, Alumni Association of the University of New South Wales: Kensington, NSW.

Encel, S. (2005) 'Sociology', in Germov, J. and McGee, T. (eds), *Histories of Australian Sociology*, Melbourne University Press: Carlton, pp. 43–55.

Engels, F. (1969 [1845]) *The Condition of the Working Class in England* (introduction by Hobsbawm, E.), Panther Books: London.

Enthoven, A. (1988) 'Managed Competition of Alternative Delivery Systems', *Journal of Health Politics, Policy and Law* 13(2): 305–21.

Evans, D. (2003) 'Taking Public Health Out of the Ghetto', *Social Science and Medicine* 57: 959–67.

Evans, M.S. (2009) 'Defining the Public, Defining Sociology', *Public Understandings of Science* 18: 5–22.

Faris, R.E. (ed) (1964) *Handbook of Medical Sociology*, Rand McNally: Chicago.

Faris, R. and Dunham, H.W. (1939) *Mental Disorders in Urban Areas*, University of Chicago Press: Chicago.

Field, D. (1988) 'Teaching Sociology in UK Medical Schools', *Medical Education* 22(4): 294–300.

Figlio, K. (1987) 'The Lost Subject of Medical Sociology', in Scambler, G. (ed), *Sociological Theory and Medical Sociology*, Tavistock: London, pp. 77–109.

Fitzgerald, T.; Fothergill, A.; Gilmore, K.; Irwin, K.; Kunkel, C.A.; Leahy, S.; Nielsen, J.M.; Passerini, E.; Virnoche, M.E. and Walden, G. (1995) 'What's Wrong Is Right', *Sociological Forum* 10(3): 493–8.

Fleck, L. (1979 [1935]) *The Genesis and Development of a Scientific Fact*, University of Chicago Press: Chicago.

Fletcher, R. (1971) *The Making of Sociology* (Volume Two, Developments), Michael Joseph: London.

Flexner, A. (1910) *Medical Education in the United States and Canada*, Bulletin No. 4, Carnegie Foundation for the Advancement of Teaching: New York.

Flood, A.B. and Fennell, M.L. (1995) 'Through the Lenses of Organisational Sociology', *Journal of Health and Social Behavior* 35(extra issue 1): 154–69.

Foucault, M. (1965) *Madness and Civilization* (Translated Howard, R.), Pantheon: New York.

Foucault, M. (1970) *The Order of Things*, Tavistock: London.

Foucault, M. (1972) *The Archaeology of Knowledge* (Translated by Sheridan Smith, A.M.), Pantheon: New York.

Foucault, M. (1973) *The Birth of the Clinic*, Tavistock: London.

Foucault, M. (1977) *Discipline and Punish*, Tavistock: London.

Foucault, M. (1980) 'The Politics of Health in the Eighteenth Century', in Gordon, C. (ed), *Power/Knowledge*, Harvester: Brighton.

Foucault, M. (1991) 'Questions of Method', in Burchell, G.; Gordon, C. and Miller, P. (eds), *The Foucault Effect*, Harvester Wheatsheaf: London.

Fourcade-Gourinchas, M. (2001) 'Politics, Institutional Structures, and the Rise of Economics', *Theory and Society* 30(3): 397–447.

Fox, D.M. (1996) *Power and Illness*, University of California Press: Berkeley.

Fox, N. and Ward, K. (2008) 'Pharma in the Bedroom... and the Kitchen... The Pharmaceuticalisation of Daily Life', *Sociology of Health and Illness* 30(6): 856–68.

Frank, A. (1998) 'Stories of Illness as Care of the Self: A Foucauldian Dialogue', *Health* 2(3): 329–48.

Freeman, H.; Levine, S. and Reeder, L. (1963) 'Present Status of Medicine Sociology', in Freeman, H.; Levine, S. and Reeder, L. (eds), *Handbook of Medical Sociology*, Prentice-Hall: Englewood Cliffs, NJ, pp. 476–9.

Freeman, H.E. and Reeder, L.G. (1957) 'Medical Sociology', *American Sociological Review* 22(1): 73–81.

Freidson, E. (1961) *Patients' Views of Medical Practice*, Russell Sage: New York.

Freidson, E. (1970a) *Profession of Medicine*, Dodd and Mead: New York.

Freidson, E. (1970b) *Professional Dominance*, Atherton Press: New York.

Freidson, E. (1975) *Doctoring Together*, Elsevier: New York.

Freidson, E. (1978) 'The Development of Design by Accident', in Elling, R. and Sokolowska, M. (eds), *Medical Sociologists at Work*, Transaction Books: New Brunswick, pp. 115–34.

Freidson, E. (1983) 'Viewpoint', *Sociology of Health and Illness* 5(2): 208–19.

Freidson, E. (1986a) 'Knowledge and the Practice of Sociology', *Sociological Forum* 1(4): 684–700.

Freidson, E. (1986b) *Professional Powers*, University of Chicago Press: Chicago.

Freidson, E. (1994) *Professionalism Reborn*, University of Chicago Press: Chicago.

Frenk, J. and Duran-Arenas, L. (1993) 'The Medical Profession and the State', in Hafferty, F.W. and McKinlay, J.B. (eds), *The Changing Medical Profession*, Oxford University Press: New York, pp. 25–42.

Freud, S. (1938) *Basic Writings*, Modern Library: New York.

Fuchs, S. (1993) 'A Sociological Theory of Scientific Change', *Social Forces* 71(4): 933–53.

Fuchs, S. and Ward, S. (1994) 'What Is Deconstruction, and Where and When Does It Take Place?' *American Sociological Review* 59: 481–500.

Fuller, S. (1995) 'Is There Life for Sociological Theory after the Sociology of Scientific Knowledge?' *Sociology* 29(1): 159–66.

Fulton, O. and Holland, C. (2001) 'Profession or Proletariat', in Enders, J. (ed), *Academic Staff in Europe*, Greenwood Press: Connecticut.

Gabe, J.; Calnan, M. and Bury, M. (eds) (1991) *The Sociology of the Health Service*, Routledge: London.

Gaffney, D.; Pollock, A.M.; Price, D. and Shaoul, J. (1999a) 'The Private Finance Initiative', *British Medical Journal* 319(7204): 249–53.

Gaffney, D.; Pollock, A.M.; Price, D. and Shaoul, J. (1999b) 'The Private Finance Initiative', *British Medical Journal* 319(7202): 116–19.

Gallagher, A.P. (1982) *Coordinating Australian University Development*, University of Queensland Press: St. Lucia.

Gaziano, E. (1996) 'Ecological Metaphors as Scientific Boundary Work', *American Journal of Sociology* 101(4): 874–907.

Genoni, P. and Haddow, G. (2009) 'ERA and the Ranking of Humanities Journals', *Australian Humanities Review* 46: 1–12.

Genoni, P.; Haddow, G. and Dumbell, P. (2009) 'Assessing the Impact of Australian Journals in the Social Sciences and Humanities', http://www.conferences.alia.org.au/online2009/docs/PresentationC16.pdf [accessed December 2010].

George, V. (1984) 'Class Inequalities in Education and Health', *Australian Journal of Social Issues* 19(3): 184–95.

George, J. and Davis, A. (1998) *States of Health*, Addison Wesley Longman: Melbourne.

Gerhardt, U. (1989) *Ideas about Illness: An Intellectual and Political History of Medical Sociology*, Palgrave Macmillan: London.

Germov, J. (1995) 'Medi-Fraud, Managerialism and the Decline of Medical Autonomy', *Australian and New Zealand Journal of Sociology* 31(3): 51–66.

Germov, J. and McGee, T. (eds) (2005) *Histories of Australian Sociology*, Melbourne University Press: Carlton.

Gibson, D. and Boreham, P. (1981) 'Managing Communications', *Australian Journal of Social Issues* 16(1): 52–66.

Gieryn, T.F. (1983) 'Boundary-Work and the Demarcation of Science from Non-Science', *American Sociological Review* 48: 781–95.

Gieryn, T.F. (1999) *Cultural Boundaries of Science*, The University of Chicago Press: Chicago.

Gilding, M. (2006) 'DNA Paternity Tests', *Health Sociology Review* 15(1): 84–95.

Glaser, B. and Strauss, A. (1967) *The Discovery of Grounded Theory*, Aldine: Chicago.

Glaser, B. and Strauss, A. (1968) *Time for Dying*, Aldine: Chicago.

Glasner, H. (1979) 'Professional Power and State Intervention in Medical Practice', *Australian and New Zealand Journal of Sociology* 15(3): 20–9.

Glazer, M.P. and Glazer, P.M. (1989) *The Whistleblowers*, Basic Books: New York.

Goffman, E. (1961) *Asylums*, Doubleday and Anchor: New York.

Gold, M. (1977) 'A Crisis of Identity', *Journal of Health and Social Behavior* 18: 160–8.

Goldberg, T. (1958) *Family Influences and Psychosomatic Illness*, Tavistock: London.

Good, J.M.M. (2000) 'Disciplining Social Psychology', *Journal of the History of the Behavioural Sciences* 36(4): 383–403.

Gouldner, A.W. (1970) *The Coming Crisis of Western Sociology*, Heinemann: London.

Gouldner, A.W. (1979) *The Future of Intellectuals and the Rise of the New Class*, Seabury: New York.

Gouldner, A.W. and Miller, S.M. (1965) *Applied Sociology*, Free Press: New York.

Graham, W. (2000) 'Academic Freedom or Commercial Licence?' in Turk, J.L. (ed), *The Corporate Campus*, James Lorimer: Toronto, pp. 23–30.

Graham, S. (1964) 'Sociological Aspects of Health and Illness', in Faris, R.E. (ed), *Handbook of Medical Sociology*, Rand McNally: Chicago, pp. 310–47.

Gramsci, A. (1971) *Selections from the Prison Notebook*, Lawrence and Wishart: London.

Gray, D.E. (2005) *Health Sociology*, Pearson: Frenchs Forest.

Gray, B.H. and O'Leary, J. (2000) 'The Evolving Relationship between Medical Sociology and Health Policy', in Bird, C.; Conrad, P. and Fremont, A. (eds), *Handbook of Medical Sociology*, Prentice Hall: New Jersey, pp. 258–70.

Grbich, C. (1999) *Qualitative Research in Health*, Allen and Unwin: St Leonards.

Grbich, C. (ed) (1996) *Health in Australia: Sociological Concepts and Issues*, Prentice Hall: Sydney.

Green, J. and Armstrong, D. (1993) 'Controlling the Bed State', *Sociology of Health and Illness* 15(3): 337–52.

Greene, M. (1978) 'The Crisis in Medical Sociology?' *Journal of Health and Social Behavior* 19(1): 117.

Groenewegen, P. (2002) 'Accommodating Science to External Demands', *Science, Technology and Human Values* 27(4): 479–98.

Guillemin, M. (1996) 'Constructing Menopause Knowledge Through Socio-Material Practices', *Annual Review of Health Social Science* 6: 40–56.

Hackett, E.J. (2005) 'Essential Tensions', *Social Studies of Science* 35: 787–826.

Hafferty, F.W. and Light, D.W. (1995) 'Professional Dynamics and the Changing Nature of Medical Work', *Journal of Health and Social Behavior* (extra issue): 132–53.

Halsey, A.H. (1985) 'Provincials and Professionals', in Bulmer, M. (ed), *Essays on the History of British Sociological Research*, Cambridge University Press: Cambridge, pp. 151–64.

Halsey, A.H. (2004) *A History of Sociology in Britain*, Oxford University Press: Oxford.

Hamilton, P. (1997) 'The Enlightenment and Social Science', in Boudon, R.; Cherkaoui, M. and Alexander, J. (eds), *The Classical Tradition in Sociology. The European Tradition*, Volume 1, Sage: London, pp. 17–48.

Haney, C.A.; Zahn, M.A. and Howard, J. (1983) 'Applied Medical Sociology', *Teaching Sociology* 11: 92–104.

Harley, K.; Willis, K.; Gabe, J.; Short, S.; Collyer, F.M.; Natalier, K. and Calnan, M. (2011) 'Constructing Health Consumers: Private Health Insurance Discourses in Australia and the United Kingdom', *Health Sociology Review* 20(3): 306–20.

Hart, N. (1977) 'Parenthood and Patienthood', in Davis, A. and Horobin, G.(eds), *Medical Encounters*, Croom Helm: London.

Hatty, S. (1987) 'Woman Battering as a Social Problem', *Australian and New Zealand Journal of Sociology* 23(1): 36–46.

Haug, M.R. (1973) 'Deprofessionalisation', *Sociological Review Monograph* 20: 195–211.

Hawkins, N. (1958) *Medical Sociology*, Charles Thomas: Springfield, IL.

Hayes, D. and Ross, C.E. (1986) 'Body and Mind', *Journal of Health and Social Behavior* 27(4): 3874–900.

Henderson, L.J. (1917) *The Order of Nature*, Harvard University Press: Cambridge.

Henderson, L.J. (1935) 'The Physician and Patient as a Social System', *New England Journal of Medicine* 212: 819–23.

Henderson, S. and Petersen, A.R. (ed) (2002), *Consuming Health*, Routledge: London.

Hepburn, L. (1992) *Ova-Dose? Australian Women and the New Reproductive Technology*, North Sydney: Allen and Unwin.

Hetzel, B.S. (1974) *Health and Australian Society*, Penguin: Victoria.

Hicks, N. (1976) 'Introduction (Editorial)', in Hicks, N. (ed), *Proceedings of the Annual Meeting of the Australian and New Zealand Society for Eidemiology and Research in Community Health*, May 1976, University of Queensland. ANZSERCH: North Adelaide, pp. 1–3.

Hicks, N. (1977) 'Medicine, Politics and a Healthy Society', in Hicks, N. (ed), *Proceedings of the Annual Meeting of the Australian and New Zealand Society for Eidemiology and Research in Community Health*, May 1977, University of Adelaide. ANZSERCH: North Adelaide, pp. 133–8.

Hindess, B. (1987) *Freedom, Equality, and the Market*, Tavistock: London.

Hodder, I. (1994) 'The Interpretation of Documents and Material Culture', in Denzin, N.K. and Lincoln, Y.N. (eds), *Handbook of Qualitative Research*, Sage: Thousand Oaks, pp. 393–402.

Hollingshead, A.B. (1973) 'Medical Sociology', *Milbank Memorial Fund Quarterly* 51: 531–42.

Hollingshead, A.B. and Redlich, F.C. (1958) *Social Class and Mental Illness*, Wiley: New York.

Holmwood, J. (2007) 'Sociology as Public Discourse and Professional Practice', *Sociological Theory* 25(1): 46–66.

Holmwood, J. and Scott, S. (2010) (Chairs), *International Benchmarking Review of UK Sociology*, The Economic and Social Research Council, the British Sociological Association, and the Heads and Professors of Sociology Group, www.britsoc.co.uk.

Homer, A.R. (1977) 'Women and the Politics of "Psychotheraphy" ', *Australian Journal of Social Issues* 12(2): 120–9.

Hopkins, A. (1984) 'Blood Money? The Effect of Bonus Pay on Safety in Coal Mines', *Australian and New Zealand Journal of Sociology* 20(1): 23–46.

Hopkins, A. (1989) 'The Social Construction of Repetition Strain Injury', *Journal of Sociology* 25(2): 239–59.

Horobin, G. (1973) *Experience with Abortion*, Cambridge University Press: Cambridge.

Horobin, G. (1985) 'Medical Sociology in Britain', *Sociology of Health and Illness* 7(1): 94–107.

House, J.S.; Strecher, V.; Metzner, H.L. and Robbins, C.A. (1986) 'Occupational Stress and Health among Men and Women in the Tecumseh Community Health Study', *Journal of Health and Social Behavior* 27: 62–77.

Howarth, G. (1998) 'What's Emotion Got to Do with It?' *Annual Review of Health Social Science* 8: 2–7.

Hughes, D. (1977) 'Everyday and Medical Knowledge in Categorising Patients', in Dingwall, R.; Heath, C.; Reid, M. and Stacey, M. (eds), *Health Care and Health Knowledge*, Croom Helm: London.

Hughes, D. (1988) 'When Nurse Knows Best', *Sociology of Health and Illness* 10(1): 1–23.

Hughes, D. and Griffiths, L. (1999) 'On Penalties and the Patient's Charter', *Sociology of Health and Illness* 21(1): 71–94.

Hughes, D.; May, D. and Harding, S. (1987) 'Growing Up on Ward Twenty', *Sociology of Health and Illness* 9(4): 378–410.

Hughes, D.; Petsoulas, P.; Allen, P.; Doheny, S. and Vincent-Jones, P. (2011) 'Contracts in the English NHS: Market Levers and Social Embeddedness', *Health Sociology Review* 20(3): 321–37.

Hunt, L. (1996) 'Social Movements and the Construction of Health Knowledge', *Annual Review of Health Social Science* 6: 173–202.

Hunt, G.J. and Sobal, J. (1990) 'Teaching Medical Sociology in Medical Schools', *Teaching Sociology* 18: 319–28.

Hunter, T. (1963) 'Some Thoughts on the Pharmaceutical Benefits Scheme', *Australian Journal of Social Issues* 1(4): 32–42.

Huyard, C. (2009) 'How Did Uncommon Disorders Become "Rare Diseases"?' *Sociology of Health and Illness* 31(4): 463–77.

Huxley, J. (1936) 'Eugenics and Society' Galton Lecture', *Eugenics Review* 27(1): 11–31.

Idler, E. (1979) 'Definitions of Health and Illness and Medical Sociology', *Social Science and Medicine* 13A: 723–31.

Idler, E. (2001) 'Religion, Health, and Nonphysical Senses of Self', in Cockerham, W. and Glasser, M. (eds), *Readings in Medical Sociology*, Prentice Hall: New Jersey, pp. 171–87.

Ilerbaig, J. (1999) 'Allied Sciences and Fundamental Problems', *Journal of the History of Biology* 32: 439–69.

Illich, I. (1977) *Limits to Medicine*, Penguin: Harmondsworth.

Illsley, R. (1975) 'Promotion to Observer Status', *Social Science and Medicine* 9: 63–7.

Iphofen, R. and Poland, F. (1997) 'Professional Empowerment and Teaching Sociology to Health Care Professionals', *Teaching Sociology* 25(1): 44–56.

Jackson, J.A. (1975) 'Sociology in Contemporary Britain', in Mohan, R.P. and Martindale, D. (eds), *Handbook of Contemporary Developments in World Sociology*, Greenwood Press: Westport, CT.

Jaco, E.G. (ed) (1958) *Patients, Physicians, and Illness*, Free Press: New York.

James, C. (1987) 'Occupational Injury', *Australian and New Zealand Journal of Sociology* 23(1): 47–64.

Jasso-Aguilar, R. and Waitzkin, H. (2011) 'Multinational Corporations, the State, and Contemporary Medicine', *Health Sociology Review* 20(3): 245–57.

Jefferys, M. (1973) The selection of students for medical education: report on a working group convened by the Regional Office for Europe of the World Health Organization, Bern, 21–25 June 1971, Copenhagen: Regional Office for Europe, World Health Organization.

Jefferys, M. (1986) 'The Transition from Public Health to Community Medicine', *Social History of Medicine Bulletin (London)* 39: 47–63.

Jefferys, M. (1991) 'Medical Sociology and Public Health', *Public Health* 105: 15–21.

Jefferys, M. (1997) 'Social Medicine and Medical Sociology 1950–1970', *Clio Medica* 43: 120–36.

Jefferys, M. (2001) 'The Development of Medical Sociology in Theory and Practice in Western Europe 1950–1990', in Matcha, D. (ed), *Readings in Medical Sociology*, Allyn and Bacon: Boston, pp. 14–19.

Jewson, N. (1976) 'The Disappearance of the Sick Man from Medical Cosmologies: 1770–1870', *Sociology* 10: 225–44.

Jobling, R. (1977) 'Learning to Live with It', in Davis, A. and Horobin, G. (eds), *Medical Encounters*, Croom Helm: London, pp. 72–86.

Johnson, M. (1975) 'Medical Sociology and Sociological Theory', *Social Science and Medicine* 9: 227–32.

Johnson, T. (1972) *Professions and Power*, Palgrave Macmillan: London.

Jones, F.L. (1973) 'Editorial', *Australian and New Zealand Journal of Sociology* 9(1): 1–2.

Jones, R.A. (1978) 'Subjectivity, Objectivity, and Historicity', *American Journal of Sociology* 84(1): 175–81.

Jones, R.A. (1997) 'The Other Durkheim', in Camic, C. (ed), *Reclaiming the Sociological Classics*, Blackwell: Oxford, pp. 142–72.

Jones, R.K. and Jones, P.A. (1975) *Sociology in Medicine*, English Universities Press: London.

Kaplan, G.A.; Haan, M.N. and Syme, S.L. (1987) 'Socioeconomic Status and Health', *American Journal of Preventative Medicine* 3(Supplement): 125–9.

Keim, W. (2011) 'Counterhegemonic Currents and Internationalisation of Sociology', *International Sociology* 26(1): 123–45.

Kellehear, A. (1990) *Dying of Cancer*, Harwood: New York.

Kellehear, A. (ed) (2000) *Death and Dying in Australia*, Oxford University Press: South Melbourne.

Kelly, M. and Field, D. (1996) 'Medical Sociology, Chronic Illness and the Body', *Sociology of Health and Illness* 18: 241–57.

Kinsey, A.; Pomeroy, W.B. and Martin, C.E. (1948) *Sexual Behavior in the Human Male*, W.B. Saunders: Philadelphia, pA.

Kippax, S.; Connell, R.W.; Dowsett, G.W. and Crawford, J. (1993) *Sustaining Safe Sex*, Falmer: London.

Kirkman, M. (1999) 'I Didn't Interview Myself', *Annual Review of Health Social Science* 9: 32–41.

Klein, R. (ed) (1989) *Infertility*, Allen and Unwin: Sydney.

Kleinman, A. (1978) 'Concepts and a Model for the Comparison of Medical Systems as Cultural Systems', *Social Science and Medicine* 12: 85–95.

Knorr Cetina, K.D. (1981a) *The Manufacture of Knowledge*, Pergamon Press: Oxford.

Knorr Cetina, K.D. (1981b) 'The Micro-Sociological Challenge of Macro-Sociology', in Knorr Cetina, K.D. and Cicourel, A.V. (eds), *Advances in Social Theory and Methodology*, Routledge: London.

Knorr Cetina, K.D. (1982) 'Scientific Communities or Transepistemic Arenas of Research?' *Social Studies of Science* 12: 101–30.

Knorr Cetina, K.D. (1999) *Epistemic Cultures*, Harvard University Press: Cambridge.

Knudsen, H.K.; Roman, P.M.; Johnson, J.A. and Ducharme, L.J. (2005) 'A Changed America?' *Journal of Health and Social Behavior* 46(3): 260–73.

Kohler, R.E. (1982) *From Medical Chemistry to Biochemistry*, Cambridge University Press: Cambridge.

Konrad, G. and Szelényi, I. (1979) *The Intellectuals on the Road to Class Power*, Harcourt Brace Jovanovich: New York.

Krupinski, J. and Stoller, A. (1968) 'Occupational Hierarchy of First Admissions to the Victorian Mental Health Department, 1962–1965', *Australian and New Zealand Journal of Sociology* 4(1): 55–63.

Krupinski, J. and Stoller, A. (eds) (1971) *The Health of a Metropolis, the Findings of the Melbourne Metropolitan Health and Social Survey*, Heinemann Educational Australia: Melbourne.

Krupinski, J. and Stoller, A. (eds) (1974) *The Family in Australia*, Pergamon Press: Rushcutters Bay, NSW.

Kuhn, T.S. (1970) *The Structure of Scientific Revolutions*, Chicago University Press: Chicago.

Kurasawa, F. (2002) 'Which Barbarians at the Gates?' *The Canadian Review of Sociology and Anthropology* 39(3): 323–47.

Kurzman, C. and Owens, L. (2002) 'The Sociology of Intellectuals', *Annual Review of Sociology* 28: 63–90.

Lamont, M. and Molnár, V. (2002) 'The Study of Boundaries in the Social Sciences', *Annual Review of Sociology* 28: 167–95.

Lane, K. (1996) 'Birth as Euphoria', in Colquhoun, D. and Kellehear, A. (eds), *Health Research in Practice*, Chapman and Hall: London, pp. 153–73.

Langer, J. (1992) 'Emergence of Sociology', in Langer, J. (ed), *Emerging Sociology*, Avebury: Aldershot and Sydney, pp. 1–18.

Lantz, H.R. (1984) 'Continuities and Discontinuities in American Sociology', *The Sociological Quarterly* 25: 581–96.

Larson, M. (1977) *The Rise of Professionalism*, University of California Press: Berkeley.

Lasch, C. (1965) *The New Radicalism in America, 1889–1963*, Alfred A. Knopf: New York.

Lawler, J. (1991) *Behind the Screens: Nursing, Somology, and the Problem of the Body*, Churchill Livingstone: Melbourne.

Lawrence, C. (1985) 'Incommunicable Knowledge', *Journal of Contemporary History* 20: 503–20.

Lawrence, C. (1994) *Medicine in the Making of Modern Britain, 1700–1920*, Routledge: New York.

Lawton, J. (1998) 'Contemporary Hospice Care', *Sociology of Health and Illness* 20(2): 121–43.

Lawton, J. (2003) 'Lay Experiences of Health and Illness', *Sociology of Health and Illness* 25: 23–40.

Lazarsfeld, P.F. and Reitz, J.G. (1975) *An Introduction to Applied Sociology*, Elsevier: New York.

Lazarsfeld, P.F.; Sewell, W.H. and Wilensky, H.L. (eds) (1967) *The Uses of Sociology*, Basic Books: New York.

Leahey, E. (2007) 'Not by Productivity Alone', *American Sociological Review* 72(4): 533–61.

Legge, D. (1977) 'Cost Control and Quality Assurance', in Hicks, N. (ed), *Proceedings of the Annual Meeting of the Australian and New Zealand Society for Eidemiology and Research in Community Health*, May 1977, University of Adelaide. ANZSERCH: North Adelaide, pp. 7–13.

Leicht, K. and Fennell, M. (1997) 'The Changing Organisational Context of Professional Work', *Annual Review of Sociology* 23: 215–31.

Lengermann, P.M. (1979) 'The Founding of the *American Sociological Review*', *American Sociological Review* 44(2): 185–98.

Leontini, R. (2006) 'Looking Forward, Looking Back: The Narrative of Testing Positive to Huntington's Disease', *Health Sociology Review* 15(2): 144–55.

Lesky, E. (ed) (1976) *A System of Complete Medical Police: Selections from Johann Peter Frank*, Johns Hopkins University Press: Baltimore.

Levine, S. (1987) 'The Changing Terrains in Medical Sociology', *Journal of Health and Social Behavior* 28(1): 1–6.

Levine, S. (1991) 'Medical Sociology Provides New Perspectives', *Contemporary Sociology* 20(6): 827–8.

Levine, S. (1995) 'Time for Creative Integration in Medical Sociology', *Journal of Health and Social Behavior* 35(extra issue): 1–4.

Levine, S. and Croog, S.H. (1984) 'What Constitutes Quality of Life?' in Wenger, N.K.; Mattson, M.E.; Furberg, C.D. and Elinson, J. (eds), *Assessment of Quality of Life in Clinical Trials of Cardiovascular Therapies*, LeJacq Communications: Greenwich, pp. 46–66.

Liang, H.; Saraf, N.; Hu, Q. and Xue, Y. (2007) 'Assimilation of Enterprise Systems', *MIS Quarterly* 31(1): 59–87.

Liberatos, P.; Link, B.G. and Kelsey, J.L. (1988) 'The Measurement of Social Class in Epidemiology', *Epidemiological Reviews* 10: 87–121.

Light, D.W. (1992) 'Introduction: Strengthening Ties between Specialities and the Discipline', *American Journal of Sociology* 97(4): 909–18.

Light, D.W. (2000) 'Sociological Perspectives on Competition in Health Care', *Journal of Health Politics Policy and Law* 25(5): 969–74.

Light, D.W. (2001) 'Comparative Institutional Response to Economic Policy Managed Competition and Governmentality', *Social Science and Medicine* 52(8): 1151–66.

Light, D.W. and Levine, S. (1988) 'The Changing Character of the Medical Profession', *The Milbank Quarterly* 66(Supplement 2): 10–32.

Line, J. (1976) 'Crossing Traditional Boundaries', in Hicks, N. (ed), *Proceedings of the Annual Meeting of the Australian and New Zealand Society for Eidemiology and Research in Community Health*, May 1976, University of Queensland. ANZSERCH: North Adelaide, pp. 219–21.

Link, B.G. and Phelan, J. (1995) 'Social Conditions as Fundamental Causes of Disease', *Journal of Health and Social Behavior* 35(extra issue): 80–94.

Link, B.G.; Dohrenwend, B.P. and Skodol, A.E. (1986) 'Socioeconomic Status and Schizophrenia', *American Sociological Review* 51(April): 242–58.

Lipset, S.M. (1959) 'Political Sociology', in Merton, R.K.; Broom, L. and Cottrell, L.(eds), *Sociology Today*, Basic Books: New York, pp. 81–114.

Lipset, S.M. (1994) 'The State of American Sociology', *Sociological Forum* 9(2): 199–220.

Lipsett, A. (2008) 'More Female Academics Working in Universities', *Education Guardian*, 28 February.

Livingstone, D.N. (1992) *The Geographical Tradition*, Blackwell: Oxford.

Lopez, F. (1982 [1979]) *Sociology and the Nurse*, W.B. Saunders: Sydney.

Lorber, J. (1997) *Gender and the Social Construction of Illness*, Sage: Thousand Oaks, CA.

Loubser, J. (1988) 'The Need for the Indigenisation of the Social Sciences', *International Sociology* 3(2): 179–87.

Luft, H.S. (1981) *Health Maintenance Organisations*, Wiley: New York.

Lupton, D. (1993) 'Is There Life After Foucault?' *Australian Journal of Public Health* 17(4): 298–300.

Lupton, D. (1994) *Medicine as Culture*, Sage: Thousand Oaks.

Lupton, D. (2005) 'Medicine and Health Care in Australia', in Cockerham, W.C. (ed), *The Blackwell Companion to Medical Sociology*, Blackwell: Carlton, pp. 429–40.

Lupton, G.M. and Najman, J.M. (1989) 'The Sociology of Health and Illness', in Lupton, G. and Najman, J. (eds), *Sociology of Health and Illness*, Palgrave Macmillan: South Melbourne, pp. 365–78.

Lupton, G. and Najman, J.M. (eds). (1995) *A Sociology of Health and Illness*, Palgrave Macmillan: Melbourne.

Lynch, M. and Bogen, D. (1997) 'Sociology's Asociological "Core" ', *American Sociological Review* 62(3): 481–93.

Lynd, R.S. and Lynd, H.M. (1929) *Middletown*, Harcourt Brace: New York.

McDonald, L. (1994) *Women Founders of the Social Sciences*, Carleton University Press: Ottawa.

McEwan, E.D. (1977) 'A Dollar's Worth of Health', in Hicks, N. (ed), *Proceedings of the Annual Meeting of the Australian and New Zealand Society for Eidemiology and Research in Community Health*, May 1977, University of Adelaide. ANZSERCH: North Adelaide, pp. 155–66.

McGrath, G.M. (1977) 'Sociologist Heal Thyself', *Australian and New Zealand Journal of Sociology* 13(3): 254–6.

McIntire, C. (1894) 'The Importance of the Study of Medical Sociology', *Bulletin of the American Academy of Medicine* 1: 425–34.

MacIntyre, S. (1973) 'The Medical Profession and the 1967 Abortion Act in G.B.', *Social Science and Medicine* 7: 121–34.

MacIntyre, S. (2009) 'ERA, Overview and Implications', *National Academies Forum (NAF) Workshop on Excellence in Research Evaluation*, Seminar on Excellence in Research Evaluation, Canberra, 8–9 September.

McIntyre, S. and Oldman, D. (1977) 'Coping with Migraine', in Davis, A. and Horobin, G. (eds), *Medical Encounters*, Croom Helm: London, pp. 55–71.

McKeown, T. (1979) *The Role of Medicine*, Blackwell: Oxford.

McKinlay, J.B. (1975) 'Some Issues Associated with Migration, Health Status and Use of Health Services', *Journal of Chronic Diseases* 28(11–12): 579–92.

McKinlay, J.B. (1981) 'From "Promising Report" to "Standard Procedure" ', *Milbank Memorial Fund Quarterly* 59(3): 374–411.

McKinlay, J.B. and Arches, J. (1985) 'Toward the Proletarianisation of Physicians', *International Journal of Health Services* 15: 161–95.

McLachlan, G. (ed.) (1977) *Framework and Design for Planning*, 10th Series. Nuffield Provincial Hospitals Trust: London.

McLaughlin, I.C. (1926) 'History and Sociology', *American Journal of Sociology* 32(3): 379–95.

MacPherson, C.B. (1997) 'Hobbes', in Boudon, R.; Cherkaoui, M. and Alexander, J. (eds), *The Classical Tradition in Sociology. The European Tradition*, Volume 1, Sage: London, pp. 49–65.

Manderson, L. (1998) 'Health, Illness and the Social Sciences', in The Academy of Social Sciences (ed), *Challenges for the Social Sciences and Australia*, RC and NBEET: Canberra.

Mannheim, K. (1960 [1936]) *Ideology and Utopia*, Routledge and Kegan Paul.

Mannheim, K. (1971) 'The Problem of a Sociology of Knowledge', in Wolff, K.H. (ed), *From Karl Mannheim*, Oxford University Press: New York, pp. 59–115.

Marmot, M.G.; Kogevinas, M. and Elston, M.A. (1987) 'Social/Economic Status and Disease', *Annual Review of Public Health* 8: 111–35.

Marshall, H.; Robinson, P.; Germov, J. and Clark, E. (2009) *Teaching Sociology in Australia*, Education, Employment and Workplace Relations: Canberra.

Martin, B. (1991) *Scientific Knowledge in Controversy*, State University of New York Press: Albany, NY.

Martin, B. (1992) 'Scientific Fraud and the Power Structure of Science', *Prometheus* 10(1): 83–98.

Martin, B. and Richards, E. (1995) 'Scientific Knowledge, Controversy, and Public Decision-Making', in Jasanoff, S.; Markle, G.; Petersen, J. and Pinch, T. (eds), *Handbook of Science and Technology Studies*, Sage: Newbury Park, pp. 506–26.

Martin, E. (1987) *The Woman in the Body*, Beacon Press: Boston.

Martin, G.P.; Currie, G. and Finn, R. (2009) 'Reconfiguring or Reproducing Intra-Professional Boundaries?' *Social Science and Medicine* 68: 1191–8.

Martindale, D. (1976) 'American Sociology before World War II', *Annual Review of Sociology* 2: 121–43.

Marx, K. and Engels, F. (1976 [1845–6]) *German Ideology*, Progress Publishers: Moscow.

Maxwell, V. (1975) 'Organisation Interaction Patterns in the Rehabilitation of the Physically Disabled', *Australian and New Zealand Journal of Sociology* 11(2): 68–9.

Mayer, K.B. (1964) 'Sociology in Australia and New Zealand', *Sociology and Social Work* 49(1): 27–31.

Mayhew, H. (1985 [1861]) *London Labour and the London Poor*, Penguin Books: Harmondsworth, Middlesex, England.

Mayo, E. (1920) 'The Australian Political Consciousness', in Atkinson, M. (ed), *Australia*, Palgrave Macmillan: Melbourne.

Mechanic, D. (1967) *Medical Sociology*, Free Press: New York.

Mechanic, D. (1978) *Medical Sociology*, 2nd edition, Free Press: New York.

Mechanic, D. (1983) *Handbook of Health, Health Care and the Health Professions*, Free Press: New York.

Mechanic, D. (1989) 'Medical Sociology', *Journal of Health and Social Behavior* 30(2): 147–60.

Mechanic, D. (1993) 'Social Research in Health and American Socio-Political Context', *Social Science and Medicine* 36(2): 95–102.

Mechanic, D. (1996) 'Changing Medical Organisation and the Erosion of Trust', *The Milbank Quarterly* 74: 171–89.

Mechanic, D. and Levine, S. (eds) (1977) 'Issues in Promoting Health', *Medical Care* 15(5). Supplement.

Melnick, G.A.; Zwanziger, J. and Bradley, T. (1989) 'Competition and Cost Containment in California: 1980–1987', *Health Affairs* 8(2): 129–36.

Merton, R.K. (1959) 'Introduction', in Merton, R.K.; Broom, L. and Cottrell, L. (eds), *Sociology Today*, Basic Books: New York, pp. ix–xxxiv.

Merton, R.K. (ed) (1968 [1949]) 'Sociological Theories of the Middle Range', *Social Theory and Social Structure*, Free Press: New York, pp. 39–72.

Merton, R.K. (1971 [1961]) 'Social Problems and Sociological Theory', in Merton, R.K. and Nisbet, R. (eds), *Contemporary Social Problems*, Harcourt Brace Jovanovich: New York, pp. 793–845.

Merton, R.K. (1977) 'The Sociology of Science', in Merton, R.K. and Gaston, J. (eds), *The Sociology of Science in Europe*, Southern Illinois Press: Carbondale, IL.

Merton, R.; Broom, L. and Cottrell, L. (1959) *Sociology Today*, Basic Books: New York.

Merton, R.K.; Reeder, G.G. and Kendall, P. (1957) *The Student Physician*, Harvard University Press: Cambridge, MA.

Meyer, J.W. and Rowan, B. (1977) 'Institutionalised Organisations', *American Journal of Sociology* 83(2): 340–63.

Mills, C.W. (1956) *The Power Elite*, Oxford University Press: New York.

Minichiello, V. (1989) 'The Regular Visitors of Nursing Homes', *Journal of Sociology* 25(2): 260–77.

Ministry of Health (1944) *Report of the Interdepartmental Committee on Medical Schools*, The Goodenough Report, HMSO: London.

Mitropoulos, A. (2005) 'Discipline and Labour: Sociology, Class Formation and Money in Australia at the Beginning of the Twentieth Century', in Germov, J. and McGee, T. (eds), *Histories of Australian Sociology*, Melbourne University Press, 101–21.

Mizrachi, N. and Shuval, J. (2005) 'Between Formal and Enacted Policy', *Social Science and Medicine* 60: 1649–60.

Monaghan, L.F. (2001) 'Looking Good, Feeling Good', *Sociology of Health and Illness* 23: 330–56.

Montague, M. (1980) 'Are More Teenagers Having Babies?' *Australian and New Zealand Journal of Sociology* 16(3): 76–80.

Moscucci, O. (2005) 'Gender and Cancer in Britain, 1860–1910', *American Journal of Public Health* 95(8): 1312–21.

Moss, J. and Piggott, B. (1976) 'Foundation for Multi-Disciplinary Education in Community Health', in Hicks, N. (ed), *Proceedings of the Annual Meeting of the Australian and New Zealand Society for Eidemiology and Research in Community Health*, May 1976, University of Queensland. ANZSERCH: North Adelaide, pp. 209–12.

Mugford, S. and Lally, J. (1980) 'Socioeconomic Status, Gender Inequality and Women's Mental Health', *Australian Journal of Social Issues* 15(1): 30–42.

Murcott, A. (1977) 'Blind Alleys and Blinkers', *The Scottish Journal of Sociology* 1: 155–71.

Murcott, A. (2001) 'Sociology and Health', in Burgess, R. and Murcott, A. (eds), *Developments in Sociology*, Prentice-Hall: Harlow.

Murphy, J. (1986) 'The Voice of Memory', *Historical Studies* 22(87): 157–75.

Murtagh, M.J. and Hepworth, J. (2003) 'Menopause as a Long-Term Risk to Health', *Sociology of Health and Illness* 25(2): 185–207.

Naegele, K. (1965a) 'Some Observations on the Scope of Sociological Analysis', in Parsons, T.; Shils, E.; Naegele, K. and Pitts, J. (eds), *Theories of Society* (Combined Volumes), Free Press: New York, pp. 3–29.

Naegele, K. (1965b) 'Editorial Foreword', in Parsons, T.; Shils, E.; Naegele, K. and Pitts, J. (eds), *Theories of Society* (Combined Volumes), Free Press: New York, pp. 147–57.

Najman, J.M. (1979) 'Patterns of Morbidity, Health Care Utilisation and Socio-Economic Status in Brisbane 1', *Australian and New Zealand Journal of Sociology* 15(3): 55–63.

Najman, J.M. and Hewitt, B. (2003) 'The Validity of Publication and Citation Counts for Sociology and Other Selected Disciplines', *Journal of Sociology* 39(1): 62–80.

Najman, J.M.; Gibson, D.; Jones, J.; Lupton, G.; Sheehan, M.; Sheehan, P. and Western, J.S. (1983) 'Politics, Policy and Performance', *Australian and New Zealand Journal of Sociology* 19(3): 476–90.

Najman, J.M.; Jones, J.; Gibson, D.; Lupton, G.; Sheehan, M.; Sheehan, P. and Western, J.S. (1981) 'The Impact of Community Health Centres on Community Medication Use', in Sheppard, J.L. (ed), *Advances in Behavioural Medicine*, Volume 1, Cumberland College of Health Sciences: Sydney, pp. 175–200.

Navarro, V. (1976) *Medicine Under Capitalism*, Neale Watson: New York.

Nazroo, J. (1998) 'Genetic, Cultural or Socio-Economic Vulnerability?' *Sociology of Health and Illness* 20: 710–30.

Neil, C.C. and Jones, J.A. (1988) 'Environmental Stressors and Mental Health in Remote Resource Boom Communities', *Australian and New Zealand Journal of Sociology* 24(3): 437–58.

Nelkin, D. and Lindee, S. (1996) *The DNA Mystique*, Freeman: New York.

Nettleton, S. (1995) *The Sociology of Health and Illness*, Polity Press: Cambridge.

Neuendorff, D.J. (1986) 'Teenage Awareness of Family Planning Matters', *Australian Journal of Social Issues* 21(1): 57–66.

Neuman, W.L. (2000) *Social Research Methods*, 4th edition, Allyn and Bacon: London.

Nicolson, M. and McLaughlin, C. (1987) 'Social Constructionism and Medical Sociology', *Sociology of Health and Illness* 9(2): 107–26.

Nightingale, F. (1871) *Introductory Notes on Lying-in Institutions*, Longmans, Green and Co: London.

Nisbet, R.A. (1943) 'The French Revolution and the Rise of Sociology in France', *American Journal of Sociology* 49(2): 156–64.

Nisbet, R.A. (1967 [1966]) *The Sociological Tradition*, Heinemann: London.

Norris, P. (2001) 'How "We" Are Different from "Them" ', *Sociology of Health and Illness* 23(1): 24–43.

Oakley, A. (1975) 'The Trap of Medicalised Motherhood', *New Society*, 18 December, p. 639.

Oakley, A. (1976) 'The Family, Marriage and Its Relationship to Illness', in Tuckett, D. (ed), *An Introduction to Medical Sociology*, Tavistock: London.

Oakley, A. (1991) 'Eugenics, Social Medicine and the Career of Richard Titmuss in Britain 1935–50', *British Journal of Sociology* 42(2): 165–94.

Oberschall, A. (ed) (1972) *The Establishment of Empirical Sociology*, Harper and Row: New York.

Ogburn, W. (1922) *Social Change with Respect to Culture and Original Nature*, B.W. Huebsch: New York.

Ogburn, W. and Nimkoff, M. (1964 [1947]) *A Handbook of Sociology*, Routledge and Kegan Paul: London.

Olesen, V. (1974) 'Convergences and Divergences', *Medical Anthropology Newsletter* 6(1): 6–10.

Olesen, V. and Woods, N.F. (1986) *Culture, Society, and Menstruation*, Hemisphere Publishing Corporation: Washington, DC.

Orr, J.B. (1936) *Fodd, Health and Income*, Palgrave Macmillan: London.

Osborne, L.W. (1984) 'The Ethical Review of Medical Research', *Australian Journal of Social Issues* 19(3): 155–60.

Packman, J. (1968) *Child Care*, Allen and Unwin: London.

Palmer, D. (2000) 'Identifying Delusional Discourse', *Sociology of Health and Illness* 22(5): 661–78.

Palmer, G.R. and Short, S. (2010) *Health Care and Public Policy*, Palgrave Macmillan: South Yarra, VIC.

Parodi, A.; Neasham, D. and Vineis, P. (2006) 'Environment, Population and Biology', *Perspectives in Biology and Medicine* 49(3): 357–68.

Parry, R.H. (2004) 'The Interactional Management of Patients' Physical Incompetence', *Sociology of Health and Illness* 26(7): 976–1007.

Parsons, T. (1959) 'Some Problems Confronting Sociology as a Profession', *American Sociological Review* 24(4): 547–69.

Parsons, T. (1965) 'An Outline of the Social System', in Parsons, T.; Shils, E.; Naegele, K. and Pitts, J. (eds), *Theories of Society* (Combined Volumes), Free Press: New York, pp. 30–79.

Parsons, T. (1968 [1937]) *The Structure of Social Action, Volume 1: Marshall, Pareto, Durkheim*. Free Press: New York.

Parsons, T. (1970 [1951]) *The Social System*, Routledge and Kegan Paul: London.

Patrick, D. and Scambler, G. (eds) (1982) *Sociology as Applied to Medicine*, Bailliere Tindall: London.

Pauly, P. (1984) 'The Appearance of Academic Biology in Late Nineteenth-Century America', *Journal of the History of Biology* 17: 369–97.

Pearlin, L.I. (1992) 'Structure and Meaning in Medical Sociology', *Journal of Health and Social Behavior* 33(1): 1–9.

Peek, C.W. (1971) 'The Sociology of Sociologists', in Tiryakian, E. (ed), *The Phenomenon of Sociology*, Meredith: New York, pp. 442–51.

Pels, D. (1999) 'Privileged Nomads', *Theory, Culture and Society* 16(1): 63–86.

Pels, D. (2000) *The Intellectual as Stranger*, Routledge: London.

Pemberton, J. (1934) 'Malnutrition in England', *University College Hospital Magazine* 191: 53–9.

Pemberton, J. (2002) 'Origins and Early History of the Society for Social Medicine in the UK and Ireland', *Journal of Epidemiology and Community Health* 56: 342–6.

Pescosolido, B. and Kronenfeld, J. (1995) 'Health, Illness, and Healing in an Uncertain Era', *Journal of Health and Social Behavior* (extra issue): 5–33.

Petersdorf, R. and Feinstein, A. (1980) 'An Informal Appraisal of the Current Status of "Medical Sociology" ', in Eisenberg, L. and Kleinman, A. (eds), *The Relevance of Social Science for Medicine*, Reidel: Dordrecht, Holland, pp. 27–48.

Petersen, A.R. (1998) *Unmasking the Masculine*, Sage: London.

Petersen, A.R. (2007) *The Body in Question*, Routledge: New York.

Petersen, A.R. and Bunton, R. (eds) (1997) *Foucault, Health and Medicine*, Routledge: London.

Petersen, A. and Waddell, C. (eds) (1998) *Health Matters*, Allen and Unwin: Sydney.

Phelan, T.J. (2000) 'Bibliometrics and the Evaluation of Australian Sociology', *Journal of Sociology* 36(3): 345–63.

Pieris, R. (1969) 'The Implantation of Sociology in Asia', *International Social Science Journal* 21(3): 433–44.

Pike, R.M. (1963) 'The Professions', *Australian Journal of Social Issues* 1(3): 2–10.

Platt, J. (1985) 'Weber's *Verstehen* and the History of Qualitative Research', *British Journal of Sociology* 36(3): 448–66.

Platt, J. (1992) ' "Case Study" in American Methodological Thought', *Current Sociology* 40(1): 17–48.

Platt, J. (2002) 'The History of the British Sociological Association', *International Sociology* 17(2): 179–98.

Platt, J. (2010) 'Sociology', in Backhouse, R.E. and Fontaine, P. (eds), *The History of the Social Sciences since 1945*, Cambridge University Press: Cambridge, pp. 102–35.

Pollock, A.M. (1993) 'The Future of Health Care in the United Kingdom', *British Medical Journal* 306(6894): 1703–4.

Pollock, A.M. (2000) 'Will Intermediate Care Be the Undoing of the NHS?' *British Medical Journal* 321(7258): 393–4.

Pollock, A.M.; Dunnigan, M.; Gaffney, D.; Macfarlane, A. and Majeed, F.A. (1997) 'What Happens When the Private Sector Plans Hospital Services for the NHS', *British Medical Journal* 314(7089): 1266–71.

Pollock, A.M. and Price, D. (2011) 'The Final Frontier: The UK's New Coalition Government Turns the English National Health Service Over to the Global Health Care Market', *Health Sociology Review* 20(3): 294–305.

Posner, T. (1977) 'Magical Elements in Orthodox Medicine', in Dingwall, R.; Heath, C.; Reid, M. and Stacey, M. (eds), *Health Care and Health Knowledge*, Croom Helm: London.

Pringle, R. (1998) *Sex and Medicine*, Cambridge University Press: Cambridge.

Propper, C.; Burgess, S. and Gossage, D. (2003) *Competition and Quality*, CMPO Working Paper Series No. 03/077, University of Bristol: Bristol.

Pyett, P.; Waples-Crowe, P.; Hunter Loughron, K. and Gallagher, J. (2008) 'Healthy Pregnancies, Healthy Babies for Koori Communities', *Aboriginal and Islander Health Worker Journal* 32(1): 30–2.

Quah, S. (2005) 'Health and Culture', in Cockerham, W. (ed), *The Blackwell Companion to Medical Sociology*, Blackwell: Victoria, pp. 23–42.

Rawlings, B. (1989) 'Coming Clean', *Sociology of Health and Illness* 11(3): 279–94.

Reader, G. and Goss, M.E.W. (1959) 'The Sociology of Medicine', in Merton, R.K.; Broom, L. and Cottrell, L.S. (eds), *Sociology Today, Problems and Prospects*, Basic Books: New York, pp. 229–46.

Reed, M. (1996) 'Organisational Theorising', in Clegg, S.R.; Hardy, C. and Nord, W. (eds), *Handbook of Organisational Studies*, Sage: London, pp. 31–56.

Reeder, S.J. and Mauksch, H. (1979) 'Nursing', in Freeman, H.; Levine, S. and Reeder, L. (eds), *Handbook of Medical Sociology*, Prentice-Hall: Englewood Cliffs, NJ, pp. 209–29.

Rees, S. and Emerson, A. (1983) 'Confused and Confusing', *Australian Journal of Social Issues* 18(1): 46–54.

Reid, J. and Trompf, P. (1991) *The Health of Aboriginal Australia*, Harcourt Brace Jovanovich: Sydney.

Reid, M. (1976) 'The Development of Medical Sociology in Britain', *Discussion Paper in Social Research No. 13*, University of Glasgow: Glasgow.

Reiger, K. (1999) "'Sort of Part of the Women's Movement. But Different" Mothers' Organisations and Australian Feminism', *Women's Studies International Forum* 22(6): 585–95.

Reissman, C.K. (1983) 'Women and Medicalisation', *Social Policy* 14: 3–18.

Relman, A. (1980) 'The New Medical-Industrial Complex', *New England Journal of Medicine* 303: 963–70.

Revans, R.W. (ed). (1972) *Hospitals*, Tavistock: London.

Reznik, D.L.; Murphy, J.W. and Belgrave, L.L. (2007) 'Globalisation and Medicine in Trinidad', *Sociology of Health and Illness* 29(4): 536–50.

Rhoades, L.J. (1981) *A History of the American Sociological Association 1905–1980*, American Sociological Association: Washington, DC.

Rhoades, G. and Slaughter, S. (1998) 'Academic Capitalism, Managed Professionals, and Supply-Side Higher Education', in Martin, R. (ed), *Chalk Lines: The Politics of Work in the Managed University*, Duke University Press: Durham, pp. 33–68.

Richards, L. (2005) *Handling Qualitative Data*, Sage: London.

Richards, L. and Richards, T. (1981) *NUDIST: A Computer Assisted Technique for Thematic Analysis of Unstructured Data*, Department of Sociology, La Trobe University: Bundoora.

Richmond, K. (2005) 'Sociology's Roller-Coaster Ride in Australia', in Germov, J. and McGee, T. (eds), *Histories of Australian Sociology*, Melbourne University Press: Carlton, pp. 57–64.

Richmond, K. (2010) 'Early Health Sociology', Unpublished Paper, Personal communication with the author, November 2010.

Rigney, A. (1992) 'Time for Visions and Revisions', *Storia della Storiografia* 22: 85–92.

Ripper, M. (2008) 'Australian Sperm Donors', *Health Sociology Review* 17(3): 313–25.

Ritchey, F.J. and Raney, M.R. (1981) 'Medical Role-Task Boundary Maintenance', *Medical Care* 19(1): 90–103.

Ritzer, G. (1990) 'The Current Status of Sociological Theory', in Ritzer, G. (ed), *Frontiers of Social Theory*, Columbia University Press: New York, pp. 1–30.

Rivett, G. (1986) *The Development of the London Hospital System 1823–1982*, The King's Fund: London.

Roach Anleu, S. (2005) 'Refashioning Sociology', in Germov, J. and McGee, T. (eds), *Histories of Australian Sociology*, Melbourne University Press, Carlton, pp. 307–19.

Roberts, H. and Woodward, D. (1981) 'Changing Patterns of Women's Employment in Sociology: 1950–80', *British Journal of Sociology* 32(4): 531–46.

Robinson, D. (1973) *Patients, Practitioners, and Medical Care*, Heinemann Medical Books: London.

Roemer, M.I. (1976) *Health Care Systems in World Perspective*, Health Administration Press: Ann Arbor.

Ross, C.E. and Mirowsky, J. (1999) 'Refining the Association between Education and Health', *Demography* 36(4): 445–60.

Ross, D. (1979) 'The Development of the Social Sciences', in Oleson, A. and Voss, J. (eds), *The Organisation of Knoweldge in Modern America, 1860–1920*, Johns Hopkins Press: Baltimore, pp. 107–38.

Ross, D. (1991) *The Origins of American Social Science*, Cambridge University Press: Cambridge.

Ross, E.A. (1969 [1901]) *Social Control*, Case Western Reserve University Press: Cleveland.

Ross, M.W. (1988) 'AIDS and the Pursuit of Happiness', *Australian Journal of Social Issues* 23(2): 103–11.

Rothenberg, A. (1990) *Creativity and Madness*, Johns Hopkins University Press: Baltimore.

Rothwell, R. and Zegveld, W. (1985) *Reindustrialisation and Technology*, Longman: London.

Rowland, D.; Pollock, A.M. and Vickers, N. (2001) 'The British Labour Government's Reform of the National Health Service', *Journal of Public Health Policy* 22(4): 403–14.

Rowse, T. (2002) *Nugget Coombs*, Cambridge University Press: Melbourne.

Rubinstein, A. (1982) 'Mediterranean Back and Other Stereotypes', *Australian Journal of Social Issues* 17(4): 295–303.

Ruffini, J.L. (ed) (1983) *Advances in Medical Social Science*, Volume 1, Gordon and Breach Science Publishers: New York.

Ruffini, J.L. (ed) (1984) *Advances in Medical Social Science*, Volume 2, Gordon and Breach Science Publishers: New York.

Russell, C. and Schofield, T. (1986) *Where It Hurts: An Introduction to Sociology for Health Workers*, Allen and Unwin: Australia.

Ryan, J. and Dent, O. (1984) 'An Introduction to Survival Analysis', *Australian and New Zealand Journal of Sociology* 20(2): 183–96.

Ryle, J.A. (1948) *Changing Disciplines*, Oxford University Press: Oxford.

SAANZ (1970) *SAANZ Membership Directory 1970* (Compiled and edited by R. Nies). The Sociological Association of Australian and New Zealand, and the Clarendon Press: Kensington.

Saggers, S. and Gray, D. (2001) 'Theorising Indigenous Health', *Health Sociology Review* 10(2): 21–32.

Saint, E.G. (1963) 'The Evolution of Medical Training', *Australian Journal of Social Issues* 1(3): 11–16.

Sanda, A. (1988) 'In Defence of Indigenisation in Sociological Theories', *International Sociology* 3(2): 189–99.

Sargent, M.J. (1968) 'Heavy Drinking and Its Relation to Alcoholism', *Australian and New Zealand Journal of Sociology* 4(2): 146–57.

Sargent, M.J. (1973) *Alcoholism as a Social Problem*, University of Queensland Press: St. Lucia.

Sax, S. (1967) 'The Need for Infirmary Accommodation', *Australian Journal of Social Issues* 3(1):33–40.

Sax, S. (1972) *Medical Care in the Melting Pot*, Angus and Robertson: Sydney.

Scambler, G. (1987) 'Introduction', in Scambler, G. (ed), *Sociological Theory and Medical Sociology*, Tavistock: London, pp. 1–8.

Scambler, G. (2005) 'General Introduction', in Scambler, G. (ed), *Medical Sociology*, Volume One, Routledge: London, pp. 1–11.

Schrecker, C. (2008) 'Textbooks and Sociology', *Current Sociology* 56(2): 201–19.

Schultz, A. (1967) *The Phenomenology of the Social World*, Northwestern Press: Evanston, IL.

Scott, J. (2005) 'Some Principle Concerns in the Shaping of Sociology', in Halsey, A.H. and Runciman, W.G. (eds), *British Sociology Seen from Without and Within*, Oxford University Press: Oxford, pp. 136–44.

Scott, W.H. (1979) *Australian and New Zealand Sociology 1971–78. An Introduction*, Monograph Series Number 3. Anthropology and Sociology, Monash University, and The Sociological Association of Australia and New Zealand.

Scott, W.R. and Backman, E.V. (1990) 'Institutional Theory and the Medical Care Sector', in Mick, S. and Associates (eds), *Innovations in Health Care Delivery*, Jossey-Bass: San Francisco, pp. 20–52.

Scotton, R.B. (1969) 'The Nimmo Report', *Australian Journal of Social Issues* 4(2): 85–7.

Scotton, R.B. (1974) *Medical Care in Australia*, Sun Books and the Institute of Applied Economic and Social Research, University of Melbourne: South Melbourne.

Scotton, R.B. (1977) 'Health Costs and Health Policy', in Hicks, N. (ed), *Proceedings of the Annual Meeting of the Australian and New Zealand Society for Eidemiology and Research in Community Health*, May 1977, University of Adelaide. ANZSERCH: North Adelaide, pp. 61–70.

Scull, A.T. (1975) 'Medical Men as Moral Entrepreneurs', *European Journal of Sociology* 16(2): 218–61.

Scully, D. and Bart, P. (1973) 'A Funny Thing Happened on the Way to the Oriface', *American Journal of Sociology* 78: 1045–50.

Seale, C. (2008) 'Mapping the Field of Medical Sociology', *Sociology of Health and Illness* 30(5): 677–95.

Seidman, S. (1983) 'Beyond Presentism and Historicism', *Sociological Inquiry* 55: 79–94.

Seidman, S. (1985) 'The Historicist Controversy', *Sociological Theory* 3(1): 13–16.

Selznick, P. (1957) *Leadership in Administration*, Evanston: Illinois.

Selznick, P. (1959) 'The Sociology of Law', in Merton, R.K.; Broom, L. and Cottrell, L. (eds), *Sociology Today*, Basic Books: New York, pp. 115–27.

Sheff, T.J. (1967) *Mental Illness and Social Processes*, Harper and Row: New York.

Shepherd, N. (2003) 'State of the Discipline: Science, Culture and Identity in South African Archaeology, 1870–2003', *Journal of South African Studies* 29(4): 823–44.

Sheridan, S. and Dally, S. (2006) *Twenty Years: Women's Studies at Flinders, 1986–2006*, Department of Women's Studies, Flinders University of South Australia, Lythrum Press: Adelaide.

Shils, E. (1965) 'The Calling of Sociology', in Parsons, T.; Shils, E.; Naegele, K. and Pitts, J. (eds), *Theories of Society* (Combined Volumes), Free Press: New York, pp. 1405–48.

Shils, E. (1982) 'Knowledge and the Sociology of Knowledge', *Knowledge, Creation, Diffusion, Utilisation* 4: 7–32.

Shumway, D.R. and Messer-Davidow, E. (1991) 'Disciplinarity', *Poetics Today* 12(2): 201–25.

Sica, A. (2010) 'Merton, Mannheim, and the Sociology of Knowledge', in Calhoun, C. (ed), *Robert K. Merton: Sociology of Science and Sociology as Science*, Columbia University Press: New York, pp. 164–81.

Sigerist, H.E. (1937) *Socialised Medicine in the Soviet Union*, Norton: New York.

Simpson, G. and Yinger, J.M. (1959) 'The Sociology of Race and Ethnic Relations', in Merton, R.K.; Broom, L. and Cottrell, L. (eds), *Sociology Today*, Basic Books: New York, pp. 376–99.

Skultans, V. (1975) *Madness and Morals: Ideas on Insanity in the 19th Century*, Routledge and Kegan Paul: London.

Slaughter, S. and Leslie, L.L. (1997) *Academic Capitalism*, Johns Hopkins University Press: Baltimore, MD.

Small, A. (1903) 'What Is a Sociologist?' *American Journal of Sociology* 8(4): 468–77.

Small, A. (1923) 'Some Contributions to the History of Sociology', *American Journal of Sociology* 28(4): 385–418.

Small, A. (1924) *Origins of Sociology*, University of Chicago Press: Chicago.

Smith, R.J. (1977) 'Creative Penmanship in Animal Testing Prompts FDA Controls', *Science* 198: 1227–9.

Snyder, C.R. (1958) *Alcohol and the Jews*, Free Press: Glencoe.

Spencer, L. (2006) *Cultural Keyline: The Life Work of Dr Neville Yeomans*, Unpublished PhD Dissertation, James Cook University: Townsville, Australia.

Spruit, I.P. and Kromhout, D. (1987) 'Medical Sociology and Epidemiology', *Social Science and Medicine* 25(6): 579–87.

Stacey, M. (ed) (1976) *The Sociology of the NHS*, Sociological Review Monograph Number 22, University of Keele: Keele.

Stacey, M. (1980) 'Charisma, Power and Altruism', *Sociology of Health and Illness* 2(1): 64–91.

Stacey, M. (1988) *The Sociology of Health and Healing: A Textbook*, Unwin Hyman: London.

Stacey, M. with Homans, H. (1978), 'The Sociology of Health and Illness', *Sociology* 12(1): 281–307.

Stacey, M.; Reid, M.; Heath, C. and Dingwall, R. (eds) (1977) *Health and the Division of Labour*, Croom Helm: London.

Stanton, P.; Willis, E.; and Young, S. (eds) (2005) *Workplace Reform in the Healthcare Industry*, Palgrave Macmillan: Basingstoke.

Star, S.L. and Griesemer, J.R. (1989) 'Institutional Ecology, "Translations" and Boundary Objects', *Social Studies of Science* 19(3): 387–420.

Stark, E.; Flitcraft, A. and Frazier, W. (1979) 'Medicine and Patriarchal Violence', *International Journal of Health Services* 9(3): 461–93.

Stark, W. (1961) 'Herbert Spencer's Three Sociologies', *American Sociological Review* 26(4): 515–21.

Starr, P. (1983) *The Social Transformation of American Medicine*, Basic Books: New York.

Steele, C.; Butler, L. and Kingsley, D. (2006) 'The Publishing Imperative', *Learned Publishing* 19(4): 277–90.

Stein, N.W. (1977) 'Just What Is Sociology?', *Teaching Sociology* 5(1): 15–36.

Stern, B. (1927) *Social Factors in Medical Progress*, AMS Press: New York.

Stern, B. (1941) *Society and Medical Progress*, Princeton University Press: Princeton.

Stevens, R. (1971) *American Medicine and the Public Trust*, Yale University Press: New Haven.

Stimson, G. and Webb, B. (1975) *Going to See the Doctor*, Routledge and Kegan Paul: London.

Stinchcombe, A.L. (1994) 'Disintegrated Disciplines and the Future of Sociology', *Sociological Forum* 9(2): 279–91.

Stocking, G.W. (1995) 'Delimiting Anthropology', *Social Research* 62(4): 933–66.

Stokes, J.; Strand, P. and Jaffe, C. (1984) 'Distribution of Behavioural Science Faculty in U.S. Medical Schools', *Social Science and Medicine* 18: 753–6.

Storz, M.L. (1978) 'Effects of Official Labelling on Husband's Perceptions of Their Wives', *Australian and New Zealand Journal of Sociology* 14(1): 346–50.

Straus, R. (1957) 'The Nature and Status of Medical Sociology', *American Sociological Review* 22(2): 200–4.

Straus, R. (1999) 'Medical Sociology', *Journal of Health and Social Behavior* 40(2): 103–10.

Straus, A.; Fagerhaugh, S.; Suczec, B. and Wiener, C. (1982) 'Sentimental Work in the Technologised Hospital', *Sociology of Health and Illness* 4(3): 254–79.

Streek, W. and Thelen, K. (2005) 'Institutional Change in Advanced Political Economies', in Streek, W. and Thelen, K. (eds), *Beyond Continuity*, Oxford University Press: Oxford, pp. 1–57.

Strong, P. (1977) 'Medical Errands', in Davis, A. and Horobin, G. (eds), *Medical Encounters*, Croom Helm: London, pp. 38–54.

Strong, P. and Robinson, J. (1990) *The NHS – Under New Management*, Open University Press: Buckingham.

Sturdy, S. and Cooter, R. (1998) 'Science, Scientific Management, and the Transformation of Medicine in Britain c.1870–1950', *History of Science* 36: 421–66.

Sullivan, L. (1989) 'Social Legislation for the Reproductive Technologies', *Australian Journal of Social Issues* 24(1): 33–43.

Sumner, W.G. and Keller, A.G. (1927) *The Science of Society*, Yale University Press: New Haven.

Susser, M. and Watson, W. (1971) *Sociology in Medicine*, Oxford University Press: London.

Sutton, C. and Beran, R.G. (1983) 'The Role of the Health System in Reducing the Stigma Attached to Epilepsy', *Australian Journal of Social Issues* 18(3): 203–8.

Swain, C. and Harrison, J. (1979) 'The Nursing Home as Total Institution', *Australian Journal of Social Issues* 14(4): 274–84.

Syme, S.L. (1998) 'Social and Economic Disparities in Health', *The Milbank Quarterly* 76(3): 493–505.

Syme, S.L. (2000) 'Social Epidemiology and Medical Sociology', in Bird, C.; Conrad, P. and Fremont, A. (eds), *Handbook of Medical Sociology*, Prentice Hall: New Jersey, pp. 365–76.

Szasz, T.S. (1971) *The Manufacture of Madness*, Routledge and Kegan Paul: London.

Taylor, D. and Bury, M. (2007) 'Chronic Illness, Expert Patients and Care Transition', *Sociology of Health and Illness* 29(1): 27–45.

Therborn, G. (1976) *Science, Class and Society*, NLB: London.

Thomas, S.; Steven, I.; Browning, C.; Dickens, E.; Eckermann, L.; Carey, L. and Pollard, S. (1992) 'Focus Groups in Health Research', *Annual Review of Health Social Science* 2: 7–20.

Thompson, E.C. (2006) 'Internet-Mediated Networking and Academic Dependency in Indonesia, Malaysia, Singapore and the United States', *Current Sociology* 54(1): 41–61.

Timmermans, S. (1998) 'Resuscitation Technology in the Emergency Department', *Sociology of Health and Illness* 20(2): 144–67.

Tiryakian, E. (ed) (1971) *The Phenomenon of Sociology: A Reader in the Sociology of Sociology*, Meredith: New York.

Titmuss, R.M. (1943) *Birth, Poverty and Wealth*, Hamish Hamilton: London.

Titmuss, R.M. and Titmuss, K. (1942) *Parents Revolt*, Secker and Warburg: London.

Todd Report (1968) *Report of the Royal Commission on Medical Education* (Cmnd.3569), HM Stationery Office: London.

Tolbert, P.S. and Zucker, L.G. (1996) 'The Institutionalisation of Institutional Theory', in Clegg, S.R.; Hardy, C. and Nord, W. (eds), *Handbook of Organisation Studies*, Sage: London, pp. 175–90.

Touraine, A. (1971) *The Post-Industrial Society*, Random House: New York.

Towell, D. and Harries, C. (eds) (1979) *Innovation in Patient Care*, Croom Helm: London.

Townsend, P. (1962) *The Last Refuge*, Routledge and Kegan Paul: London.

Tuckett, D. (ed). (1976) *An Introduction to Medical Sociology*, Tavistock: London.

Tuckett, D. and Kaufert, J. (eds) (1978) *Basic Readings in Medical Sociology*, Tavistock: London.

Turner, B.S. (1986a) 'Sociology as an Academic Trade', *Journal of Sociology* 22(2): 272–82.

Turner, B.S. (1986b) 'The Vocabulary of Complaints', *Australian and New Zealand Journal of Sociology* 22(3): 368–86.

Turner, B.S. (1987) *Medical Power and Social Knowledge*, Sage: London.

Turner, B.S. (1990) 'The Interdisciplinary Curriculum', *Sociology of Health and Illness* 12(1): 1–23.

Turner, B.S. (1992) *Regulating Bodies*, Routledge: London.

Turner, B.S. (1995 [1987]) *Medical Power and Social Knowledge*, Sage: London.

Turner, B.S. (2000) 'The History of the Changing Concepts of Health and Illness', in Albrecht, G.; Fitzpatrick, R. and Scrimshaw, S. (eds), *The Handbook of Social Studies in Health and Medicine*, Sage: London, pp. 9–23.

Turner, R.J. and Lloyd, D. (1999) 'The Stress Process and the Social Distribution of Depression', *Journal of Health and Social Behavior* 40(4): 374–404.

Turner, S.P. and Turner, J.H. (1990) *The Impossible Science*, Sage: London.

Twaddle, A.C. (1974) 'The Concept of Health Status', *Social Science and Medicine* 8(1): 29–38.

Twaddle, A.C. and Hessler, R.M. (1977) *A Sociology of Health*, Mosby: St. Louis.

Umberson, D.; Williams, K. and Sharp, S. (2000) 'Medical Sociology and Health Psychology', in Bird, C.; Conrad, P. and Fremont, A. (eds), *Handbook of Medical Sociology*, Prentice Hall: New Jersey, 353–64.

van Krieken, R. (2002) 'The Paradox of the "Two Sociologies" ', *Journal of Sociology* 38(3): 255–73.

Veit-Brause, I. (2001) 'Scientists and the Cultural Politics of Academic Disciplines in Late 19th-Century Germany', *History of the Human Sciences* 14(4): 31–56.

Virchow, R.L.K. (1978 [1859]) *Cellular Pathology as Based upon Physiological and Pathological Histology*, John Churchill: London.

Waddington, I. (1973) 'The Role of the Hospital in the Development of Modern Medicine', *Sociology* 7: 213.

Wadsworth, Y. (1984) *Do It Yourself Social Research*, Victorian Council of Social Service and Melbourne Family Care Organisation: Collingwood.

Wadsworth, Y. (1991) *Everyday Evaluation on the Run*, Action Research Issues Association: Melbourne.

Wadsworth, M. and Robinson, D. (1976) *Studies in Everyday Medical Life*, Martin Robertson: London.

Wagner, P. (2001) *A History and Theory of the Social Sciences*, Sage: London.

Waitzkin, H. (1981) 'The Social Origins of Illness', *International Journal of Health Services* 11: 77–103.

Waitzkin, H. (1983) *The Second Sickness*, Free Press: New York.

Waitzkin, H. (1998) 'Is Our Work Dangerous? Should It Be?' *Journal of Health and Social Behavior* 39(1): 7–17.

Wajcman, J. (1991) *Feminism Confronts Technology*, Allen and Unwin: North Sydney.

Wallace, R. (1993) 'Social Disintegration and the Spread of AIDS-2', *Social Science and Medicine* 37(7): 887–96.

Walsh, A. and Walsh, P.A. (1989) 'Love, Self-Esteem, and Multiple Sclerosis', *Social Science and Medicine* 29(7): 793–8.

Warbasse, J. (1909) *Medical Sociology*, Appleton and Company: Haverhill.

Ward, J. (1979) 'Symposium on the Sociology of Medicine', *Australian and New Zealand Journal of Sociology* 15(3): 18–19.

Ward, L.F. (1968 [1883]) *Dynamic Sociology* (2 volumes), Greenwood Press: New York.

Wardell, M. and Turner, S. (1986) 'Introduction', in Wardell, M. and Turner, S. (eds), *Sociological Theory in Transition*, Allen and Unwin: Boston, pp. 11–18.

Wardwell, W.I. (1982) 'The State of Medical Sociology – A Review Essay', *The Sociological Quarterly* 23(4): 563–71.

Waring, J. (2007) 'Adaptive Regulation or Governmentality', *Sociology of Health and Illness* 29(2): 163–79.

Warner, J. (1992) 'The Fall and Rise of Professional Mystery', in Cunningham, A. and Williams, P. (eds), *The Laboratory Revolution in Medicine*, Cambridge University Press: Cambridge, pp. 110–41.

Warner, J. (1995) 'The History of Science and the Sciences of Medicine', *Osiris* 10: 164–93.

Warner, R. (1976) 'Sociological Theory in Historical Context', in Smelser, N. and Warner, R. (eds), *Sociological Theory*, Learning Press: New Jersey, pp. 3–133.

Webb, S. and Webb, B. (1910) *English Poor Law Policy*, Longmans Green: London.

Webb, S. and Webb, B. (1916) *The Prevention of Destitution*, S. Webb and B. Webb: London.

Webb, S. and Webb, B. (1968 [1932]) *Methods of Social Study*, A.M. Kelley: New York.

Weber, M. (1930) *The Protestant Ethic and the Spirit of Capitalism*, Unwin University Books: London.

Weber, M. (1948) *From Max Weber*, Routledge and Kegan Paul: London.

Weber, M. (1949 [1922]) *The Methodology of the Social Sciences*, Free Press: New York.

Weed, F.J. (2005) 'The Sociological Department at the Colarado Fuel and Iron Company, 1901 to 1907', *Journal of the History of the Behavioral Sciences* 41(3): 269–84.

Weedon, C. (1997) *Feminist Practice and Poststructuralist Theory*, Oxford: Blackwell.

Weerakkody, V.; Dwivedi, Y.K. and Irani, Z. (2009) 'The Diffusion and Use of Institutional Theory', *Journal of Information Technology* 24(4): 354–68.

Weingast, B. (2002) 'Rational-Choice Institutionalism', in Katznelson, I. and Milner, H. (eds), *Political Science*, Norton: New York.

Wen, M.; Cagney, K.A. and Christakis, N.A. (2005) 'Effect of Specific Aspects of Community Social Environment on the Mortality of Individuals Diagnosed with Serious Illness', *Social Science and Medicine* 61: 1119–34.

Western, J. (2005) 'Some Notes on the History of Sociology', in Germov, J. and McGee, T. (eds), *Histories of Australian Sociology*, Melbourne University Press, pp. 49–55.

Western, J.S. (1963) 'Social Work and Professional Socialisation', *Australian Journal of Social Issues* 1(4): 53–65.

Western, J.S. (1976) 'Prospects for the Improvement of Health in Australia', in Smithurst, B.A. (ed), *The Gordon Symposium*, University of Queensland Press: St. Lucia, pp. 48–54.

Western, J.S. (1998) 'Sociology', in *Challenges For The Social Sciences and Australia*, Volume 1, The Academy of the Social Sciences in Australia, the Australian Research Council, and the National Board of Employment, Education and Training: Canberra, pp. 223–32.

Western, J.S. and Wilson, P.R. (1968) 'Conscription', in Forward, R. (ed), *Conscription in Australia*, University of Queensland Press: St. Lucia, pp. 223–241.

White, K.N. (2002) *An Introduction to the Sociology of Health and Illness*, Sage: London.

White, K.N. and Collyer, F.M. (1997) 'To Market To Market: Corporatisation, Privatisation and Hospital Costs', *Australian Health Review* 20(2):13–25.

White, K.N. and Collyer, F.M. (1998) 'Health Care Markets in Australia', *International Journal of Health Services* 28(3): 487–510.

Whitlam, G. (1968) 'The Alternative Health Program', *Australian Journal of Social Issues* 3(4): 33–50.

Whitley, R. (1977) 'The Sociology of Scientific Work and the History of Scientific Developments', in Blume, S. (ed), *Perspectives in the Sociology of Science*, Wiley: London, pp. 21–50.

Whitlock, F.A. (1979) 'Witch Crazes and Drug Crazes', *Australian Journal of Social Issues* 14(1): 43–54.

Wieland, G. and Leigh, H. (1971) *Changing Hospitals*, Tavistock: London.

Wild, R.A. (1977) 'Social Stratification and Old Age', *Australian Journal of Social Issues* 12(1): 19–32.

Wilkinson, R. (1996) *Unhealthy Lifestyles*, Routledge: London.

Williams, G. (1984) 'The Genesis of Chronic Illness', *Sociology of Health and Illness* 6(2): 175–200.

Williams, R.M. (2006) 'The Long Twentieth Century in American Sociology: A Semiautobiographical Survey', *Annual Review of Sociology* 32:1–23.

Williams, S.J. (2000) 'Chronic Illness as Biographical Disruption or Biographical Disruption as Chronic Illness?' *Sociology of Health and Illness* 22(1): 40–67.

Williams, S.J. (2001) 'Sociological Imperialism and the Profession of Medicine Revisited', *Sociology of Health and Illness* 23(2): 135–58.

Willis, Evan. (1979) 'Sister Elizabeth Kenny and the Evolution of the Occupational Division of Labour in Health Care', *Australian and New Zealand Journal of Sociology* 15(3): 30–8.

Willis, Evan. (1982) 'Research and Teaching in the Sociology of Health and Illness', *Community Health Studies* 6(2): 144–53.

Willis, Evan. (1983) *Medical Dominance*, George Allen and Unwin: Melbourne.

Willis, Evan. (ed) (1988) *Technology and the Labour Process*, Allen and Unwin: Sydney.

Willis, Evan. (1991) 'The Sociology of Health and Illness in Australia', *Annual Review of Health Social Science* 1: 46–53.

Willis, Evan. (1994) *Illness and Social Relations*, Allen and Unwin: Sydney.

Willis, Evan. (1998) 'The "New Genetics" and the Sociology of Medical Technology', *Journal of Sociology* 34(2): 170–83.

Willis, Evan. (2005) 'The First Sociology Doctorate in Australia', *Nexus* 17(1): 11–13.

Willis, Evan. and Broom, A. (2004) 'State of the Art', *Health Sociology Review* 13(2): 122–44.

Willis, Eileen.; Reynolds, L. and Keleher, H. (2009) *Understanding the Australian Health Care System*, Churchill Livingstone Elsevier: Sydney.

Willis, K. and Elmer, S. (2007) *Society, Culture and Health*, Oxford University Press: South Melbourne.

Willmott, P. (1985) 'The Institute of Community Studies', in Bulmer, M. (ed), *Essays on the History of British Sociological Research*, Cambridge University Press: Cambridge, pp. 137–50.

Wilson, L. and Kolb, W. (1949) *Sociological Analysis*, Harcourt, Brace and World: New York.

Wilson, P.R. and Gorring, P. (1985) 'Social Antecedents of Medical Fraud and Overservicing', *Australian Journal of Social Issues* 20(3): 175–87.

Wilson, P.R. and Western, J.S. (1972) *The Policeman's Position Today and Tomorrow*, University of Queensland Press: St. Lucia.

Wolff, K. (1970) 'The Sociology of Knowledge and Sociological Theory', in Reynolds, L. and Reynolds, J. (eds), *The Sociology of Sociology*, David McKay: New York, pp. 31–67.

Wolinsky, F.D. and Marder, W.D. (1985) *The Organisation of Medical Practice and the Practice of Medicine*, Health Administration Press: Ann Arbor.

Wootton, B. (1959) *Social Science and Social Pathology*, Allen and Unwin: London.

Wright, P. and Treacher, A. (eds) (1982) *The Problem of Medical Knowledge*, Edinburgh University Press: Edinburgh.

Yeomans, N. (1966) 'Collective Therapy', *Australian Journal of Social Issues* 2(4): 2–12.

Yoxen, E. (1983) *The Gene Business*, Oxford University Press: New York.

Yang, Y. (2007) 'Is Old Age Depressing?' *Journal of Health and Social Behavior* 48(1): 16–32.

Yeomans, N. (1965) *Collected Papers on Fraser House and Related Healing Gatherings and Festivals*, Mitchell Library Archives, State Library of New South Wales: Sydney.

Zadoroznyj, M. (1999) 'Social Class, Social Selves and Social Control in Childbirth', *Sociology of Health and Illness* 21(3): 267–89.

Zaret, D. (1980) 'From Weber to Parsons and Schutz', *American Journal of Sociology* 85(5): 1180–201.

Zola, I.K. (1991) 'Bringing Our Bodies and Ourselves Back In', *Journal of Health and Social Behavior* 32(1): 1–16.

Zubrzycki, J. (1979) 'The Challenge of Change', *Australian and New Zealand Journal of Sociology* 15(3): 83–9.

Zubrzycki, J. (2005) 'The Teaching of Sociology in Australian Universities, Past and Present', in Germov, J. and McGee, T. (eds), *Histories of Australian Sociology*, Melbourne University Press: Carlton, pp. 219–44.

Zucker, L. (1987) 'Institutional Theories of Organisation', *Annual Review of Sociology* 13: 443–64.

Index